ECGs for Beginners

ECGs for Beginners

Antoni Bayés de Luna

Emeritus Professor of Cardiology, Autonomous University of Barcelona
Senior Investigator, Institut Català Ciències Cardiovasculars
Hospital Sant Pau
Senior Consultant, Hospital Quiron
Barcelona, Spain

WILEY Blackwell

Published by John Wiley & Sons, Inc., Hoboken, New Jersey
Published simultaneously in Canada

For general information on our other products and services or for technical support, please contact our Customer Care Department within the United States at (800) 762-2974, outside the United States at (317) 572-3993 or fax (317) 572-4002.

Wiley also publishes its books in a variety of electronic formats. Some content that appears in print may not be available in electronic formats. For more information about Wiley products, visit our web site at www. wiley.com.

Library of Congress Cataloging-in-Publication Data:

Bayés de Luna, Antoni, 1936– author.
  ECGs for beginners / Antoni Bayés de Luna.
    p. ; cm.
  Includes bibliographical references and index.
  ISBN 978-1-118-82131-2 (pbk.)
  I. Title.
  [DNLM: 1. Electrocardiography–methods.   2. Heart Diseases–diagnosis.   WG 330]
  RC683.5.E5
  616.1'207547–dc23
                                                    2014012635

Cover image courtesy of the author
Printed and bound in Malaysia by Vivar Printing Sdn Bhd

1 2014

Contents

Preface

It is my pleasure to present this ECG book for beginners, a book that I would have liked to own when I began to study electrocardiography. It has been written with beginners in mind, therefore it is a book for 'readers with little knowledge of the subject' who want to learn 'quickly and didactically', uncovering what appears to be complex or mysterious because in fact it is an essential part of their professional work. Figures and diagrams, many of them already published in my previous books, in combination with a succinct text have been carefully put together for this purpose.

I am proud to be able to help these readers so that the study of the ECG may be easier for them. It is something I have always tried to do in my nearly 50 years as a university professor, and something my students have often remarked on. I have written previous and more extensive ECG books in English, Catalan and Spanish in the last 40 years, which have been translated into eight languages with more than 20 editions. However, this new book is special because it contains the essentials of the ECG: the cheapest, the quickest and most useful technique that has existed in medicine for over 100 years.

This book contains text in bold that indicates certain points that I feel are especially important. The reader will also find letters in the margins that refer to key concepts for a correct understanding of the ECG. At the end of each chapter, these reference points are used in a short quiz for self-assessment. In this way, residents of any medical specialization, not only cardiology, but also general practitioners, intensivists, anesthesiologists, pediatricians, medical students, and nurses will be able to understand normal and pathologic ECG morphologies, recognizing the patterns and understanding how they originate.

My objective has been to decode the electrocardiographic curve into an understandable sequence representing the electrical activation of the heart so that it may be followed step-by-step, from the initial stimulus in the sinus node to the ventricular myocardium. I explain how the P wave, the QRS complex, and the T wave morphologies originate, and how they occur in both normal and pathologic conditions. It is not advisable to memorize the ECG patterns, but rather understand deductively how they occur. With this in mind, I have included more figures and less text.

The book is comprised of four parts and 18 chapters. The first part outlines the basic normal ECG; the second the typical morphologies in different pathologies; the third the ECG patterns of arrhythmias and the fourth part deals with the important to use correctly the ECG in the clinical context of the patient. This is really the most important aim of modern clinical electrocardiography.

If a certain concept is not fully understood, the reader should not despair. A second reading is often all that is needed. I am also happy to help through internet correspondence. Complementary resources are available as well, including our recent volumes 'Clinical Arrhythmology' and 'Clinical Electrocardiography' (Wiley-Blackwell, 2011 and 2012, respectively). These books are more extensive and include exhaustive reference sections, while this book lists only the essential references.

Finally, I would like to add one important last piece of advice. The clinical context is extremely relevant in the interpretation of ECGs, and is often the deciding factor when interpreting a case. As a rule we should not assume that if a normal ECG is present we can rule out heart disease, just as we should not become too alarmed with certain isolated pathological ECG patterns because they may represent something nonspecific.

I would like to thank each and every reader for their interest in this book. I would also like to express my respect and admiration for those authors whose books helped in my training: Drs. Grant and Marriot in the U.S., Dr. Stock in the U.K., Drs. Sodi and Cabrera in Mexico, Dr. Tranchesi in Brazil, and Drs. Rosenbaum and Elizari in Argentina and others whom I have consulted, and who are listed in the Bibliography. I am very grateful to my close collaborators: Drs. J. Riba, M. Fiol, A. Bayés-Genís, and also to J. Guindo, D. Goldwasser, A. Baranchuk, J. García Niebla and D. Conde, as well as my previous fellows W. Zareba, R. Brugada, I. Cygankiewicz, P. Iturralde, R. Baranowski and X.

Viñolas and many others, because all of them have been my greatest source of inspiration and support. I also thank Montserrat Saurí and Joan Crespo and in the last period Esther Gregoris, my secretariat team, who are so hard-working and always cheerful. I would also lie to thank the Menarini Co, namely and especially Dr. M. Ballarin, for their logistical support. I lovingly thank my wife Maria Clara, who has always tolerated my hectic pace, as well as my five children and 13 grandchildren, who know that I will always be there for them ... albeit with pen in hand.

Antoni Bayés de Luna
Cathedral Square. Vic. Christmas 2014
abayes@csic-iccc.org

Forewords to Previous Editions

Textbook of Clinical Electrocardiography, Martinus Nijhoff Publishers, 1993

Dr. Antonio Bayés de Luna is not only an expert in the use of the electrocardiogram as a diagnostic tool, but as clearly demonstrated in this text, he is a highly skilled teacher of its appropriate use. This text provides this knowledge in a clear manner at all levels of sophistication.

Hein J.J. Wellens, Maastricht, 1993

Basic Electrocardiography, Futura Blackwell, 2007

Prof. Antoni Bayes de Luna, the author of this textbook, is a world-wide renowned electrocardiographer and clinical cardiologist who has contributed to our knowledge and understanding of electrocardiography over the years. This textbook is an asset for every cardiologist, internist, primary care physician as well as medical students interested in broadening their skills in electrocardiography.

Yochai Birnbaum, Texas, 2007

Clinical Arrhythmology, Wiley Blackwell, 2011

I felt that this book demonstrated the great authority of the author as well as his deep knowledge of clinical arrhythymology and electrocardiography, great didactic capabilities and many years of experience in this field. I am sure that it will be extremely useful for readers.

Valentí Fuster, New York, 2011

Clinical Arrhythmology, Wiley Blackwell, 2011

His various books on electrocardiography, published in the most common languages are known by every admirer of the electrical activity of the heart. No cardiologist has described the ECG in as much detail as he. His detailed work has consisted of the nearly impossible job of dissecting the electrical activity of the heart.

Pere Brugada, Brussels, 2011

Clinical Electrocardiography: A Textbook, Wiley Blackwell, 2012

Professor Antoni Bayes de Luna is a master cardiologist who is the most eminent electrocardiographer in the world today. As a clinician he views the electrocardiogram as the means to an end, the evaluation of a patient with known or suspected heart disease, rather than as an end in itself. In an era of multi-authored texts which are often disjointed and present information that is repetitive and even contradictory, it is refreshing to have a body of information which speaks with a single authoritative respected voice. Clinical Electrocardiography is such a book.

Eugene Braunwald, Boston, 2011

Foreword

This new edition, the 12th, of Prof. Antoni Bayés de Luna's classic book on clinical electrocardiography, is especially important 'for beginners' and reinforces the clinical utility of the surface electrocardiogram. It is quite evident that ECG patterns cannot be memorized without a clear clinical understanding of the subject. This is different from other textbooks on electrocardiography. Notably, Prof. A. Bayés de Luna has presented up-to-date, well explained concepts as well as new evidence to explain the pathophysiology of ECG patterns.

Prof. Bayés has worked tirelessly to research the electrophysiological mechanisms that explain electrical changes and has systematically organized these ideas. The reader will find an explanation and the clinical relevance of the significant diagnostic and therapeutic repercussions in any abnormality seen in the ECG. As his pupils and collaborators for many years, we greatly value his teachings, which have reached many countries throughout the world; since the publication of the first edition in 1977, the book has been translated into more than 10 languages.

While this book has already become classic ECG reading material around the world, this new edition stands out because of its particularly large quantity of figures, more than in previous editions, and because of the importance placed on the correlation between ECG findings and those obtained by cardio MRI. At the same time, the book contains new tables that summarize important aspects and mistakes typically made when first learning ECG interpretation or when the latest electrocardiographic information has not been made available.

This book represents 40 years of meticulous, innovative, and even obsessive study by its author. As his fellows, we are extremely proud to present this work and recommend it to all who wish to understand the complexity of ECG recordings. After so many years on the front line, Prof. A. Bayés de Luna continues to surprise us with new ideas and possible new explanations for difficult ECG tracings. He is a very gifted specialist in this field. His tenacity and discipline in writing this work on his own has allowed the text to be agile and flow easily from one section to another. Like Braunwald or Hurst, Bayés de Luna is classic reading.

The four parts allow the reader to become familiar with the normal ECG and the various pathologic patterns, including ventricular enlargement, ventricular block, and arrhythmias.

Antoni Bayés de Luna is *Professor Emèritus* in Cardiology at the Universitat Autònoma de Barcelona. Since 2006 his research group has published 59 articles and nine books, all during a period in his life when many of his fellow professionals are considering retirement. He has lectured internationally on 20 occasions and has recently overseen the 51st annual clinical electrocardiography course. Congratulations Professor, and please, never slow down!

Miquel Fiol Sala
Cap de l'Unitat Coronària i
Director de l'Institut de Biomedicina
Hospital Son Espases, Palma

Antoni Bayés Genis
Cap Servei de Cardiologia
H. Germans Trias i Pujol. Badalona
Professor Titular de Cardiologia, UAB

PART I

The Normal Electrocardiogram

In the first chapter the anatomical and electro-physiological bases essential to understanding the human electrocardiogram (ECG), are outlined. Chapter 2 explains how the ECG records the path of cardiac activation through the heart from the sinus node to the ventricular muscle in the form of activation curves (depolarization and repolarization) of the atria (P waves) and ventricles (the QRS-T complex). Chapter 3 describes ECG devices and recording techniques. Lastly, Chapter 4 explains in detail the process for interpreting normal and pathologic ECG recordings, including the normal characteristics of each parameter studied.

A full understanding of these concepts is essential before continuing on to the other parts of the book. Please start the first four chapters again if necessary.

ECGs for Beginners, First Edition. Antoni Bayés de Luna.
© 2014 John Wiley & Sons, Inc. Published 2014 by John Wiley & Sons, Inc.

CHAPTER 1

Anatomical and Electrophysiological Bases

1.1. The heart walls

The heart has four cavities, two atria and two ventricles, comprised mainly of contractile cells called cardiomyocytes. The electrical stimulus originating in the sinus node (SN) is distributed through the entire heart by means of a specific conduction system (SCS).

The left ventricle (LV) has four walls: anterior, septal, inferior, and lateral. Figure 1.1 shows the three segments of the anterior and inferior walls, the five segments of the septal and lateral walls, and the apex segment (segment 17). Magnetic resonance imaging has now shown that the previously-named posterior wall corresponds to the inferobasal segment of the inferior wall (segment 4 in Fig. 1.1) (Bayés de Luna et al., 2006a; Bayés de Luna A and Fiol-Sala, 2008).

1.2. Coronary circulation (Fig. 1.2)

Based on coronary perfusion, the heart is divided into two zones: the anteroseptal zone, perfused by the left anterior descending artery (LAD) (Fig. 1.2A) and the inferolateral zone, perfused by the right coronary artery (RCA) and circumflex artery (CX) (Figs 1.2C and 1.2D). The heart has areas of shared perfusion (shown in grey in Fig. 1.2A) in which one of the two arteries dominates. For example, segment 17 (apex) is perfused by the LAD, if long; otherwise by the RCA and even partially by the CX.

1.3. The specific conduction system (Fig. 1.3)

Electrical stimuli pass through the internodal pathways (Bachmann, Wenckebach and Thorel bundles), from the sinus node to the AV node and the His bundle. From there stimuli reach the ventricles through the ventricular conduction system: the right branch (RB) and the trunk of the left branch (LB), and its divisions (superoanterior and inferoposterior fascicles and the middle fibers that exist between them) (Figs 1.3A and 1.3B).

Figure 1.3C shows in grey the structures that the AV junction encompass. Figure 1.3D shows the three activation entry points in the left ventricle (LV) (Durrer et al., 1970).

1.4. The ultrastructure of cardiac cells

- There are two types of cell in the heart:
  1. Contractile cells or cardiomyocytes, which are responsible for cardiac pump function (contractile). Under normal conditions these cells do not have automatic capacity and cannot generate stimuli.

ECGs for Beginners, First Edition. Antoni Bayés de Luna.
© 2014 John Wiley & Sons, Inc. Published 2014 by John Wiley & Sons, Inc.

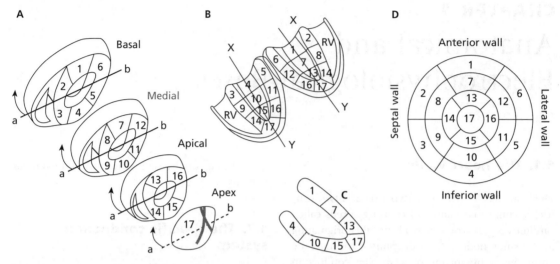

Figure 1.1 (A) Segments into which the left ventricle is divided according to the transverse (short-axis) sections performed at the basal (B), medial (M), and apical (A) levels. The basal and medial sections delineate into six segments each, while the apical section shows four segments. Together with the apex, they constitute the 17 segments into which the left ventricle can be divided, according to the classification performed by the American Imaging Societies (Cerqueira et al., 2002). Also shown is the view of the 17 segments with the heart open in a horizontal long-axis plane (B) and vertical long-axis (sagittal-like) plane (C). In D, the 17 segments and the four walls of the heart are shown in a 'bull's-eye view'. RV = right ventricle.

2. Specific cells (cells of specific system of conduction), which are in charge of impulse formation (automaticity) and impulse transmission to the contractile myocardium.

• **Contractile cells** (Fig. 1.4) are comprised of the following:

1. **The contractile system** made up of myofibers in which the contractile unit is the sarcomere (Figs 1.4A, 1.4B2, and 1.4B3), a structure that can contract and relax. The energy for this activity is provided by mitochondria.

2. **The cellular activation–relaxation system** consisting of the cellular membrane formed by a lipid bilayer (sarcolemma) (Figs 1.4B1 and 1.4B2). Ions (Na^+, K^+, and especially Ca^{++}), responsible for activation, depolarization and repolarization, systole, and cellular rest (diastole) phases, flow through channels that exist in this membrane.

3. The transverse tubular (T) system (Fig. 1.4B2), which allows electrical excitation to enter the cell, and the sarcoplasmatic reticulum (Fig. 1.4

B2) which contains the calcium necessary for cellular contraction.

4. **The specific cells,** non-contractile, are of three types: (a) **P cells**, the ones with more automaticity, located especially in sinus node 4; (b) **Purkinje cells,** with less automaticity, located especially in the His bundle, bundle branches and Purkinje network; and (c) **transitional cells.**

1.5. The electrophysiology of cardiac cells

1.5.1. Transmembrane diastolic potential (TDP) and transmembrane action potential (TAP) in automatic and contractile cells

All contractile cardiac cells at rest show equilibrium between the external electrical charges and the internal negative charges (Fig. 1.5A). When a micro-electrode is located inside a contractile cell at rest while a second micro-electrode remains in

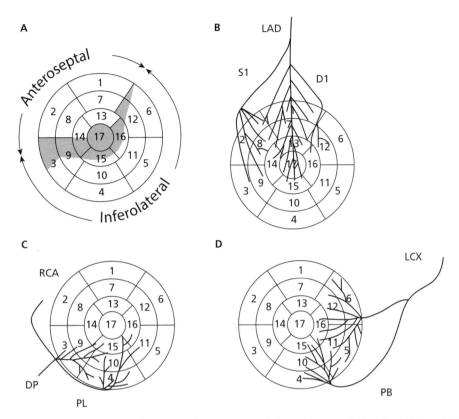

Figure 1.2 According to the anatomical variants of coronary circulation, the areas of shared variable perfusion are shown in grey (A). The perfusion of these segments by the corresponding coronary arteries (B–D) can be seen in the 'bull's-eye' images. For example, the apex (segment 17) is usually perfused by the LAD but sometimes by the RCA, or even the LCX. Segments 3 and 9 are shared by LAD and RCA, and also the small part of the mid-low lateral wall is shared by LAD and LCX. Segments 4, 10 and 15 correspond to the RCA or the LCX, depending on which of them is dominant (the RCA in >80% of the cases). Segment 15 often receives blood from LAD.

the exterior (Fig. 1.5B), a difference in transmembrane potential, called the transmembrane diastolic potential (TDP), is produced. Under normal conditions the voltage is −90 mV (Fig. 1.5B).

As contractile cells are not automatic; TDP is rectilinear (Fig. 1.6). This means that during the diastolic phase, an equilibrium between the potassium outward ionic current, and the sodium and calcium inward ionic current takes place.

When the contractile cell receives a stimulus transmitted from a neighboring cell, sodium current enters the cell rapidly. This creates a stimulus upon reaching the threshold potential, which forms the transmembrane action potential (TAP) (Fig. 1.6).

Thus, in the contractile cells the formation of TAP (Fig. 1.6), which is the basis of cellular activation (depolarization and repolarization), takes place because a stimulus (a) transmitted from a neighboring cell, originating from a rapid entry of sodium, reaches the threshold potential (TP) and results in a TAP (b and c are stimuli under threshold potential) (Fig. 1.8B). The TAP has four phases: phase 0 that is the depolarization, the loss of external electrical charges, and phases 1 to 3 involve repolarization, the recovery of these charges.

Cells of the specific conduction system (SCS) have an ascending TDP, because they present some diastolic depolarization due to a rapid

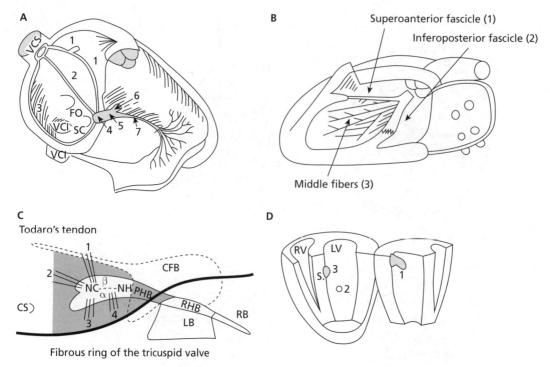

Figure 1.3 (A) Right lateral view of the specific conduction system. 1, 2 and 3: internodal tracts; 4: AV node; 5: bundle of His; 6: left branch; 7: right branch with its ramifications; Ao: aorta; AVN: AV node; CS: coronary sinus; FO: fossa ovalis; IVC: inferior cava vein; SN: sinus node; SVC: superior cava vein. (B) Left lateral view of LV: see the superoanterior (SA) division (1), the inferoposterior (IP) division (2) and the middle fibers (3) (quadrifascicular theory) or rather a quadruple input of ventricular activation theory. (C) Structure of the AV junction extending further than the AV node (the compact node). The zone shaded in gray is included in the AV junction, and may be involved in the reentry circuits exclusive to the AV junction: CFB: central fibrous body; N: compact AV node; PHB: bundle of His—penetrating portion; RHB: bundle of His—ramifying portion; LB: left branch; RB: right branch. Slow conduction (α) and rapid conduction (β) pathways; 1–4: entry of fibers of internodal pathways into the AV node: NH: nodal-His transition zone; CS: coronary sinus. (D) The open left ventricle shows the three points of LV activation according to Durrer (see text).

inactivation of the potassium outward currents. The sinus node (SN) is the SCS structure with the greatest ascending TDP, and thus it presents the greatest automaticity, and is the physiological pacemaker of the heart.

The TAP in automatic cells (Fig. 1.7) takes place when the TDP reaches the threshold potential. This occurs at the exact point when the ionic curves of sodium (arising) and potassium (decreasing) cross (Fig. 1.8), resulting in the entry of sodium into the cell. This occurs more rapidly when the TDP curve is sharper, as in SN automatic cells.

SCS cells after cellular depolarization (TAP) that present slow ascent (phase 0) (contractile cells) experience shorter repolarization phases (2 and 3).

1.5.2. Electroionic correlation in TAP formation (Figs 1.8 and 1.9)

In both contractile (Fig. 1.6) and automatic cells (Fig. 1.7) TAP curves originate because first a rapid entry of sodium occurs, followed by sodium and calcium, into the cell during phase 0, or cellular depolarization. Later this is followed by a slow exit of potassium, resulting in the repolarization process

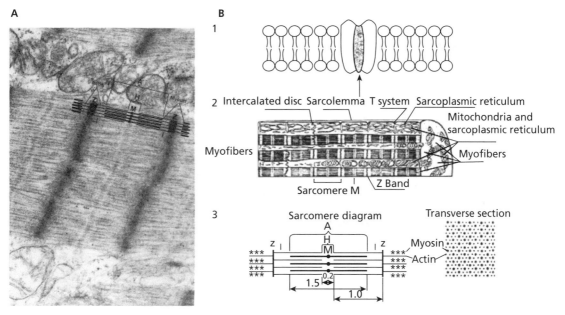

Figure 1.4 (A) Microphotography of a sarcomere where actin and myosin filaments are observed (see B-3). (B-1) Structure of the cellular membrane (or sarcolemma) showing an ionic channel. (B-2) Section of a myocardial contractile cell including all different elements. (B-3) Enlarged sarcomere scheme.

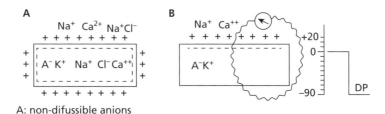

Figure 1.5 (A) The predominant negative charges inside the cell are due to the presence of significant non-diffusible anions which outweigh the ions with a positive charge, especially K^+. (B) Two microelectrodes placed at the surface of a myocardial fiber record a horizontal reference line during the resting phase (zero line), signifying no potential differences on the cellular surface. When one of the two electrodes is introduced inside the cell, the reference line shifts downwards ($-90\,mV$). This line (the DP) is stable in contractile cells and has a more or less ascending slope in the specific conduction system cells (Figs 1.6 and 1.7).

(phases 2 and 3). Figure 1.8 shows this process in a contractile cell through the formation of the depolarization and repolarization dipoles, which will be explained in the next chapter (Bayés de Luna, 2012a). Figure 1.9 shows the most relevant ionic current in automatic (A), and contractile cells (B) during systole.

1.5.3. Stimuli transmission from the sinus node to the contractile myocardium

Figure 1.10 shows how stimuli are transmitted from the SN (the most automatic cells) to the AV node, branches and ventricular Purkinje fibers, which present progressively less automatism, and

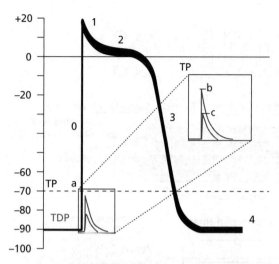

Figure 1.6 Transmembrane diastolic or resting potential (TDP) and transmembrane action potential (TAP) of contractile cells.

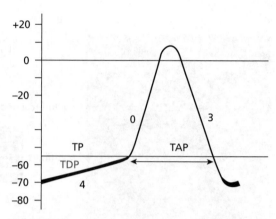

Figure 1.7 Transmembrane diastolic or resting potential (TDP) and transmembrane action potential (TAP) of automatic cells.

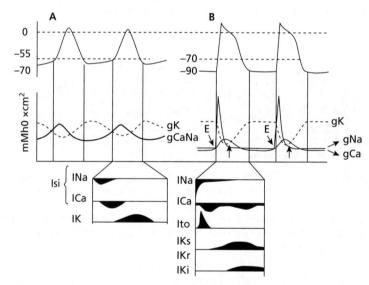

Figure 1.8 The most relevant ionic currents in automatic (A) and contractile (B) cells during systole. Contractile cells are characterized by an early and abrupt Na$^+$ inward flow and an initial and transient K$^+$ outward flow (*I*to). These are not present in automatic cells.

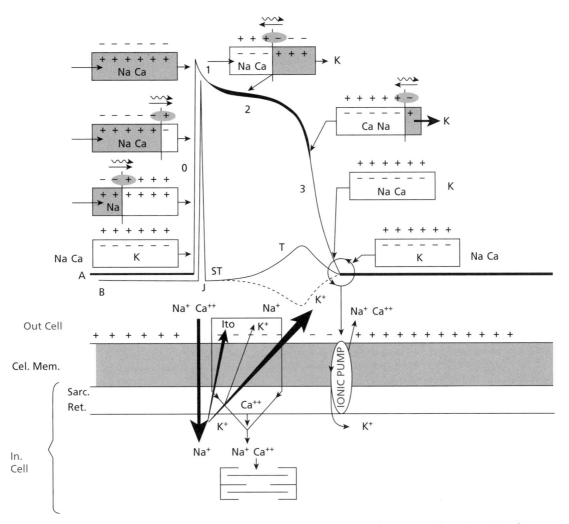

Figure 1.9 Diagram of the electro-ionic changes occurring during cellular depolarization and repolarization of contractile myocardium cells. In phase 0, when the Na inward flow occurs, the depolarization dipole ($-+$) is formed. In phase 2, when an important and constant K outward flow is observed, the repolarization dipole is formed ($+-$). Depending on whether we examine a single cell or the whole left ventricle, a negative repolarization wave (broken line) or a positive repolarization wave (continuous line) is recorded respectively (see Section 2.1.2 in Chapter 2).

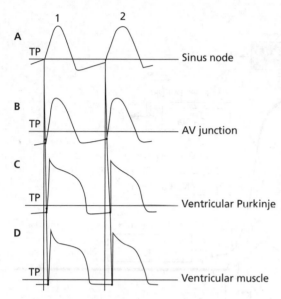

Figure 1.10 Sinus node AP (A) transmitted to the AV junction (B), the ventricular Purkinje (C) and ventricular muscle (D) (TP: threshold potential).

finally to the ventricular muscles (nonautomatic contractile cells). This process is explained in the next chapter in the section on heart activation and the domino theory.

Self-assessment

A. Which segment of the LV does the area previously known as the posterior wall correspond to?

B. Which artery perfuses the LV apex?

C. How many activation entry points are in the LV?

D. How many types of cardiac cells exist?

E. What is TDP?

F. What is TAP?

G. What role do ions play in the formation of TAP?

CHAPTER 2

The ECG Curve: What Is It and How Does It Originate?

2.1. How does the TAP of a myocardiac cell become the curve of the cellular electrogram?

The electrical activity (depolarization and repolarization) of a contractile cell (or wedge preparation) is recorded when a microelectrode is located outside the cell and another inside, as a steep positive curve followed by a plateau with a descending slope, called the transmembrane action potential (TAP) (see Figs 2.1A and 1.6).

A However, if the deflection of this electrical activity is recorded by an electrode located on the opposite side of the cell (or wedge preparation), it shows one curve, called the **cellular electrogram**, formed by a sharp, high-voltage positive wave (QRS) (⋀) followed by an isoelectric space, and then a more gradual, wide negative wave with a lower voltage, known as the T wave (⌣), results (Fig. 2.1).

We will now look at the formation process of the cellular electrogram curve (Fig. 2.1B and C) (see Bayés de Luna, 2012a; Macfarlane et al., 2011).

2.1.1. The formation process of the cellular electrogram (cellular activation) (Fig. 2.1)

2.1.1.1. Cellular depolarization (Fig. 2.1B)
B When a cell (wedge preparation) is activated, it receives an electrical impulse and depolarizes. During this phenomenon the surface of the cell that was full of positive charges becomes negative,

starting in the place where the stimulus is applied, with the formation of a **dipole of depolarization** that is a pair of charges, namely, −+. This dipole advances along the surface of the cell to the area where the electrode is located, that is on the opposite side. **The depolarization dipole has a vectorial expression**, with the head of the vector located on the positive side of the dipole.

As it advances, a progressively more positive deflection is detected, until finally it is completely positive (⋀) (equivalent to QRS complex). An electrode located in the central part of the cell records first positively and later negatively (⋀ᵣ), because it first faces the head of the depolarization dipole (head of the vector), and then the tail of the vector, which is negative.

2.1.1.2. Cellular repolarization (Fig. 2.1C)
Once the cell (or wedge preparation) is depolarized, the process of repolarization takes place. This process starts by means of the **repolarization dipole** (+−), originating on the same side as the depolarization dipole. The repolarization dipole advances in the surface of the cell and progressively recovers the lost positive charges, slowly reaching C the recording electrode, producing a slow and gradual negative curve (T wave).

Cellular activation may be compared to a car passing by in the dark, going towards the recording electrode. The lights of the car, as it moves closer, are facing the electrode which records positivity (depolarization). Afterwards, the car starting from the original point advances in reverse towards the

ECGs for Beginners, First Edition. Antoni Bayés de Luna.
© 2014 John Wiley & Sons, Inc. Published 2014 by John Wiley & Sons, Inc.

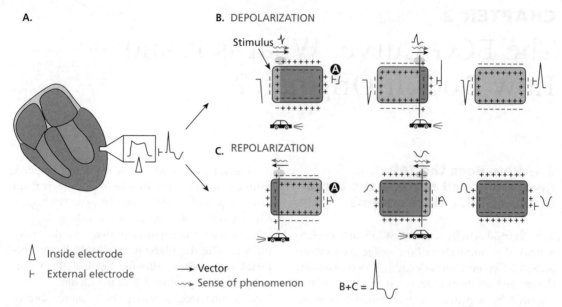

A.

B. DEPOLARIZATION

Stimulus

C. REPOLARIZATION

△ Inside electrode

⊢ External electrode

→ Vector

⤳ Sense of phenomenon

B+C =

Figure 2.1 (A) An electrode located in a wedge section of myocardial tissue records TAP curve similar to the TAP recorded when a microelectrode is located inside the cell (Fig. 1.6). When one electrode is placed outside a curve, the so-called 'cellular electrogram' is recorded. (B and C) Diagram showing how the curve of the cellular electrogram originates, based on the dipole theory (B depolarization and C repolarization). (See Plate 2.1.)

same electrode. However, as the car approaches the electrode, because the lights are facing the opposite side, it records negativity (repolarization) (Fig. 2.1B and C).

> Both dipoles have a vectorial expression. The head of the vector ⇄ is located at the positive charge, even when the sense of the phenomenon is different (Fig. 2.1).

2.1.2. Why is the T wave in the human ECG positive, while in the cellular electrogram it is negative?

This may be explained by two theories.

2.1.2.1. The theory of the depolarization and the repolarization dipole (Fig. 2.2)

If we look at the left ventricle, which is responsible for the human ECG to a large degree, acting as an enormous cell, it is possible to see how depolarization starts in the endocardium, where the electrical stimulus arrives from the Purkinje fibers. An electrode (⊢ A), located on the epicardium on the oppo-

site side, meanwhile detects that the depolarization dipole is approaching; this is a positive complex because this electrode faces the positive charge of the depolarization dipole (the vector head).

However, repolarization does not begin in the same location as that of the isolated cell. Repolarization in the heart begins in the most perfused area: the subepicardium. The subendocardium is an area of terminal perfusion, and physiologically it is less perfused than the subepicardium. The subendocardium may be considered to have some physiologic ischemia. Thus the repolarization dipole advances from the subepicardium to the subendocardium, like a car passing by in reverse with the front lights visible (positive charge of the dipole, or vector head), facing the subepicardium. Thus a positive charge is detected there.

In summary: The path of the electrical activity in the LV of the human heart is determined by depolarization and repolarization dipoles as previously described. These dipoles have a vectorial expression, with the head of the vector located at the positive charge.

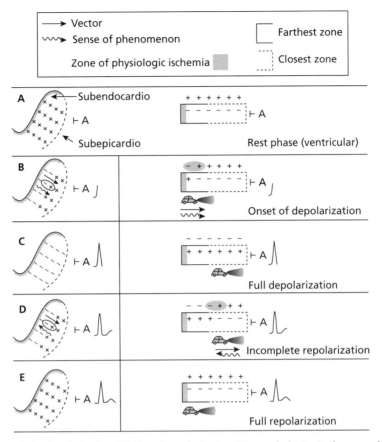

Figure 2.2 Diagram of the depolarization (QRS) and repolarization (T) morphologies in the normal human heart. The figures to the left show a view of the free left ventricular wall from above, and we see only the distribution of the charges on the external surface of this 'enormous left ventricular cell.' In the right column we see a lateral view in which the changes in the electrical charges can be appreciated. With electrode A in the epicardium, a normal ECG curve is recorded.

Figure 2.3 outlines the sense (〰➤) of the depolarization and repolarization phenomenon, the dipoles, and its vector ⇉ expression during depolarization and repolarization (activation) of the heart, namely of the LV, which is considered to be mostly responsible for this process.

2.1.2.2. The theory of the sum of TAP of the subendocardium and subepicardium

E This is an alternative theory that may explain the formation of a human ECG curve. The human ECG recorded from an electrode (⊢) located on the LV epicardium (largely responsible for the ECG curve) may be considered, according to Ashman (Bayés de Luna, 2012a), the sum of the TAP of the subendocardial area and the TAP of the subepicardial area of the LV wall. As the TAP of the subepicardium is recorded as negative and starts and ends before the TAP of the subendocardium, which is recorded as positive, the sum of both explains the recording of a positive deflection (QRS), an isoelectric space (ST) and a terminal positive wave (T) (see legend, Fig. 2.4).

2.2. The activation of the heart

• **Only activation** (depolarization and repolarization) **of the atrial and ventricular myocardial**

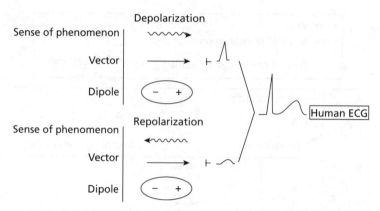

Figure 2.3 Ventricular depolarization and repolarization dipoles, with the corresponding vectors and direction of the phenomenon and resulting human ECG curve (QRS–T curve).

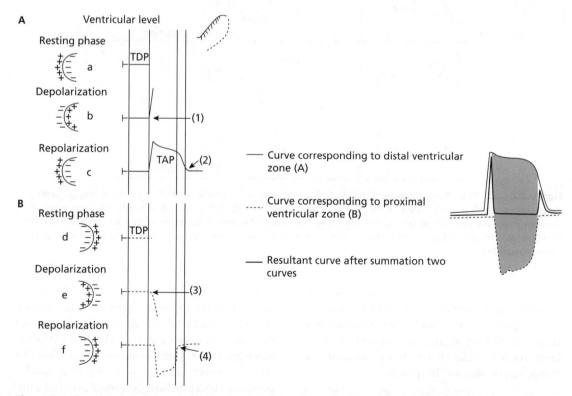

Figure 2.4 The subendocardial zone distal to the electrode depolarizes before (Ab-1) and repolarizes later (Ac-2) than the subepicardial zone (Be and Bf and 4). The electrode in Ab faces the positive charges of opposed part and records a positive PAT, that later during repolarization returns to the isoelectric line because the electrode faces the negative charges (Ac). The depolarization of the subepicardial zone starts later and is recorded as negative because the electrode faces the outside negative charges of the subepicardium. Therefore, the TAP of the subepicardium is recorded as negative and starts before and also finishes before the TAP of the subendocardium, because the repolarization in humans starts in the subepicardium (see Section 2.1.2). Therefore, the sum of both TAPs explains the positive initial (QRS) and final (T) positive deflexion and in between an isoelectric line (ST).

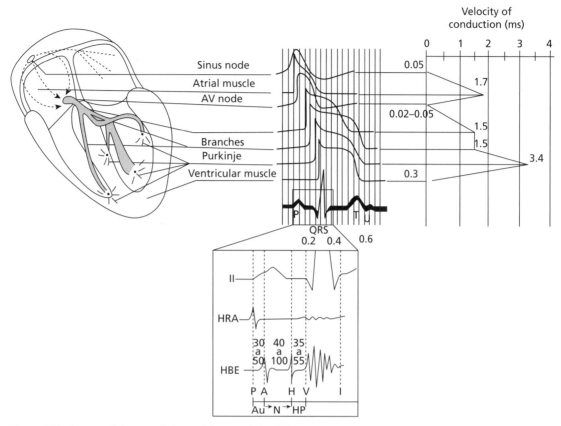

Figure 2.5 Diagram of the morphology of the AP of the different specific conduction system structures as well as the different conduction speeds (ms) through these structures. Below is an enlarged depiction of the PR interval with a histogram recording. HRA: High right atria; HBE: ECG of the bundle of His; PA: from start of the P wave to the low right atrium; AH: from low right atrium to the bundle of His; HV: from the bundle of His to the ventricular Purkinje.

mass (contractile cells) **is detected in the ECG (P QRS-T).**

• The electrical activation of the sinus node (SN) and the passing of the stimulus through the SCS are not recorded on a surface ECG, because the electrical potential they generate is too low. The lower part of Figure 2.5 shows how these potentials may be detected as short, sharp deflections in a recording of intracavitary ECG.

• Figure 2.5 shows the correlation between the action potential (TAP) generated by cells in specific areas of the heart and the surface ECG, as well as the stimulus conduction speed as it passes through these areas.

• The global depolarization vector of the atria (P wave) and ventricles (QRS) is the sum of many successive, instantaneous depolarization vectors in these structures, configuring the P and QRS loops (see below) (Figs 2.6 and 2.9).

2.2.1. Atrial activation (Fig. 2.6)

Atrial depolarization (Figs 2.6 and 2.7) begins in the SN and goes first to the right atrium, spreading in concentric curves to the septum and left atrium mainly through the Bachmann bundle.

The sum of multiple instantaneous vectors in the atria originates a curve called the atrial depolarization loop, which represents the path followed by

F

the stimulus following depolarization of both atria. Due to the fact that this begins in the right atrium, it follows a spatial anti-clockwise direction. This atrial depolarization loop can express itself with a maximum or global vector, that is the sum of all instantaneous atrial depolarization vectors and, ultimately, the sum of the depolarization vectors of the right and left atria. The positive part of the atrial depolarization global dipole is located at the head of this global vector. Thus, on the surface of the body (left thorax) a positive curve, called the **P loop or wave**, is recorded.

Depolarization of atrial muscle, which has a very thin wall, starts in the SN and continues along

the entire wall. When depolarization begins, a depolarization dipole with a vectorial expression forms, and is directed toward the electrode located in front, originating a positive wave (P wave) (Fig. 2.7A and D).

Atrial repolarization (Fig. 2.7E to G) begins in the same place (E) as depolarization, and the repolarization dipole also occupies the entire thickness of the atrial wall because, as stated previously, this is very thin. Consequently, the repolarization dipole approaches the recording electrode (left thorax), which faces the negative charge of the dipole (vector tail), resulting in the recording of a slower and longer negative curve compared to the positive P wave because the process is more lasting (F and G).

The negative wave of atrial repolarization is not generally detected, because it remains hidden in the ventricular depolarization complex (QRS) (Fig. 2.8), except when the P wave has a high voltage or when AV block occurs, which produces a delayed recording of QRS.

2.2.2. Ventricular activation

The path of the stimulus through the intraventricular SCS is recorded in the ECG as a straight line between the atrial activation P wave and the ventricular activation (QRS-T), and this corresponds to the PR segment.

The electrical stimulus reaches three areas of the LV first (Fig. 1.3D). These areas correspond to the superoanterior and the inferoposterior fascicles, and the middle fibers (also named septal fascicles).

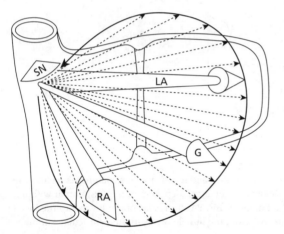

Figure 2.6 Left, right, and global (G) atrial depolarization vector and P loop. The successive multiple instantaneous vectors are also pictured.

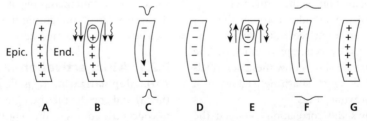

⤳ = Sense of phenomenon (depolarization B and repolarization E).
⟶ = Vector of the phenomenon of depolarization and repolarization.

Figure 2.7 (A) Atrial resting phase. (B and C) Depolarization sequence. (D) Complete depolarization. (E and F) Atrial repolarization sequence. (G) The cellular resting phase.

Ventricular depolarization: The path of the electrical activity through the ventricles, from the endocardium to the epicardium, originates a loop (Fig. 2.9A) that when recorded with an electrode located in front of it in the LV epicardial wall, may be divided into three vectors. The middle vector, or vector 2, is the most important and is the expression of most of the depolarization of the LV (R wave). An initial part, vector 1 (q wave), moves from left to right, and upwards in the intermediate and vertical heart (in the horizontal heart below), and represents the sum of the depolarization of the three small areas of initial depolarization in the LV as described by Durrer (Fig. 1.3D). Lastly, vector 3 represents the depolarization of the last parts of the septum and the right ventricle (RV) and it is also directed upward and to the right ('s' wave). By joining these three vectors, we have a loop that

represents the whole of the ventricular depolarization process known as the QRS loop or QRS complex.

The QRS loop in Figure 2.9A is that of a heart in an intermediate position with a morphology that is detected with an electrode (⊢) located in front of the main depolarization vector (vector 2) (see Figs 2.11 and 2.26).

Ventricular repolarization takes place later on, the path of which explains the formation of a loop (**T wave or loop**) with a maximal vector similar to the QRS global loop (Figs 2.9B, 2.11, and 2.28).

Naturally, the QRS and T loops, at different rotations of the heart, vary according to the different locations of the vectors and the orientation of the loops (Bayés de Luna, 2012a).

2.2.3. Domino theory

Cardiac activation can be compared to a row of dominoes as they fall. **Sinus node**, with the most automatic capacity (black domino), corresponds to the first domino, transmitting the stimulus to the neighboring structures. Figure 2.10 shows each phase, from the start of the diastole (phase 1), through all diastole (DTP) (phase 2), and then the entire activation phase (depolarization and repolarization of the atria and ventricles, phases 3 to 8). The grey dominos show decreasing automaticity.

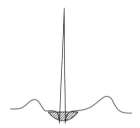

Figure 2.8 See the atrial repolarizaton wave hidden in the QRS complex.

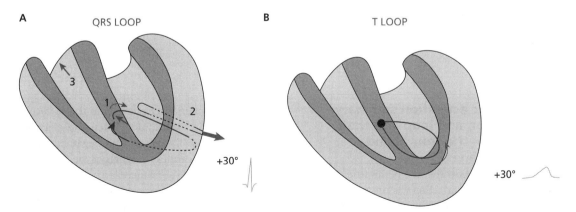

Figure 2.9 QRS (A) and T (B) loops of a heart without rotations (see Chapter 4). (See Plate 2.9.)

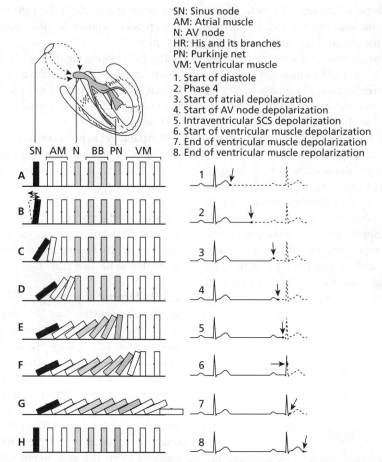

Figure 2.10 Sequence of cardiac activation: an analogy using dominoes. The first domino topples the next and so on. This occurs in the heart, when the heart structure with the most automatic capacity (the first black domino) has moved enough (C) to transmit its impulses to the neighboring cells. The black domino represents the heart pacemaker (SN: sinus node) and the gray dominoes represent cells with less automaticity, which in fact do not usually manifest, since these cells are depolarized by the propagated impulse transmitted by the black domino (SN). White dominoes usually do not feature automaticity. The point dividing the continuous line from the broken one in the ECG curve indicates the time point corresponding to these different electrophysiological situations in the cardiac cycle.

2.2.4. Cardiac activation summary: dipole, vector, and loop and their projection on the frontal and horizontal planes

Figure 2.11 shows how the sum of the atrial (A) and ventricular (B) depolarization vectors and ventricular repolarization (C) (top), with the corresponding loops (middle) can explain the morphology of an

ECG taken from an electrode (⊢) on the surface of the LV. Positivity is recorded when the electrode faces the head of the vector and negativity when facing the tail, regardless of whether the phenomenon is moving towards (depolarization) or away from (repolarization) the recording electrode. Obviously, an electrode located opposite to this location will record an inverse pattern (Figs 2.11 and 2.12).

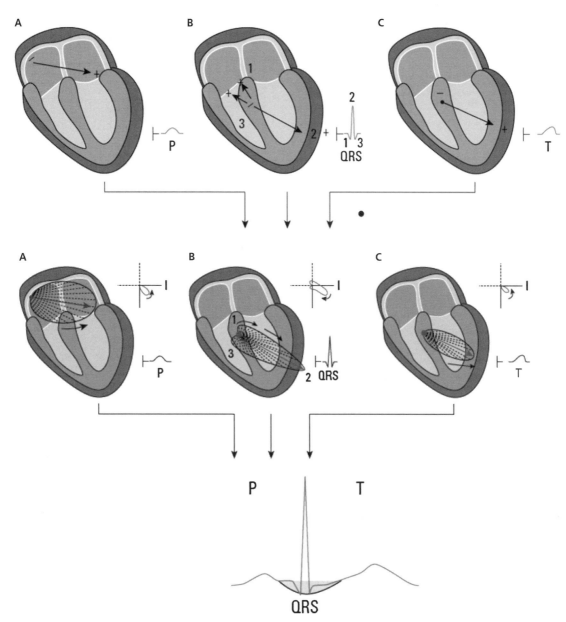

Figure 2.11 Above: Atrial depolarization (A), ventricular depolarization (B) and ventricular repolarization (C) vectors. **Middle:** Respective loops of these processes. **Below:** The resultant ECG curve.

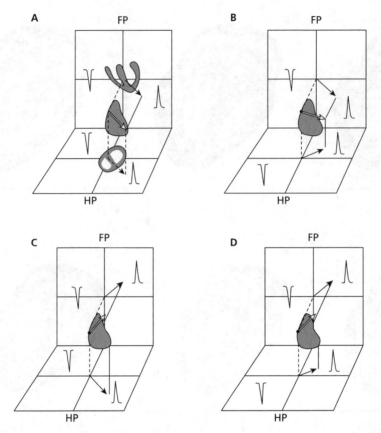

Figure 2.12 The projection of four spatial vectors in FP and HPA: (A) forwards and below; (B) backwards and below; (C) upwards and forwards; and (D) backwards and upwards) originate positive and negative complexes according to whether the recording place faces the head or the tail of the vector.

2.2.5. The projection of the electrical activity of the heart on a plane surface

Bearing in mind that the heart is a three-dimensional organ, visualizing on paper or screen the electrical activity of the heart (vector or loop) must involve two planes, the frontal plane (FP) and the horizontal plane (HP).

Figure 2.12 shows how the projection of different spacial vectors (or loops) originate positive or negative morphologies on the FP and HP according to whether the location of the recording is facing the head (+) or tail (−) of this vector.

Even before we examine specific derivations or the projection of vectors and loops in the positive and negative hemifields of these derivations, it is possible to see that positivity or negativity is recorded according to whether we face the head or tail of the vector. The projection of loops on the FP and HP that will be explained later, will clearly explain why bi or trifascicular deflections are recorded.

2.3. Lead concept

To see better landscapes, monuments and sculptures on a plane surface, we must take pictures from several angles, as seen in Figure 2.13. In the same way, to understand better the electrical activity of the heart, we have to record the ECG from various points, called leads. The ECG morphology

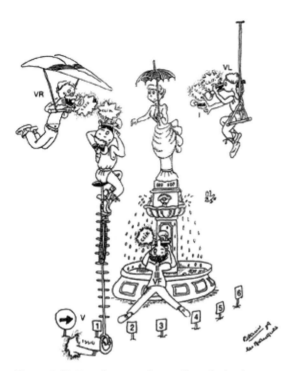

Figure 2.13 For a better understanding of a landscape, building, or statue it is necessary to contemplate or take photographs from different angles, as shown in this case with the 'Dama de la Sombrilla' (Umbrella Lady), a landmark in Barcelona. Similarly, if we want to learn about the electrical activity of the heart it is necessary to record the activation route from different angles (leads) (drawing by my sister Pilarín Bayés de Luna).

differs according to the location from which the recording takes place.

There are six leads located on the frontal plane (FP): I, II, III, VR, VL and VF. They record the electrical activity with electrodes located on the limbs. **There are also six leads on the horizontal plane** (HP): V1-V6, which record this activity with electrodes placed on the precordium (see below).

Each lead is placed in a specific place (at an angle) on the FP of HP, and each lead has a lead line that travels from the opposite side (180°) passing through the center of the heart. Each lead is also divided into positive and negative parts. The positive part goes from the point in which the lead is located to the center of the heart (a continuous line, in Figures 2.14 to 2.18). The negative part is made up from the center of the heart to the opposing pole (discontinued line, Figs 2.14, 2.15 and 2.18).

2.3.1. Frontal plane leads

There are three leads called bipolar limb leads located between two points of the body (I, II, and III) (Fig. 2.14) and three monopolar leads (VR, VL, and VF), which are in fact also bipolar because they measure the difference in potential between a point (VR on the right shoulder; VL on the left shoulder and VF on the left leg) and the central terminal connected to the center of the heart (Fig. 2.16).

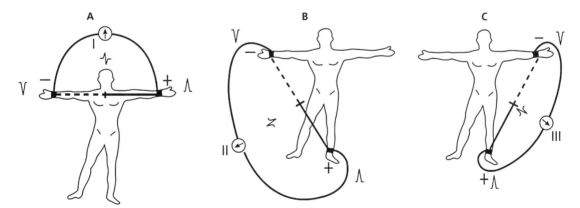

Figure 2.14 (A) Lead I records the differences in potential between the left arm (+) and right arm (−). (B) Lead II records the differences in potential between the left leg (+) and right arm (−). (C) Lead III records the differences in potential between the left leg (+) and left arm (−).

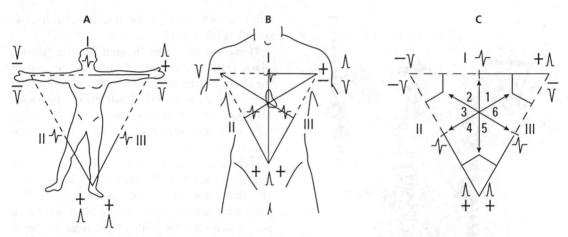

Figure 2.15 (A) Einthoven's triangle. (B) The same triangle superimposed on a human torso. Observe the positive (continuous line) and negative (dotted line) parts of each lead. (C) Different vectors (from 1 to 6) produce different projections according to their location. For example, Vector 1 has a positive projection in I, negative projection in III, and isodiphasic projection (zero) in II.

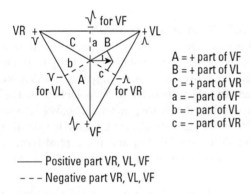

A = + part of VF
B = + part of VL
C = + part of VR
a = − part of VF
b = − part of VL
c = − part of VR

—— Positive part VR, VL, VF
- - - Negative part VR, VL, VF

Figure 2.16 Any vector projected on VR, VL, or VF produces a projection that can be positive, negative, or isodiphasic. Vector 1 has a positive projection on VL, a negative projection on VR, and an isodiphasic projection on VF.

The three bipolar leads of the limbs are recorded through electrodes located on the arms and legs. Lead I (A) obtains the difference in potential between the left arm (+) and the right arm (−), lead II (B) between the left leg (+) and the right arm (−), and lead III (C) between the left leg (+) and left arm (−) (Fig. 2.14).

These three bipolar leads constitute the Einthoven triangle, shown in Figure 2.15A. Figure 2.15B shows the triangle superimposed on the human torso (B). We can see the positive part (continuous line) and the negative part of each lead.

Different vectors (1 to 6) (Fig. 2.15C) originate different projections according to their location. For example, vector 1 has a positive projection in lead I, a negative projection in lead III, and an isodiphasic (0) in lead II. Thus, the voltage of lead II is equal to the sum of the voltages of I and III.

This sum, **II = I + III**, is called **the law of Einthoven.** This law must always be observed in order to ensure that the ECG is recorded and labeled correctly.

Leads VR, VL, and VF record the electrical activity from the right shoulder, the left shoulder, and the left leg. They also have a lead line with a positive part, which goes from the recording point to the center of the heart (continuous line) and a negative part that goes the area from the center of the heart to the opposite point (dotted line).

Any vector projected in VR, VL, or VF originates a projection that may be positive, negative, or isodiphasic. In Figure 2.16, vector 1 directed at 0°, has a positive projection in VL (B ∧), a negative projection in VR (C ∨) , and an isodiphasic projection in VF (-∿).

Bailey hexaxial system (Fig. 2.17): If we move the three leads of the Einthoven triangle, I, II, and III, to the center of the heart, we see that they are located at +0° (I), +60° (II), and +120° (III). If we do the same with the three leads VR, VL, and VF, they will be located at VR (−150°), VL (−30°), and VF (+90°). This situation constitutes the Bailey's hexaxial system in which all the distances among the positive and negative lead lines of all six leads of the FP are separated by 30°.

These spacial references among the FP leads, and also to those of the HP (see later), must be memorized. While this book is meant for deductive teaching, there are some concepts that must be retained in one's memory.

2.3.2. Horizontal plane leads

Figure 2.18 shows where the electrodes of the six precordial leads on the thorax are located (A) and the angles of the six positive poles with the separations existing between them (B). Figure 2.18 explains in detail where these six leads should be correctly placed. This is extremely important because the ECG morphologies may be modified, especially in V1–V2, with small changes in location, causing potentially dangerous confusion (see Sections 3.2 and 3.3 in Chapter 3).

Occasionally, recordings of leads in the right side of V1 (V3R, V4R) (Fig. 2.18) or the left of V6 (V7: posterior axillary line; V8: inferior angle of scapula; and V9: left paravertebral area) are made. These may be useful in some cases of ischemic heart disease (Chapter 9), but they are not used much in practice.

Figure 2.17 Bailey's hexaxial system (see text).

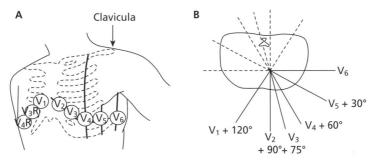

V1= 4th intercostal space (ICS) to the right of sternum
V2= 4th intercostal space (ICS) to the left of sternum
V3= between V2 and V4
V4= middle clavicular line in the 5th ICS
V5= anterior axillary line (at V4 level)
V6= middle axillary line (at V4 level)

Figure 2.18 (A) Sites where the exploring electrodes are placed in precordial leads. (B) Situation of the positive pole in the six precordial leads.

2.4. Hemifield concept

If we trace to each lead a perpendicular line
L **that passes through the center of the heart,
we will obtain one positive and one negative
hemifield.**

Figure 2.19A shows how in leads I and VF the
corresponding vector and loop fall in the positive
hemifield of each lead, and thus the morphology
in both is completely positive. In Figure 2.19B and
C we may see how an ECG morphology in a lead,
in this case VF or I, can be +− or −+, with the
same maximal vector direction, according to
whether the rotation of the loop is clockwise (a) or
anti-clockwise (b). In addition, Figure 2.19D shows
how the start and end parts of QRS originate

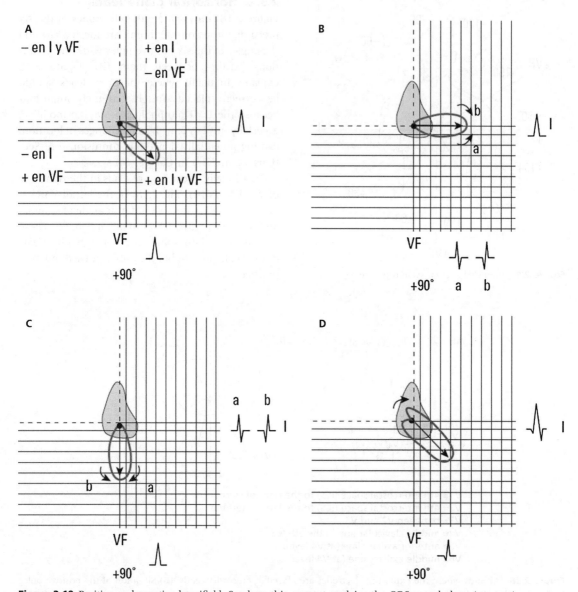

Figure 2.19 Positive and negative hemifield. See how this concept explains the QRS morphology (see text).

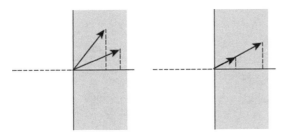

Figure 2.20 Relationship between the magnitude and direction of a vector and its positivity in a determined lead, in this case I (see text).

through the correlation of this part of the loop with the positive or negative hemifields (I and VF in D).

Figure 2.20 shows how voltage of a vector or loop is of greater or lesser importance in different leads according to the magnitude and direction of this vector or its corresponding loop, in this case in lead I. Where there are two vectors with the same direction, the voltage in this lead will only depend on the magnitude of the vector (B). However, in case of vectors with the same magnitude (A) the voltage in this lead depends on the location of the vector in its positive or negative hemifield, and consequently on the projection of this vector on the corresponding line of the lead, in this case lead I.

If a vector (Fig. 2.21) falls in the positive or negative hemifield of a particular lead, it originates a positivity or negativity in this lead. If it is located at the limit of both hemifields, the deflection will be diphasic +− or −+, according to the clockwise or counter-clockwise sense of the loop (see Figs 2.19, 2.22–2.24).

2.4.1. Vector–loop–hemifield correlation

By considering loops (global stimulus path) instead of the maximal vector, which does not include the direction of stimuli and the presence of initial and final vectors, we are able to understand the following: (1) in cases of maximal vector that falls in the limit of a positive and negative hemifield of a lead, whether the morphology will be ⋀⋁ or ⋁⋀, according

the sense of rotation of the loop; and (2) how to explain the positive or negative initial and/or final parts that many complexes present (↑, ↓).

This loop–hemifield correlation in a normal heart with a QRS loop and a maximal vector located at +60° in the FP and −20° in the HP explains the morphology recorded in these leads (Fig. 2.22).

Figure 2.23 explains how the ECG morphology allows us to estimate the stimulus path, that is the P, QRS, or T loop (in this case QRS), and vice versa. The morphologies in two leads are always correlated with the corresponding loop and vice versa; in Figure 2.23, VF and I, and V2 and V6. In this figure, in lead I and VF, firstly a small negative deflection is recorded. This indicates that the loop begins in the negative hemifield of both leads, but soon moves first toward the positive hemifield of lead I, because positivity is recorded in this lead first. Next, it enters in the positive hemifield of VF, but the initial negativity (q) in I is lower than in VF, because the greater part of the loop is in the negative hemifield of VF than of I. Finally, the QRS complex ends with a small negativity in I, but not in VF, indicating that the loop has completed its path and upon closing remains in the positive hemifield in VF and somewhat in the negative hemifield of I.

The same process in reverse produces a recording of the ECG curve through the loop. For the loop–hemifield correlation in V2 and V6 we can follow the same rule.

Figure 2.24 shows an isodiphasic deflection in a specific lead (in this case VF) that can be positive–negative (A) or negative–positive (B) according to the sense of rotation (clockwise or counter-clockwise of the loop). The area of the complex is greater if the loop is more open (C and D). Lastly, if a large part of the loop is located in the positive hemifield, the deflection is diphasic, but not iso-diphasic (E and F).

2.4.1.1. Loop-hemifield correlation: P loop
(Fig. 2.25)
Figure 2.25 shows the P loop in a heart without rotations and its projection on the FP (maximal vector at +30° in EF) and the HP. The loop–hemifield

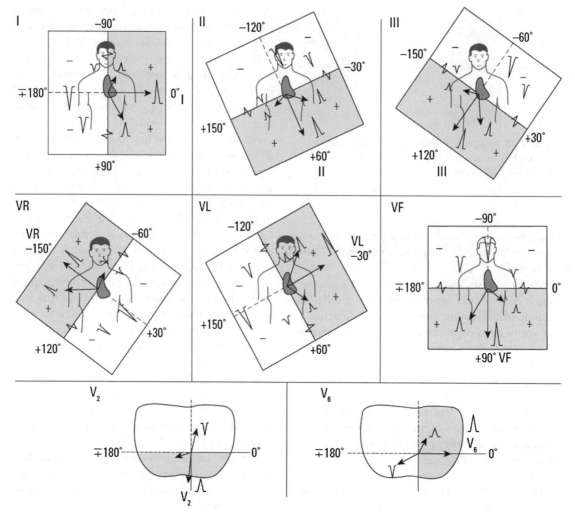

Figure 2.21 Positive and negative hemifields of the six FP leads and the V2 and V6 leads of the HP (see text).

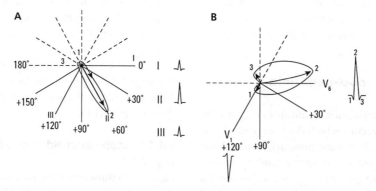

Figure 2.22 (A) Frontal plane: Relationship between the morphology of I, II, and III and the situation of the three vectors in the respective hemifields of I, II, and III. (B) Horizontal plane: Relationship between the morphology in V1 and V6 and the situation of the three vectors in the respective hemifields.

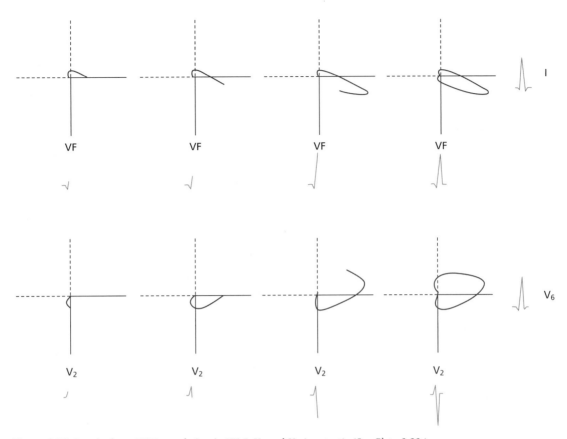

Figure 2.23 See the loop–ECG correlation in VF, I, V₂ and V₆ (see text). (See Plate 2.23.)

correlation explains the morphology of the P wave in the 12 leads and the changes that may be produced in cases of a heart with vertical or horizontal position (see Chapter 4).

2.4.1.2. Loop–hemifield correlation: QRS loop
(Fig. 2.26)
This figure shows the projection of the QRS loop in the FP and HP in a heart without rotations (intermediate position and maximal vector +30° in FP), as well as the QRS morphology in the 12 ECG leads, according to the loop–hemifield correlation (see Chapter 4). The different QRS morphologies in the six FP leads according to the projection of the QRS loop on the positive or negative hemifield of each lead can be seen in more detail in Figure 2.27.

2.4.1.3. Loop–hemifield correlation: T loop
(Fig. 2.28)
The projection of the T loop on the positive and negative hemifields of the 12 leads explains the T wave morphology. Small changes in the orientation of the loop can change the morphology, especially in V1–V2, III, VF, and VL.

To understand the electrocardiography, we must remember this sequence:

Dipole ⟶ vector ⟶ loop ⟶ hemifield

1. The dipole has a vectorial expression.
2. The sum of the various vectors of atrial and ventricular activation constitute the P, QRS, and T loops.
3. The projection of these loops on the hemifields show the ECG morphology in each lead (Figs 2.25–2.27).

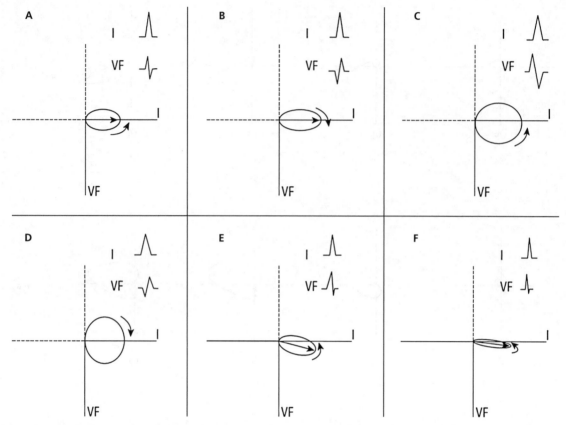

Figure 2.24 According to the direction of loop rotation, an isodiphasic deflection in a determined lead (in this case VF) is positive–negative (A) or negative–positive (B). The enclosed area is larger if the loop is more open (C and D). If more of the loop lies in the positive hemifield than in the negative hemifield, the deflection is diphasic, but not isodiphasic (E, F).

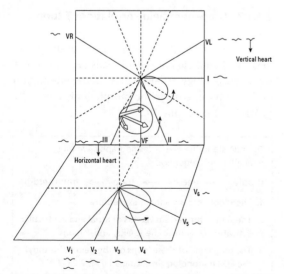

Figure 2.25 P wave morphologies in the different leads, as determined by the projection of the P loop in the positive and negative lead hemifields (see text). In a vertical heart we have a negative P wave in VL and in a horizontal heart we have a negative P wave in III.

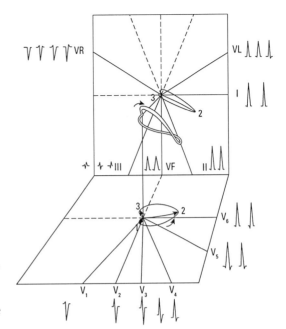

Figure 2.26 Projection of the QRS loop on the FP and HP in an intermediate heart, and morphology of the 12 ECG leads, as determined by whether the loop lies in the positive or negative hemifield of the different leads. In the case of a vertical or horizontal heart we can do the same.

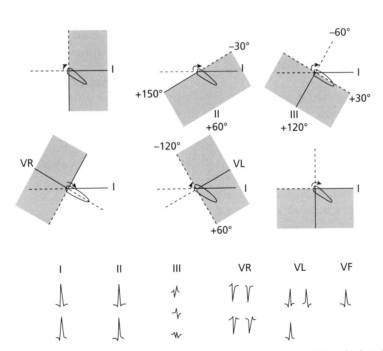

Figure 2.27 Different QRS morphologies in the six frontal plane leads, as determined by whether the QRS loop lies in the positive or negative hemifield of each lead (see text).

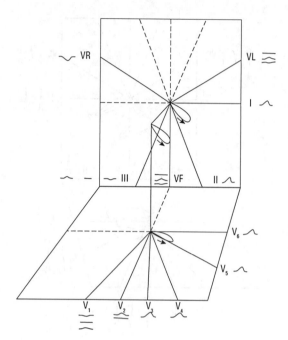

Figure 2.28 T loop and its projection on FP and HP. Observe the corresponding morphologies determined by the projection of the T loop in the positive or negative lead hemifields.

2.5. ECG wave terminology

• The P wave can be positive ($\curvearrowright$), negative ($\curvearrowright$), more/less ($\curvearrowright$) or less/more ($\curvearrowright$).
• The QRS can be diphasic ($\downarrow$, $\downarrow$), isodiphasic ($\uparrow$ $\uparrow$), triphasic ($\uparrow$ $\downarrow$), entirely positive (Λ) or entirely negative (V). The first positive component is the R wave (r if small), and the first negative component is called Q (or q if small). A negative component that follows an R/r wave is called S wave (or s if small).
• The T wave is generally positive ($\curvearrowright$) or negative ($\curvearrowright$). It is rarely more/less.
• All these morphologies depend on the location from which the electrical activity is recorded. If this happens in the epicardium of the LV (left thorax) we see the depolarization and repolarization dipoles of P, QRS, and T opposite to those from the right shoulder (right atrium) (Fig. 3.2).

• The biphasic deflections signify that the electrode is located first facing the head of the depolarization dipole and later the tail of this dipole (Fig. 2.1).
    In addition, the small positive or negative deflections at the beginning or end of QRS ($\uparrow$, $\downarrow$) indicate that although the QRS complex has a maximum vector, the ventricle depolarization generally presents small initial and final vectors at the beginning and end of depolarization that are opposing to the maximum vector, and are recorded with a small opposing deflection. However, these initial and final deflections are sometimes not reflected in the recording, because the initial or final parts of the loop fall entirely within the hemifield or remain just within its limit. This explains how, for example, the loop–hemifield correlation allows the QRS to be recorded as entirely positive in I (Λ) and presents a negative end in VF ($\downarrow$) (Fig. 2.24E and F).
• It is very important to determine whether the lack of recording of the first vectors as positive at the beginning of QRS is normal or due to a pathology (e.g. QS morphology in lead V1 or QR in lead III) (Fig. 4.22). Many of these aspects will be explained in more detail later in the book.
• Figure 2.29 shows how the P and T waves and the QRS complex are named according to morphological characteristics.

2.5.1. Normal ECG: waves and intervals

Figure 2.30 shows the waves and intervals in an ECG recorded from a derivation facing the LV.
    The measurement of the different intervals and waves is made by the graph paper of the recording (Fig. 3.3B).

Self-assessment

A. How does the TAP of a myocardial cell become the curve of the cellular electrogram?

B. How is depolarization recorded in a cellular electrogram?

C. How is repolarization recorded in the cell electrogram?

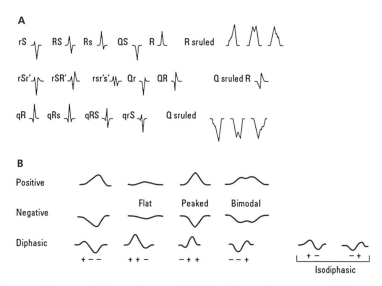

Figure 2.29 (A) The most frequent QRS complex morphologies. (B) P and T wave morphologies.

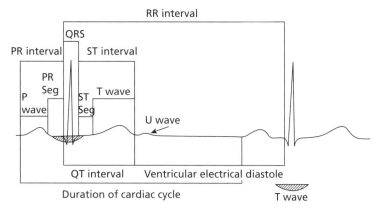

Figure 2.30 Temporal relationship between the different ECG waves and nomenclature of the various intervals and segments.

D. Why in the global heart does repolarization begin in the epicardium, and why is this relevant to how we understand the human ECG?

E. How does the sum of TAP of the subendocardium and subepicardium explain the morphology of the human ECG?

F. Describe atrial activation.

G. How does ventricular activation explain the QRS complex and the T wave?

H. What is the domino theory?

I. Describe the leads concept.

J. What are the FP leads and how do they relate to each other? (Bailey's hexaxial system).

K. What are the leads of the HP?

L. Describe the hemifield concept.

M. What is the importance of the vector–loop–hemifield correlation (P, QRS, and T loops)?

N. Why is the sequence vector–loop–hemifield so important to understanding the ECG?

O. Name the different types of morphologies for P, QRS, and T.

P. Describe the waves and intervals of a normal EC.

CHAPTER 3
Recording Devices and Techniques

3.1. Recording devices

Until recently, recording devices were analog, and recordings were generally made on thermosensitive paper.

A   Today we live in the digital age and devices are smaller, more versatile, and interactive, and may present simultaneous recordings on screen and paper (Fig. 3.1A, 1–3). There are even devices that can obtain an ECG recording by being held in the hands (Fig. 3.1A, 4).

The tracing may be sent by internet or accessed from a stored file in the hospital's computer system (Fig. 3.1B).

Figure 3.2 shows how the P wave, QRS complex, and T wave are recorded from an electrode located in a lead facing the LV, such as lead I, as well as a lead nearly opposite to it (lead VR).

3.2. The ECG recording: a step-by-step approach

B   The ECG recording must be carried out using the following steps:

1. The classic protocol involves connecting the device to an electrical source and connecting the electrodes to the device.

2. The skin of the patient is cleaned and the electrodes are placed on the appropriate areas to obtain connections with corresponding leads. Four electrodes are placed on the limbs: the red electrode on the right wrist, the yellow electrode on the left wrist, the green electrode on the left leg, and the black, or indifferent electrode on the right leg. Today the upper arms are favored over the wrists, because they provide a better recording. These electrodes are used to record the leads of the FP. Additional electrodes are placed on several places on the trunk to record the precordial leads (V1–V6). It is very important to locate the precordial leads in the appropriate location (see Chapter 2 and later).

3. The baseline should be adjusted so that the ECG recording is centered on the paper.

4. The calibration of the device is tested. In all leads the height of the calibration deflection should be 1 cm (corresponding to 1 mV) (A). The distance between the two fine horizontal lines on the recording paper is 0.1 mV (1 mm) (see later). The morphology of the calibration deflection must also be tested. The slope of the plateau must go down gradually when the calibration button is pressed (A) (Fig. 3.3A).

5. An adequate recording speed, normally 25 mm/s, must be used. In this case the distance between two vertical lines on the paper (1 mm) corresponds to 0.04 s (40 ms) and the distance between the two thick vertical lines (5 mm) corresponds to 0.2 s (200 ms) (Fig. 3.3B). A speed of 50 mm/s allows a longer distance between the intervals (QRS), but the quality of the recording, especially of the ST segment, is poorer.

6. The line of the ECG recording must be kept centered on the paper or screen.

ECGs for Beginners, First Edition. Antoni Bayés de Luna.
© 2014 John Wiley & Sons, Inc. Published 2014 by John Wiley & Sons, Inc.

A

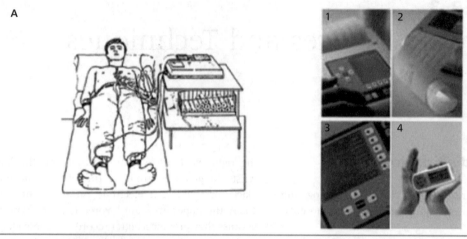

B

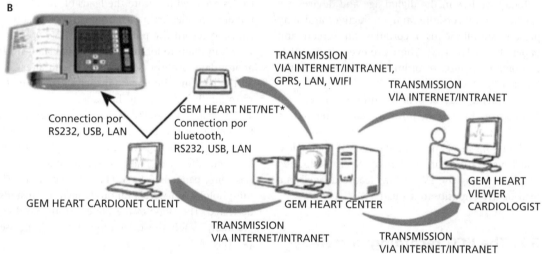

Figure 3.1 (A-1–A-3) Conventional ECG recording (see text). (A-4) Small device for self-recording an ECG strip in case of arrhythmia or precordial pain. (B) Integrated system to visualize ECG using the Internet (www.gem-med. com). (A-1–A-3) Conventional ECG recording (see text). (A-4) Small device for self-recording an ECG strip in case of arrhythmia or precordial pain (B) Integrated system to visualize ECG using the Internet (www.gem-med.com).

7. It is important to avoid artifacts (Fig. 3.3C), such as those caused by an alternate current (2) and shaking (3), which contrast with a clean recording of a normal tracing (1).

8. For each group of leads, a minimum 20 cm of tracing must be recorded. It is important to know when it is necessary to record a longer tracing (arrhythmias), or when to record during deep breathing (Q in lead III), and when to record with additional precordial leads (children, lateral or RV infarction, etc.).

9. The accuracy of the tracing must be tested (II = I + III) and the different leads must be clearly identified.

10. Today's devices usually record leads at the same time, with a minimum of six, but more often

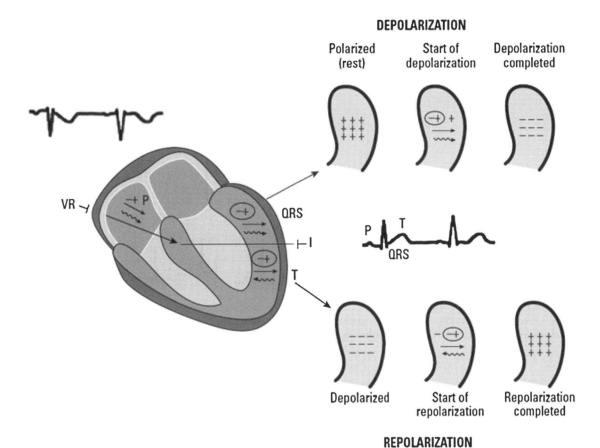

Figure 3.2 ECG recording from VR and I. Correlation with atrial depolarization and ventricular depolarization, and repolarization phenomenon (QRS and T).

12. In order to correctly measure the PR and QT intervals it is necessary to use at least three leads (see Chapter 4).

c **3.3. Recording errors**

3.3.1. Electrodes not located at an appropriate place

(see Section 4.10.4 in Chapter 4)

It is still very common to locate the electrodes inappropriately (see Figs 2.14, 2.16 and 2.18). The fol-lowing are the most frequently committed errors (Garcia-Niebla et al., 2009):

A. A high placement (2EI) of V1–V2 electrodes can result in a morphology that includes a negative P wave and often a QRS complex with r′ (Fig. 3.4) that can be confused with a partial right bundle branch block or other pathologies or vari-ants of normal ECG pattern (pectus excavatum, etc.). This disappears when the electrodes are placed on 4EI (see Chapters 2, 6 and 16).

B. The placement of leads V3–V4 too much to the right or left from the correct location

A

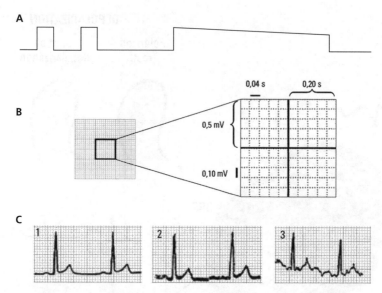

Figure 3.3 (A) Verification of proper calibration. (B) Example of a recording paper showing the distance between vertical (voltage) and horizontal (time) lines (see text). (C). 1, Normal tracing; 2, tracing with artifacts due to alternating current; 3, tracing with artifacts due to trembling.

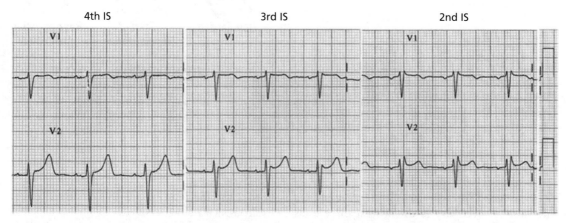

Figure 3.4 The incorrect placement of V1–V2 electrodes in the second intercostal space (2IS) instead of in 4IS explains the rSr' pattern, because the electrode in high position faces the head and not the tail of the third vector. This location also explains the negative P wave because the electrode from 2IS faces the tail of the atrial depolarization vector.

(Fig. 2.18). In patients with anteroseptal infarction, this misplacement of V3-V4 may explain an appearance (1), or not (2), of an additional involvement of the lateral wall, due to the presence, or absence, of the pathologic QRS (qrS) in V5–V6 (Fig. 3.5).

C. **Placing the electrodes on the left and right arms on the opposite side of eachother produces a morphology like dextrocardia.** See in lead I, the negative P wave and the entire inverted ECG (Fig. 3.6).

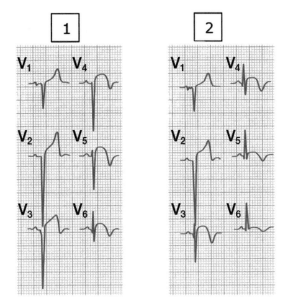

Figure 3.5 A patient with myocardial infarction of the anteroseptal zone in subacute phase. (1) Normal recording that displays extension of Q waves up to V6 (qrs). (2) Small changes in the placement of precordial V3–V6 leads have significantly modified the morphology of QRS, now being qR in lead V6.Therefore, according to the classical concept we would say that ECG 1 presents with low lateral extension of infarct, while ECG 2 does not.

D. If V1 and V2 electrodes are placed high and separate from the sternum, the recording will resemble that of VR and VL. If the VL records a qR, pattern which occurs in the case of superoanterior hemiblock, the morphology in V2 may be very similar.

3.3.2. The correct use of filters

Thanks to digital technology, filter misuse occurs rarely. However, this is still a relevant problem with analog devices. Two situations in which filter misuse can modify the true image of the recording are:

• Disappearance of an early repolarization pattern (Fig. 3.7).
• Appearance of a false Brugada pattern (Fig. 3.8).

3.3.3. Artifacts

Artifacts may arise due to patient disorder, or to malfunctions of the recording device; we present below two examples. Shaking due to Parkinson's disease is reflected in the FP leads by waves that mimic a pseudo flutter (Fig. 3.9). In a second example, a malfunction in the Holter recorder produces a false ventricular tachycardia (Fig. 3.10).

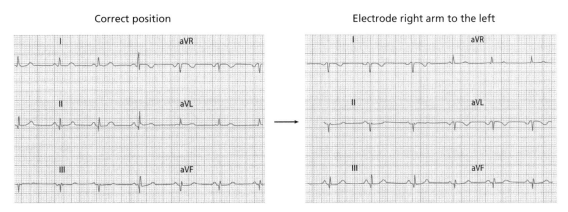

Figure 3.6 The presence of negative P wave in lead I, that has to be differentiated from dextrocardia and ectopic rhythm, is due to change of location of electrodes in the right and left arm (see text).

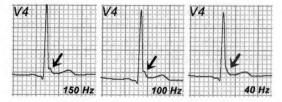

Figure 3.7 Forty-year-old patient with ECG
morphology typical for early repolarization. Observe
how a low-pass filter (40 Hz) can make the typical J
curve disappear. (See Plate 3.7.)

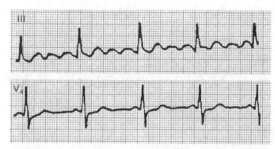

Figure 3.9 Patient with Parkinson's disease simulating
atrial flutter in some leads (in this case lead III) due to
shaking. In lead V4 we can see a normal P wave.

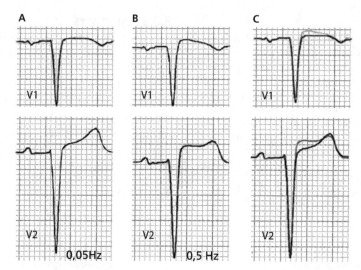

Figure 3.8 See how the devices with non-linear-phase filters may produce, when using high-pass filter of 0.5 Hz,
changes in the ECG pattern, especially in V2, in the case of left ventricular hypertrophy, which mimicks the Brugada
pattern (B). See in C the superposition of both recordings.

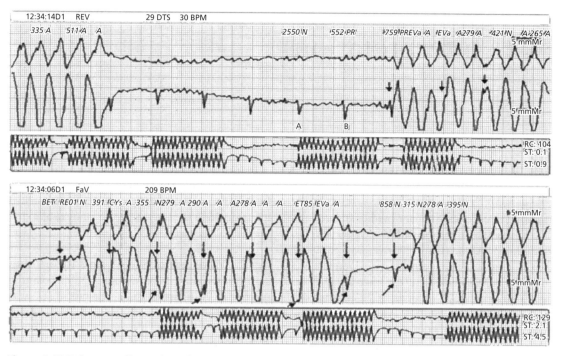

Figure 3.10 Holter recording with artifacts due to interferences that mimick runs of VT. The cadence of sinus rhythm (arrows) identify the masked QRS in the artifacts.

D 3.4. The importance of a barrier factor

The presence of any barrier factor that may affect, and generally reduce, the voltage of QRS may often be attributed to a cardiac pathology (pericardial effusion myocardial fibrosis, myocarditis, mixedema, heart failure, etc.) or an extracardiac pathology (pleural effusion, and pneumothorax). If it occurs in the left side, it may also produce a displacement of the heart.

QRS voltage is also heavily influenced by the build of the patient. Thin patients may show high voltages that simulate a left ventricular enlargement, while other patients, for example women with a large amount of breast fat, show low voltages, which can be even lower because of poor electrode placement (Bayés de Luna, 2012a).

Self-assessment

A. What are the advantages of digital ECG recording devices?

B. List the steps needed to correctly carry out an ECG recording.

C. What are the most frequent recording errors?

D. Why is the barrier factor relevant to ECG interpretation?

CHAPTER 4
ECG Interpretation

4.1. A systematic method of interpretation

The routine use of a systematic method of interpretation for both normal and pathologic ECG patterns as outlined below, is an effective way to avoid errors by ensuring that all shown parameters are checked. For example, the PR interval must be measured in the diagnosis of pre-excitation and AV block, while the QT interval is essential to the diagnosis of long and short QT syndrome.

Figures 2.29 and 2.30 show the temporal relationships between the different ECG waves and the names of intervals and segments.

4.1.1. Parameters for study
The parameters for studying normal and pathologic ECGs as the follows:
1. Heart rate and rhythm.
2. PR interval and segment.
3. QT interval.
4. P wave.
5. QRS complex.
6. ST segment and T and U waves.
7. Calculation of the electrical axes of P, QRS, or T (ÂP, ÂQRS, ÂT).
8. A normal ECG with no rotation of the heart and changes produced by rotations on the anteroposterior and longitudinal axes.
9. The evolution of normal ECG with aging.
10. Other normal ECG variants.
11. A review of abnormal findings.

In this chapter we will comment on the normal characteristics of each of these parameters. This will be helpful when we look at the abnormalities affecting these parameters in the context of different pathologies.

4.1.2. Measuring waves and intervals
Figure 4.1 shows how we measure the various waves, intervals, and segments described below.

4.2. Heart rate and rhythm

Figure 3.3B shows the distances between the vertical lines (voltage) and the horizontal ones (time). As previously described, the ECG recording device has to be calibrated, so that 1 cm in height equals 1 mV and a speed of 25 mm/s; the distance between two fine vertical lines (1 mm), corresponds to 0.04 s (40 ms); while the distance between two thick lines (5 mm) corresponds to 0.2 s (200 ms).

Using these calibrations, Table 4.1 shows a calculation of heart rate based on the RR interval.

4.2.1. Characteristics of sinus rhythm
Heart rhythm may be sinus or ectopic. Sinus rhythm is the rhythm of the sinus node, the structure with the greatest automatic capacity in the heart under normal conditions. The stimulus started in the sinus node spreads through the entire heart, originating the sinus P wave followed by the QRS complex and T wave. Nonsinus rhythms are

ECGs for Beginners, First Edition. Antoni Bayés de Luna.
© 2014 John Wiley & Sons, Inc. Published 2014 by John Wiley & Sons, Inc.

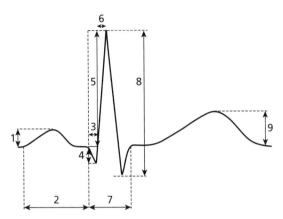

Figure 4.1 Measurement of ECG parameters: (1) voltage of the P wave: vertical intervals from the superior border of the baseline to the peak of P wave; (2) PR interval: from the onset of P wave to the onset of QRS; (3) Q-wave duration: from the point where the superior border of PR starts to descend up to the left border of the ascending arm of R wave; (4) Q-wave voltage: from the inferior border of PR to the peak of Q wave; (5) voltage of R wave: vertical distance from the superior border of PR to the peak of R wave; (6) intrinsicoid deflection: horizontal distance between the onset of QR Sand R peak; (7) QRS duration: horizontal distance from the beginning of the descent of the superior border of PR to the end of the ascendant arm of W wave or descendent arm of R wave; (8) QRS voltage: vertical distance from the most negative to the most positive peak of QRS complex; (9) voltage of T wave: vertical distance between the superior border of the baseline and the peak of T wave.

Table 4.1 Calculation of heart rate according to the RR Interval

Number of 0.20s Spaces	Heart rate
1	300
2	150
3	100
4	75
5	60
6	50
7	43
8	37
9	33

known as ectopic rhythms and are discussed in the section on cardiac arrhythmias.

4.2.1.1. Characteristics of sinus rhythm

• The normal P wave is positive in I, II, VF, and V2-V6, and negative in VR. In III and V1 the normal P wave can be ±, and −+ in VL (Figs 2.6 and 2.25). In pathologic conditions it can be ± in II, III, VF, and V2–V3 (Fig. 5.6).

• The P wave is followed by a QRS complex with a normal PR interval (0.12 s to 0.2 s) in the absence of pre-excitation or AV block.

• The heart rate at rest is usually between 50–60 to 80–100 bpm and may present a slight irregularity in the RR intervals. In children this RR irregularity can vary and may even be evident, especially with breathing.

4.2.2. Measuring heart rate and the QTc interval   C

Heart rate may be measured according to Table 4.1. However, it may also be calculated, together with the corrected QT interval (QTc), using the rule shown in Figure 4.2 (see legend).

4.3. The PR interval and the PR segment

• The PR interval is the distance from the start of P to the start of QRS. The PR segment is the distance between the end of P and the start of QRS. To measure the PR interval correctly, a minimum of three leads must be used. This allows the interval to be measured from the lead where the P wave is first recorded to the lead where the QRS is first recorded (Fig. 4.3).

• The PR segment is generally iso-electric, but includes a part of the atrial repolarization wave that even under some normal conditions (sympathetic overdrive) may be seen (Fig. 4.4). In the context of pericarditis or atrial infarction, pathologic elevations or depressions in the PR segment are present and may help for diagnosis (Fig. 5.8).

• The normal duration of the PR interval in adults ranges between 120 ms and 200 ms.

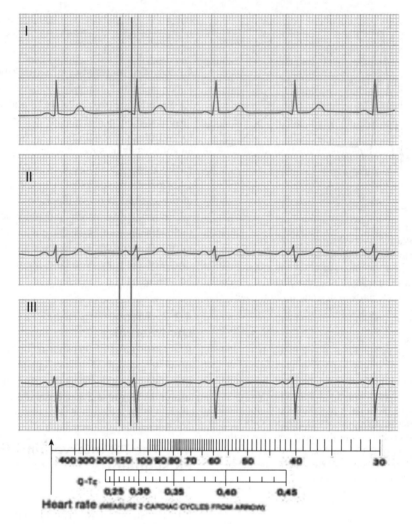

Figure 4.2 Method for measuring the heart rate and QT. (A) Heart rate: from the arrow, the rule gives the heart rate at the end of second RR. In this case 60 bpm. (B) QT interval: the corrected QT (QTc) according the heart rate corresponds to the value in the rule of QTc at the second QRS. In this case 0.39 s (390 ms) (see Table 4.2 for normal values of QT).

4.4. The QT interval

• The QT interval represents the sum of ventricle depolarization (QRS) and repolarization (ST-T).
• Sometimes it is not easy to measure. The best method is to trace a line extending the descending branch of the T wave until it crosses the iso-electric line (Fig. 4.5). This figure shows the method of measuring the QT interval in a 3-channel device. Note how the start of QRS begins in lead II.
• It is necessary to correct the value of the QT interval in relation to heart rate (QTc). There are several formulas for this measurement, the most used being those by Bazett and Fredericia. However, in practice as we said, the calculation is made as is shown in Fig. 4.2. As a general rule,

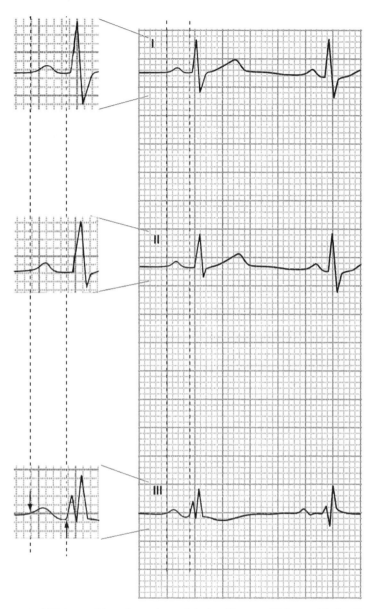

Figure 4.3 Measurement of PR interval in a three-channel device: The true PR interval is the distance between the first inscription of P wave and QRS complex in any lead. In this case (see solid lines) this happens in lead III but not in I and II. (See Plate 4.3.)

A   B

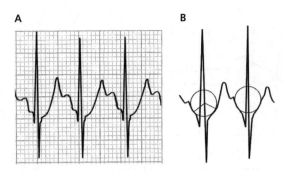

Figure 4.4 (A) A typical example of sympathetic overdrive. ECG of a 22-year-old male obtained with Holter continuous recording method during a parachute jump. (B) Drawing of the tracing that shows how the PR and ST segments form the arch of a circumference with its center located in the lower third of the R downstroke.

Table 4.2 QTc duration based on the Bazett formula in different age groups. Values are given in normal intervals, borderline, and abnormal intervals

Value	1–15 years of age	Adult male	Adult female
Normal	<440 ms	<430 ms	<450 ms
Borderline	440–460 ms	430–450 ms	450–470 ms
Permanently prolonged	>460 ms	>450 ms	>470 ms

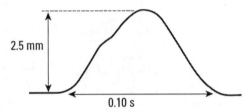

2.5 mm

0.10 s

Figure 4.6 Procedure for measuring height and width of the P wave.

QTc should always be less than 430–450 ms (Fig. 4.2).
• Abnormalities in QT (long and short QT) may be hereditary or acquired and represent a risk of arrhythmia or even sudden death (see Chapter 16).

4.5. P wave

D

• **The morphology of the P wave** in different leads during sinus rhythm is described in Chapter 2. These morphologies appear according to the projection of the P loop in the respective hemifields of the leads (Fig. 2.25).
• Normal values for height and duration are 2.5 mm and <120 ms, respectively.
• Normal P wave height and width are measured as shown in Figure 4.6.
• **Calculating the P axis (ÂP)** is carried out as with QRS (ÂQRS) (p. 49). Under normal conditions (>90% of patients), ÂP ranges between +30° and +70°, and is **never greater than +90° (negative P in lead I)**. This may only be seen in cases with electrode inversion, dextrocardia (right atrium on the left) or ectopic rhythm.

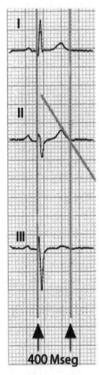

I

II

III

400 Mseg

Figure 4.5 Method of measuring the QT interval. The normal QT except in cases of a very fast heart rate, is usually less than the half RR interval. See Table 4.2 for normal values.

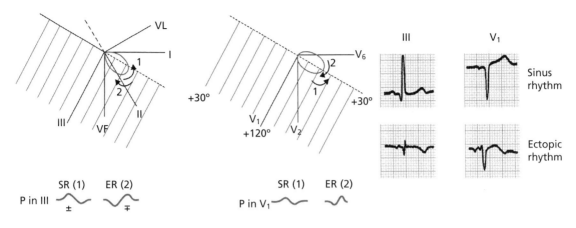

SR: Sinus rhythm   P ± o ∓, according the rotation of the loop
ER: Ectopic rhythm

Figure 4.7 According to loop rotation (counterclockwise in the FP and HP in the case of sinus rhythm and clockwise in the case of ectopic rhythm), the P wave morphology in III and V1 varies.

• **A loop-hemifield correlation** in cases of biphasic P wave (∿ or ∿) can determine whether the rhythm is sinus or ectopic (Fig. 4.7). Sinus rhythm in the P loop rotates counterclockwise in the FP and HP (Fig. 2.25).

E **4.6. The QRS complex**

• The QRS complex is abrupt and normally presents two or three deflections (Fig. 2.29). Figure 4.1 shows how ECG parameters, including those of the QRS complex, are measured.

• The normal QRS morphology in a heart with no rotations may be seen in Figure 2.26, according to the loop-hemifield correlation.

• Figures 2.26 and 2.27 show how small changes in the loop-hemifield correlation can explain slight modifications in QRS in the FP leads.

• Normal values for voltage and duration in QRS are as follows:

  – The width of a normal qRS should not exceed 100 ms.

  – The voltage of the R wave should be no greater than 25 mm for V5-V6, 29 mm in lead I, and 15 mm in VL. However, some exceptions exist,

especially in adolescent athletes and thin elderly individuals.

– The voltage in the q wave should not exceed 25% of that of the subsequent R wave, although some exceptions may occur in leads III, VL, and VF.

– The width of the q wave should be less than 40 ms and the recording should be abrupt.

– Low QRS voltage is defined by the sum of leads I, II, and II being less than 15 mm, or the sum of lead V1 or V6 as less than 5 mm, V2 or V5 as less than 7 mm, or V3 or V4 as less than 9 mm.

– The normal intrinsicoid deflection time (start of q to the peak of R) is less than 45 mm in V5-V6. This value may be greater in athletes and in presence of vagal overdrive, and sometimes in left ventricular enlargement.

– The calculation of the QRS axis (ÂQRS) is shown later (see Section 4.8). The normal value of this axis ranges between 0° and +90°, with a greater tendency toward 0° in the horizontal heart and a greater tendency toward +90° in the vertical heart. Ranges beyond +90° or +100°, or −20° or −30°, are considered pathologic.

4.7. ST segment and T wave

4.7.1. The normal ST segment and its variations (Figs 4.9 to 4.13)

The ST segment is the distance between the end of QRS (J point) and the start of the T wave. Sometimes there is a notch (J wave) or slur (J wave type) at the end of QRS (see Fig. 16.14). Under normal conditions this segment is short with a slow slope going from the end of QRS until it reaches, usually with a slight elevation, the T wave forming with its ascending slope usually a curved line slightly convex respect to isoelectric line (Fig. 4.8). The ST segment is iso-electric at the start, or only slightly above or below the iso-electric line (no more than 0.5 mm), except in V2-V3. In these leads may be elevated <2 mm in men (<2.5 cm in youngs) and <1.5 mm in women.

In vagal overdrive especially young persons, it may be elevated to 1-2 mm, or even more especially in mid/left precordial leads (Fig. 4.10B) as part of the typical early repolarization pattern, generally seen in V3-V5 (Fig. 4.10C) and less often in leads II, III, VF, I and VL.

Occasionally, including in the absence of cardio-myopathy and especially in postmenopausal women or the elderly, it may be rectified or show a slight upsloping depression (<0.5 mm) (Fig. 4.10, E and F). In these patients it is useful to make a correlation with the clinical history (hypertension, precordial pain, etc.) and perform an exercise test to confirm the significance of this pattern. Figure 6.11 shows an example of normal ST slope (A), and

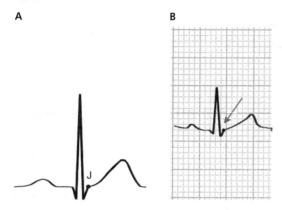

A   B

Figure 4.8 (A) Drawing showing the location of the J point. (B) The J point (arrow) in an ECG tracing. (See Plate 4.8.)

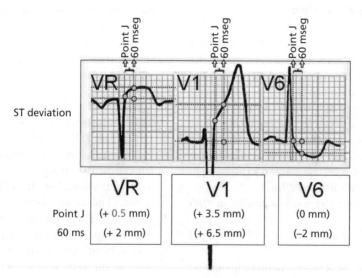

ST deviation

	VR	V1	V6
Point J	(+ 0.5 mm)	(+ 3.5 mm)	(0 mm)
60 ms	(+ 2 mm)	(+ 6.5 mm)	(–2 mm)

Figure 4.9 Method of measuring the ST shifts. The figure shows the results with the measurements at J point, and 60 ms later. (See Plate 4.9.)

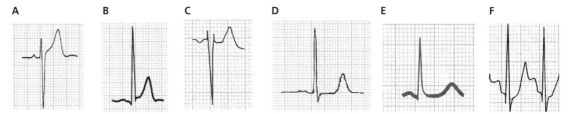

Figure 4.10 Different morphologies of atypical ST segment and T wave in the absence of heart disease. (A) ST elevation even >1 mm with mild convexity to iso-electric line that may be seen relatively often, especially in healthy young men. (B) Vagal overdrive and early repolarization in a 25-year-old man. (C) A 20-year-old man with *pectus excavatum* Normal variant of ST segment ascent (saddle morphology). (D) Straightening of ST in a healthy 45-year-old woman. (E) Flattened ST and symmetric T in a 75-year-old man without heart disease. (F) Sympathetic overdrive during a crisis of paroxysmal tachycardia in a 29-year-old woman.

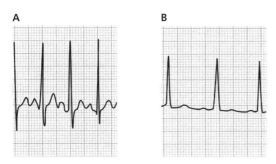

Figure 4.11 (A) Heart rate during sympathetic overdrive, and (B) after beta blockers in a case of physiological stress (parachuting). (Holter recording.) (See Plate 4.11.)

a rectified one (B), in a patient with arterial hypertension.

Lastly, it may be elevated in V1-V2, in patients with pectus excavatum and rSr' morphology (Fig. 4.10D). See the differential diagnosis with Brugada syndrome and other conditions in Chapter 16.

Figure 4.10 shows different ECG patterns that are seen in the absence of evident heart disease pattern. Some of these patterns are difficult to distinguish from pathologic ones.

The ST segment can present a small depression in normal cases, somewhat with exercise or emotional state, but it rapidly slopes up thereafter (Fig. 4.11). The ST segment responds to exercise differently in normal individuals and patients with suspected ischemic heart disease. Figure 4.12 shows pathologic ST segment responses (see legend and Fig. 9.55).

4.7.2. Measuring ST shifts

The elevation and depression of the ST segment is measured either on the J point (end of QRS) or, at different levels (+20 to +60 ms) from it. The third universal definition of myocardial infarction advises measuring the ST shifts at the J point (Thygesen et al., 2012). Figure 4.9 shows how to measure shifts (ups and downs) of the ST segment, in this case an ST elevation acute coronary syndrome (STEACS). The elevation is measured from the upper border of the PR and the depression from the lower border. If PR is not iso-electric, it is measured from the level of the start of QRS (Fig. 4.12-2B).

4.7.3. The T wave

• The T wave is positive except in VR and sometimes V1, and sometimes flat or negative in III, VF, VL, and V2. Its voltage is lower, in general much lower than that of QRS. The T wave begins at the end of the ST segment (J point) with an upward slope that is slower than the downward slope (T wave asymmetry in general) (Fig. 4.8).

• **The height of a normal T wave** does not generally exceed 6 mm in the FP and 10 mm in the HP (middle/left leads), although in vagal overdrive and early repolarization it may reach 15 to 20 mm (Fig. 4.10).

1) Normal ST after exercise

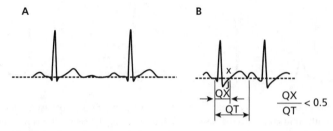

2) Pathological ST after exercise

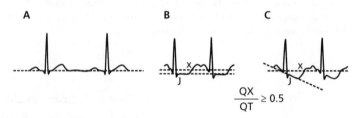

Figure 4.12 Normal ST after exercise: Although the J point and ST segments are mildly depressed, the ST segment is upsloping and the Qx/QTc 0.5. Abnormal ST after exercise: The depressed ST segment is >0.5 mm and horizontal or downsloping for at least 80 ms. Therefore the Qx/QT ≥ 0.5. For correct measurement of ST shifts see Figure 4.9.

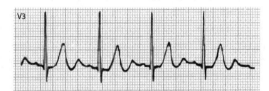

Figure 4.13 Healthy 70-year-old man (my father). Observe the rectified ST segment, peaked and symmetric T wave and the prominent U wave. Although this ECG is often seen in elderly people without evidence of ischemic heart diseases or hypertension, it is necessary to consider the clinical setting and, if necessary, to perform some complementary test (echocardiography and/or exercise testing). In this case this ECG remained unmodified for 10 years.

• **A high T wave in V1-V2**, if symmetrical especially in V1, may be seen in the hyperacute phase of STEACS due to LAD occlusion (Fig. 9.16) and chronically in the case of lateral or inferolateral infarction (Fig. 9.38).

• **A flat or negative T wave** may be seen in specific clinical situations in ischemic heart disease

(Chapter 9). It is usually not an expression of acute ischemia. It may appear:

(a) after the acute phase (post-ischemic T wave). Examples of this include cases of STEMI after percutaneous coronary interventionism (PCI), or fribrinolysis, or coronary spasm. In all these cases the T wave is very negative (Fig. 9.7);

(b) during a non-ST elevation ACS (NSTEACS). In these cases the T wave may be flat or only slightly negative) (≤2 mm) with RS or R pattern, sometimes even in leads morphology with rS; (Fig. 9.25);

(c) after Q wave-infarction: In this case the negative T wave corresponds to an intraventricular pattern (Fig. 9.30A).

• Figures 9.19 and 9.29 show other causes of high and sharp T waves and flat or negative T waves not related to myocardial ischemia.

4.7.4. The U wave

• A U wave may sometimes follow the T wave and have the same polarity but a lesser voltage.

• It is most commonly recorded in patients with bradycardia, especially those with advanced age, in leads V3-V5.

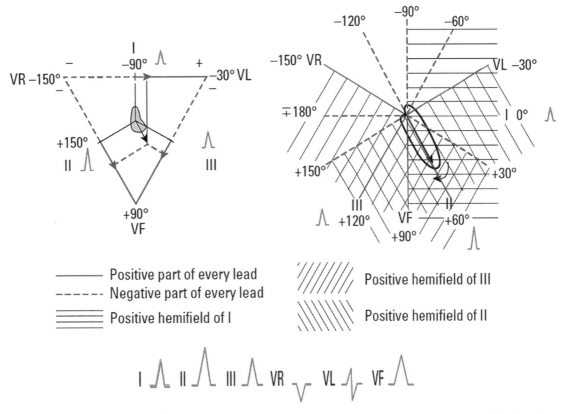

Figure 4.14 Calculation of the ÂQRS: when this is situated at +60°, the projection on I, II, and III and the situation in the positive and negative hemifields of these leads originate in I, II, and III, the morphology shown at the left of the figure. (See Plate 4.14.)

• If the polarity of the U wave is the opposite of the T wave, the cause is always pathologic (e.g. left ventricular hypertrophy, ischemia) (Fig. 9.27).

4.8. Calculating the electrical axis

The electrical axis is the resulting vector of the force generated by atrail depolarization (ÂP), ventricular depolarization (ÂQRS), and ventricular repolarization (ÂT).

The calculation of ÂQRS is explained below. ÂP and ÂT are calculated in the same way. We start at the ÂQRS located at +60° and we will see the projection of this vector on leads I, II, and III (A), and

on the hemifields of these same leads (B). Later we will do the same with ÂQRS vectors located at right and left of +60°.

A. ÂQRS +60° (Fig. 4.14)

With ÂQRS at +60° the QRS morphology is positive in leads I, II, and III, but with a higher voltage in II than in I or III (Figs 4.14 and 4.17) in accordance with Einthoven's law: II = I + III.

B. ÂQRS to the right = +90° (Fig. 4.15)

If we place ÂQRS at +90° the morphologies appear as shown in Figure 4.15 in accordance with that shown in Figure 4.14.

C. ÂQRS to the left = 0° (Fig. 4.16)

If we place ÂQRS at 0°, the morphologies in the FP appear as shown in Figure 4.16 in accordance with that shown in Figure 4.14.

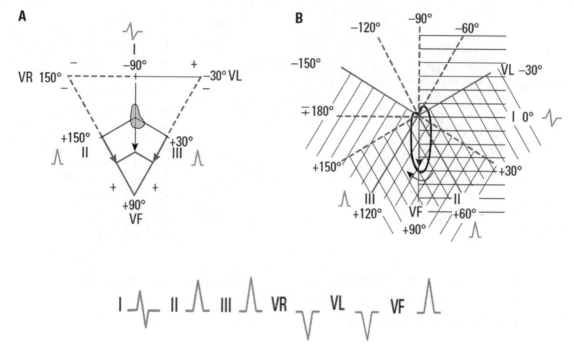

Figure 4.15 Morphologies of I, II and III with ÂQRS at +90°. (See Plate 4.15.)

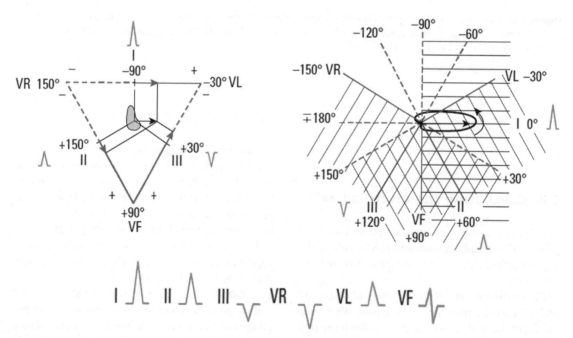

Figure 4.16 Morphologies of I, II and III with ÂQRS at 0°. (See Plate 4.16.)

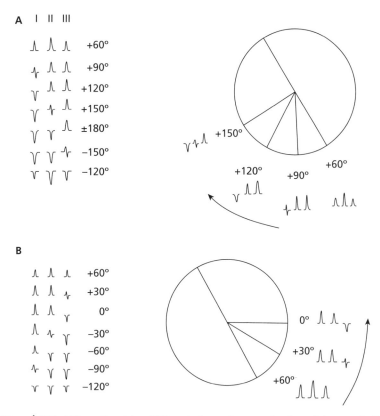

Figure 4.17 (A) When ÂQRS shifts to the right, QRS starts becoming negative from I (see text). (B) When ÂQRS deviates to the left, QRS starts becoming negative from III (see text).

H   D. Calculating ÂQRS in practice (Fig. 4.17)

– ÂQRS (and ÂP as well as ÂT) may be calculated in practice using the QRS morphologies in leads I, II, and III bearing in mind that ÂQRS at +60° has positivity in all three leads, with II equaling the sum of I and III.

– We then have to add or take away 30° for each change of morphology from positive to isodiphasic or from isodiphasic to negative. Thirty degrees are added if a change starts in I, in which case the morphology changes in I before than III. Thirty degrees are taken away if the change is initiated in III (Fig. 4.17).

– To obtain a more precise calculation for intermediate values of ÂQRS, we must proceed to the process explained below.

E. Indeterminate ÂQRS (Fig. 4.18)

When isodiphasic QRS complexes occur in I, II, and III the vectorial forces do not have a predominant direction and a GLOBAL ÂQRS cannot be calculated, although the first and second parts may be determined as shown in Figure 4.18.

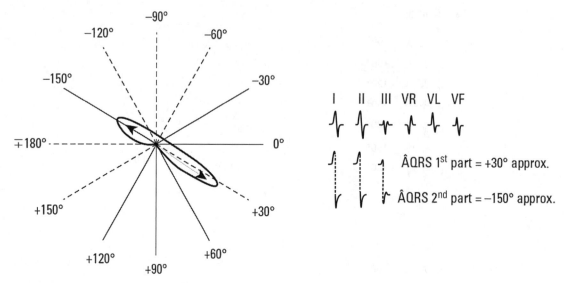

Figure 4.18 Procedure for calculating the electrical axis of the first and second parts of the QRS complex.

F. The value of measuring ÂP, ÂQRS, and ÂT

The importance of measuring these axes will become more and more apparent throughout this book, especially in the diagnosis of cavity enlargement and ventricular block. It has been recently shown that the angle formed by ÂQRS and ÂT in the frontal plane is a useful prognostic marker (see Bayés de Luna, 2012a).

4.9. Heart rotation and its repercussions on the ECG

4.9.1. The normal ECG with no rotation

• A heart with no rotation (intermediate heart) presents a ÂQRS located at about +30° and transition from the right ventricle to the left ventricle (qRs) starts in V4-V5, generally with a qR morphology (or qRs) in V6 (Fig. 4.19).

• However, a normal heart often presents some rotation on the anteroposterior and longitudinal axes which modifies the ECG; we are aware of this, but it does not indicate pathology. In different heart diseases we may see ECG patterns that are due to underlying heart disease associated or not to some rotations of the heart.

4.9.2. Heart rotation on the anteroposterior axis (Fig. 4.20)

The normal heart often presents a rotation on the anteroposterior axis. This originates a verticalization or horizontalization of the heart that is especially visible in the FP (VL and VF) (see Figure 4.20 and legend).

4.9.3. Heart rotation on the longitudinal axis (Fig. 4.21)

Rotation of this axis originates a levorotation or a dextrorotation that is especially visible in the HP (V2 and V6) (see Fig. 4.21 and legend).

4.9.4. Combined rotations (Fig. 4.22)

The vertical heart is often dextrorotated and the horizontal heart is often levorotated (Bayés de Luna, 2012a). A combined rotation, which is important to understand to avoid confusion with an inferior infarction, because in both cases may be Q in III, is the dextrorotated but horizontralized heart. The QRS loop rotates clockwise in the FP, but is oriented between 0° and 20°. This causes an S_I Q_3 morphology that disappears with breathing (change from Qr to qR). This is explained because the heart changes to a semivertical position and the loop is oriented at ≈50°) (Fig. 4.22).

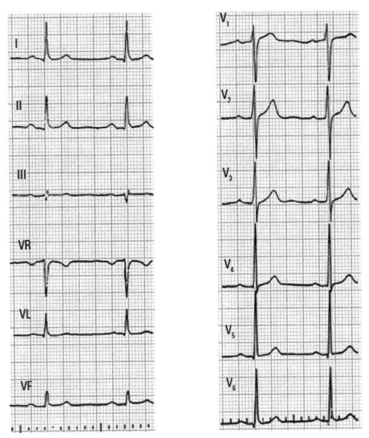

Figure 4.19 ECG of a 50-year-old male without evident heart disease and without any apparent rotation (ÂQRS = +30°, qRs in V4–V5, and qR in V6).

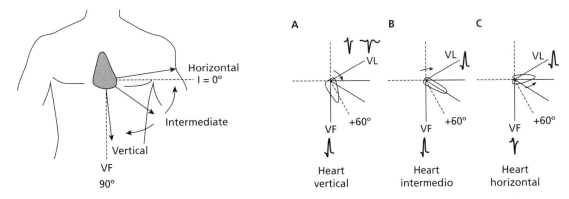

Figure 4.20 Left: ÂQRS direction in the vertical and horizontal heart. Right: QRS morphology in the vertical (A), intermediate (B), and horizontal heart (C).

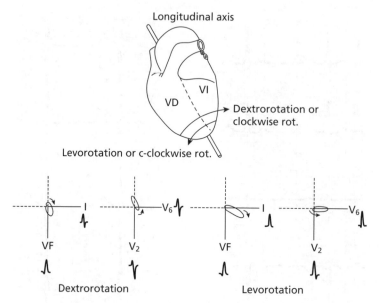

Figure 4.21 Above: Diagram to explain dextrorotation and levorotation. Below: The most common loops in the two cases and the VF, V2, and V6 morphologies.

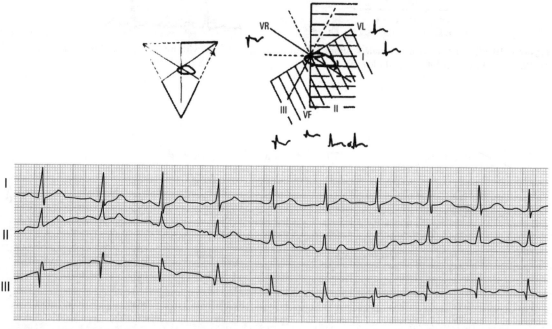

Figure 4.22 QRS loop and ECG morphologies in a case of dextrorotated and horizontalized heart. See how the Q in lead III nearly disappears with deep inspiration.

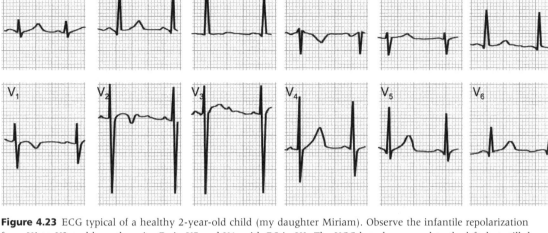

Figure 4.23 ECG typical of a healthy 2-year-old child (my daughter Miriam). Observe the infantile repolarization from V1 to V3 and how there is qRs in V5 and V6, with RS in V1. The VCG loop has moved to the left, but still does not point very far backward.

4.10. Variations of normal ECGs

4.10.1. Normal ECG changes with age

K **I. Children** (Fig. 4.23)

1. Faster heart rate
2. ÂQRS is usually to the right
3. R voltage in V1 is greater than q in V6
4. Infantile repolarization. See Fig. 4.23.
5. Adolescents occasionally show high voltage in precordial leads without left ventricular enlargement in the echocardiogram.
6. Sometimes ⋔ is recorded in V1 in children. This pattern is modified with breathing (see Bayés de Luna 2012a).

L **II. The elderly** (Fig. 4.24)

1. Greater incidence of sinus bradycardia.
2. ÂP generally >60°. Therefore $P_I < P_{III}$.
3. ÂQRS more to the left (0° or more).
4. Longer PR interval (up to 0.22 ms).
5. Frequent dextrorotation (evident S wave in V6) due to emphysema.
6. Generally lower QRS voltage. Occasionally increased voltage, especially in thin individuals.
7. Sometimes ST rectification or even small ST depression.
8. Sporadic isolated extrasystole.

4.10.2. Transitory changes in repolarization

A flattened T wave may be seen in healthy individuals following hyperventilation (Fig. 4.25), alcohol or glucose consumption, etc.

4.10.3. Other ECG patterns in the normal heart

S_1, S_2, S_3 **pattern**. This morphology may be seen in the normal heart, but also in right enlargement and peripheral right bundle branch block (Chapters 6 and 7).

Early repolarization (ER) pattern. This mor- M phology presents an abrupt wave (J wave) or slurrings at the end of QRS that is generally combined with some ST elevation. It occurs in 2% of the population, especially in the middle and left leads, often in athletes and in presence of vagal overdrive. It has been associated with the appearance of primary ventricular fibrillation (VF) (Haïsaguerre, 2008), especially when it appears in inferior leads. However cases of ER (Fig. 4.26) are not considered dangerous except in very specific circumstances, such as the presence of J waves greater than or equal to 2 mm in inferior leads (Fig. 16.14) or abrupt voltage changes of this wave or if are

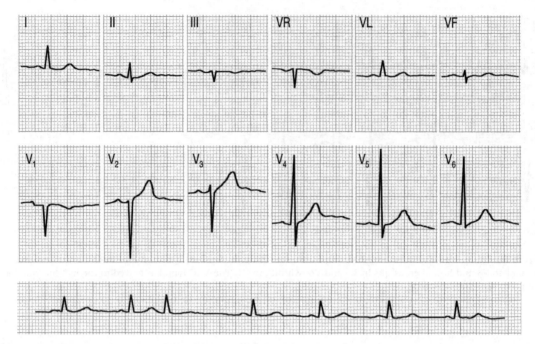

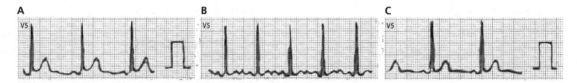

Figure 4.24 This ECG of a 90-year-old male (my grandfather Michael) is typical of the age, with low voltage on the frontal plane and poor progression of the r from V1 to V3 and Rs in V6. In the lower strip we can see an atrial premature beat, which is relatively common at this age.

Figure 4.25 (B) Changes in repolarization during exercise induced by hyperventilation in a 40-year-old healthy man (D.M.M.). (A and C) The ECG before and after hyperventilation.

followed by horizontal or descending ST segment. Furthermore, we have to be sure, in analogic not digital recording, that this pattern is not due to a recording artifact (Fig. 3.7).

Other changes related to gender or race exist, but are usually non-significant (see Bayés de Luna, 2012a).

4.10.4. Repeat the ECG recording if an ECG pattern is unusual

For instance, negative P wave in lead I; qR pattern in lead V2 with rS in V1 and RS in V3, and QR pattern in lead III. Check the recording errors and record the ECG during deep inspiration in case of QR in lead III (see Section 3.3 in Chapter 3, and Figure 4.22).

Self-assessment

A. List the study parameters in an ECG recording.

B. List the characteristics of sinus rhythm.

C. How are heart rate and the QT interval measured?

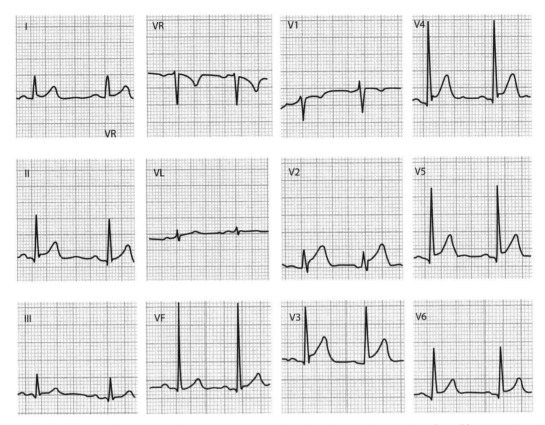

Figure 4.26 Example of an early repolarization pattern in a healthy 40-year-old man. Note the mild pattern (J wave <1 mm), seen particularly in the intermediate left precordial leads. This corresponds to a benign pattern (see Fig. 16.14).

D. List the characteristics of the normal P wave.

E. List the characteristics of the normal QRS complex.

F. How are the ST shifts measured?

G. What is the polarity and voltage of a normal T wave?

H. How is ÂQRS calculated in practice?

I. How does rotation of the heart on the anteroposterior axis affect the morphology of the ECG?

J. How does rotation of the heart on the longitudinal axis affect the morphology of the ECG?

K. What ECG changes are present in healthy children?

L. What ECG changes are present in healthy elderly individuals?

M. How does early repolarization pattern appear in the ECG?

PART II
Morphological Abnormalities in the ECG

Following the full explanation of how an ECG is produced and the characteristics of a normal ECG, this second part will outline the morphological abnormalities found in the ECG when a structural pathology is present in the heart.

Chapter 5 reviews the abnormalities in the P wave produced by atrial enlargement and atrial block and briefly explains anomalies in atrial repolarization. Chapter 6 describes ECG changes due to ventricular enlargement, and Chapter 7 explains ECG changes due to different types of ventricular block. Next, ECG patterns due to ventricular pre-excitation are outlined. Lastly, Chapter 9 describes the ECG changes produced by ischemia and necrosis, as well as the electrophysiological mechanisms behind these changes.

These chapters are aimed at providing concise information, in a practical clinical way and in the smallest possible space, of all these ECG patterns and their correlation with the heart diseases that produce them.

ECGs for Beginners, First Edition. Antoni Bayés de Luna.
© 2014 John Wiley & Sons, Inc. Published 2014 by John Wiley & Sons, Inc.

CHAPTER 5
Atrial Abnormalities

5.1. Initial considerations

This concept includes atrial enlargements and atrial blocks. These entities are different, but they are frequently associated and often have a shared ECG pattern.

Interatrial blocks, the only type of block in the atria that are well-known, are characterized in all types of heart block by the following: (1) they may have a transitory appearance; (2) they may appear without an associated pathology to explain the pattern, in this case added atrial enlargement; and (3) they may be provoked experimentally.

Patterns of atrial enlargement are due more to dilation than hypertrophy of the cavity because of the lack of thickness in the atrial wall.

Abnormalities in atrial repolarization are also briefly discussed in this chapter.

5.2. Atrial enlargements

Figures 5.1, 5.2B, and 5.2D show the P wave morphologies in cases of right atrial enlargement (RAE) and left atrial enlargement (LAE) (Bayés de Luna, 2012a).

5.2.1. Diagnostic criteria for RAE
(Fig. 5.1B and 5.2B and C)
The right atrium is enlarged mainly in some congenital (Fig. 5.2B) and valvular heart diseases, and in cor pulmonale (Fig. 5.2C).

The most common ECG criteria for the diagnosis of RAE include:
- **P wave criteria:**
  1. P wave >2.5 mm in height.
  2. Positive first part of the P wave in V1 >1.5 mm.
  3. ÂP to the right in (P pulmonale), and often even to the left (P congenitale) (Fig. 5.2).
- **QRS criteria:**
  1. Voltage in V1 < 4 mm
  2. Voltage ratio V2/V1 > 5
  3. qr or QR morphology in V1.

These criteria are very specific, and if they exist they therefore confirm the presence of the pathology in question, but they have low sensitivity. Thus, they are often not present, even when the pathology exists.

5.2.2. Diagnostic criteria for LAE
(Figs 5.1C and 5.2D)
An enlarged left atrium is mainly found in mitral stenosis and regurgitation, cardiomyopathies, arterial hypertension and ischemic heart disease. Figures 5.1C and 5.2D show examples of ECG changes in the P wave in the context of LAE.

The most commonly used ECG criteria for the diagnosis of LAE, which present generally more specificity than sensitivity, are listed below.

1. **The Morris index** = the duration and depth of the negative part of the P wave in V1 ≥40 ms × −1 mm. Figure 5.3 shows the negative component of the P wave under normal conditions (above) and in cases of LAE (below) in V1. In this example, the

ECGs for Beginners, First Edition. Antoni Bayés de Luna.
© 2014 John Wiley & Sons, Inc. Published 2014 by John Wiley & Sons, Inc.

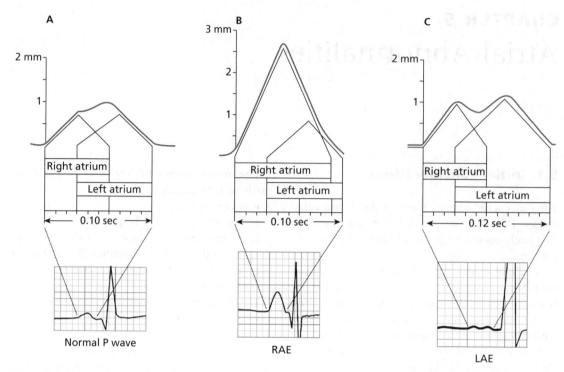

Figure 5.1 Above: diagram of atrial depolarization in a normal P wave (A); right atrial enlargement (RAE) (B); and left atrial enlargement (LAE) (C). Below: examples of the three types of P wave.

negative mode lasts 40 ms and measures −1 mm, strongly indicating LAE.

2. P wave duration in I, II and/or III ≥0.12 s + negativity of P in V1 >40 ms.

3. P wave ± in II, III, VF. Very specific but with very little sensitivity.

5.2.3. Biatrial enlargement

The diagnostic criteria are the same as in RAE and LAE, as shown in Figure 5.4.

5.3. Atrial blocks

5.3.1. Heart block

Heart block refers to a conduction disturbance or block in any part of the heart (sino-atrial junction, atria, AV junction, and ventricles) in which a stim-ulus is delayed (first-degree or partial block) or completely blocked (third-degree or advanced block). When a first or third degree block only occurs intermittently, it is referred to as second-degree block.

At the atrial level conduction only disturbances or blocks that occur between both atria (interatrial block), can be detected clearly in the ECG (Bayés de Luna, 2012a).

Furthermore, some abrupt and transitory changes in the P wave morphology that cannot be explained by any other cause (escape or fusion beats, artifacts, etc), and often without the P wave characteristics of interatrial block (see below) can correspond to some type of atrial block usually in the right atrium included in the concept of **atrial aberrancy** (see Section 10.7.3 in Chapter 10).

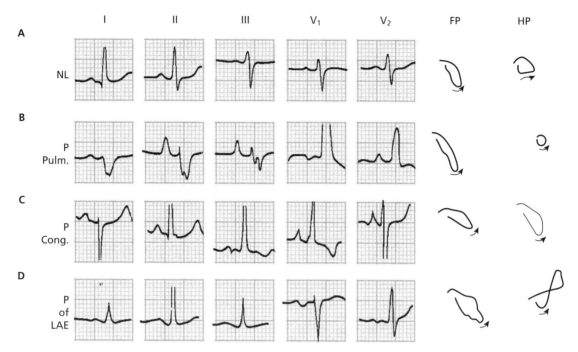

Figure 5.2 Examples of P wave morphology and loops in the following cases: (A) normal; (B) P pulmonale; (C) P congenitale; (D) Leith atrial enlargement.

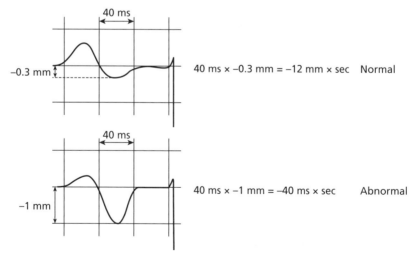

Figure 5.3 Diagram contrasting normal and abnormal negative components of the P wave in V1. When the value calculated using the width in seconds and the height in millimeters of the negative mode exceeds 40 mm × ms, it is considered abnormal.

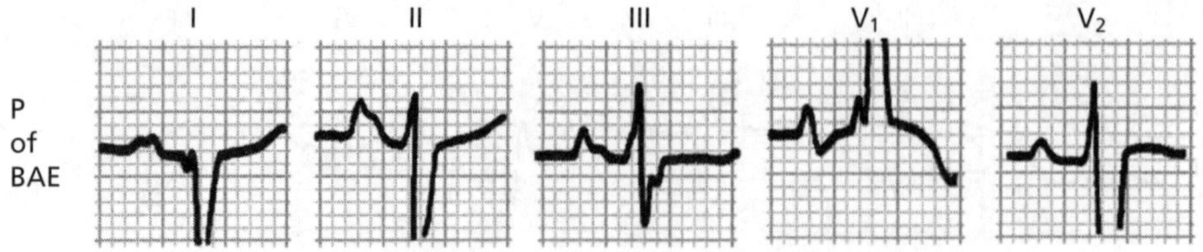

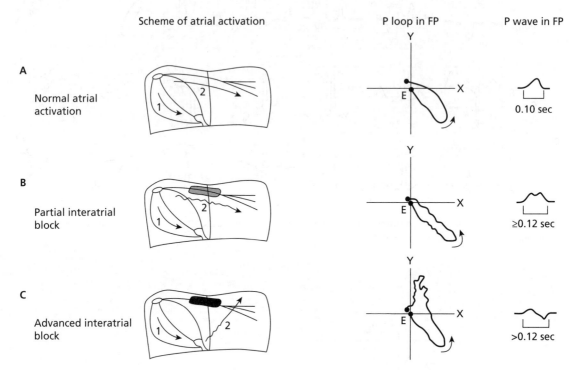

Figure 5.4 Example of P wave and loop morphology in bi-atrial enlargement (BAE).

Figure 5.5 Diagram of atrial conduction under normal circumstances (A); partial interatrial block (B); advanced interatrial block with left atrial retrograde activation (AIB with RALA) (C).

5.3.2. Interatrial block (Fig. 5.5)
Like all other types of heart block, interatrial block can be classified by three degrees (Bayés de Luna et al., 2012c).

5.3.3. ECG diagnosis
D **1. First-degree:** This type of interatrial block occurs frequently in the elderly (Spodick and Ariyarajah, 2008). The stimulus travels through the Bachmann bundle from the right atrium to the left atrium with a delay. **This generates a longer P wave** (Fig. 5.5B). LAE is often associated with first-degree interatrial block, but it may also be recorded as an isolated finding. In this case the negativity of the P wave in V1 is usually not as evident as in case of LAE.

2. Third-degree (Figs 5.6 to 5.8): This type of **E** interatrial block is less frequent and is very often associated with LAE, and paroxysmal supraventricular arrhythmia constituting a true arrhythmological syndrome (Bayés de Luna et al., 1985, Conde et al., 2014).

The stimulus is blocked in the zone of Bachmann and reaches the left atrium through a retrograde conduction from the mid-lower interatrial septum (Fig. 5.5C). This explains the presence of the longer

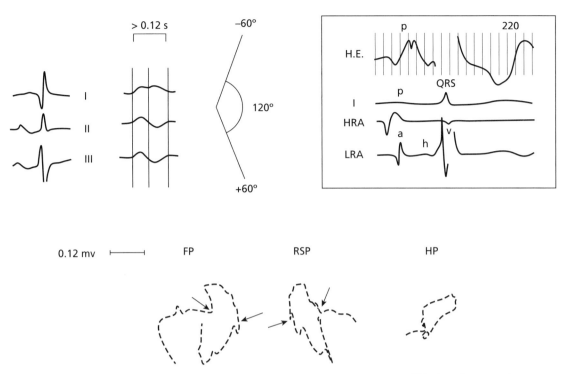

Figure 5.6 Above: P wave ± morphology in I, II, and III typical of advanced interatrial block with retrograde conduction to the left atrium. Observe how the ÂP and the angle between the direction of the activation in the first and second parts of the P wave are measured. To the right, intra-esophageal ECG (HE) and endocavitary registrations (HRA: high right atrium; LRA: low right atrium) demonstrate that the electrical stimulus moves first downwards (HRA–LRA) and then upwards (LRA–HE). Below: P loop morphology in the three planes with the inscription of the second part moving upwards.

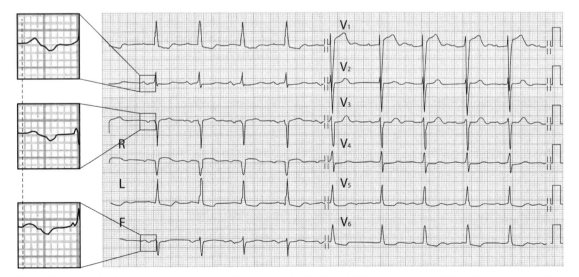

Figure 5.7 Typical ECG of advanced interatrial block (P ± in II, III, and VF and duration >120 ms) in a patient with ischemic cardiomyopathy. When amplified we can see the beginning of P in the three leads. (See Plate 5.7.)

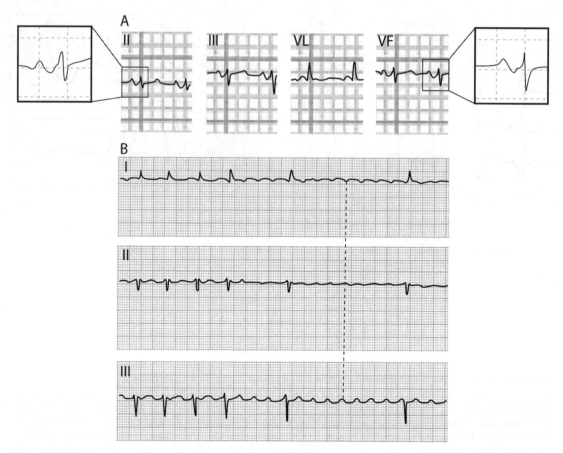

Figure 5.8 (A) Example of advanced interatrial block with retrograde conduction (P ± in II, III, and VF). (B) Associated atypical flutter.

P wave and a ± morphology in II, III, and VF, caused by the caudocranial activation of the left atrium. In V1–V3, there is also frequently a P± morphology due to associated LAE (Fig. 5.5C).

3. Second-degree: Transitory appearance of first- or third-degree interatrial block (Fig. 5.9B). This very rare pattern may be included in the concept of **atrial aberrancy**. This means, in the presence of sinus rhythm, an abnormal and transitory activation of some part of the atria; in this case the zone of Bachman's bundle exists (Fig. 5.9A)

Atrial aberrancy may also present a transient bizarre P wave without the morphology of interatrial block (Fig. 5.9B) (Chung, 1972) (see Section 10.7.3 in Chapter 10) (Bayés de Luna, 2012a).

5.4. Atrial repolarization abnormalities

The PR segment depression in II and elevation in VR as an expression of atrial injury (atrial ST-T) is an important abnormality, because it may represent the only ECG abnormality indicating acute pericarditis (Fig. 5.10).

The PR segment can also present changes in atrial infarction, but in this case other parts of the ECG will present abnormalities such as necrosis Q (acute infarction).

The typical morphology of normal atrial repolarization may be seen in cases of sympathetic overdrive (Fig. 4.4).

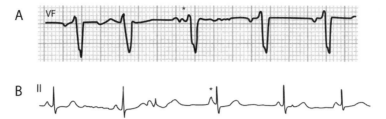

Figure 5.9 Two cases of atrial aberrancy. The first one (A) is a case of second degree interatrial block. This is a case of a patient with basal advanced interatrial block (P± with first part isoelectric that mimicks AV junction rhythm) that presents aberrant atrial conduction, ectopically induced by premature atrial complex, with a pattern, in this case, of first degree interatrial block (X). (B) A patient with aberrant atrial conduction also ectopically induced by a premature atrial complex. After this premature complex, a transitory P wave with a different morphology, but not with a pattern of first or third interatrial block appears (X). The PR interval is equal to previous PR intervals. Other explanations for this change (atrial escape, artifact, etc.) are unlikely (see Bayés de Luna, 2012a and text).

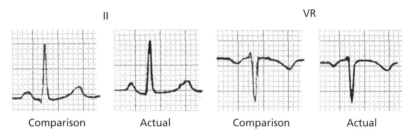

Figure 5.10 A case of recurrent pericarditis. Note the actual recording and comparison recordings, the PR elevation in VR and a "mirror" image in lead II (0.5 mm).

Self-assessment

A. What are the differentiating characteristics between atrial enlargement and interatrial block?

B. What are the diagnostic criteria for RAE?

C. What are the diagnostic criteria for LAE?

D. Outline the concept of first-degree interatrial block.

E. Outline the concept of third-degree interatrial block.

F. Explain the concepts of second degree interatrial block and the atrial aberrancy.

G. What is the most important abnormality in atrial repolarization?

CHAPTER 6
Ventricular Enlargements

6.1. Background

The term ventricular enlargement (VE) refers to both hypertrophy of the myocardial mass of the ventricles as well as dilation of the cavity, and may include a combination of both conditions.

Electrogenesis of the ECG morphology seen in VE is more frequently the result of hypertrophy than cavity dilation, the opposite of which is true in atrial enlargement. Mild or even moderate VE may not change in the ECG.

Sometimes a patient may live for many years with heart disease with VE before ECG abnormalities are present.

VE is best detected with echocardiography; however, a diagnosis of VE using ECG provides more prognostic value.

We will now outline the basic concepts and straightforward ECG criteria for the diagnosis of VE.

6.2. Right ventricular enlargement

Right ventricular enlargement (RVE) is mainly found in congenital cardiopathies, right valvular heart diseases, and chronic and acute cor pulmonale (pulmonary embolism and decompensation in chronic cor pulmonale).

A **6.2.1. Mechanisms of the electrocardiographic changes**
• Figure 6.1 shows how RVE reverses the dominant forces of left ventricle (A), changing the direc-

tion to the right and sometimes forwards, and other times backwards (B) due to the increase in RV mass and to the slowing of conduction at the level of the RV wall, because in spite of RVE the mass of LV still is greater than the RV mass.
• Often it is associated with a delayed activation of the right ventricle due to the block of impulse at the proximal level (classic right bundle branch block [RBBB]).
• Changes in repolarization in the form of negative ST-T are seen in some severe cases of RVE. Cases of decompensation of chronic cor pulmonale or pulmonary embolism are often mostly secondary to right ventricular dilation, which modifies the direction of the repolarization

6.2.2. Repercussions of these changes in the ECG

6.2.2.1. Horizontal plane
The modification in the QRS loop due to vectorial changes induced by RVE explain the QRS morphology in the HP, which moves either forwards and to the right, or backwards and to the right.

In the former (Fig. 6.2), vectorial changes induced by RVE cause the QRS loop to move forwards while maintaining the same rotation (I), then it rotates in 8 (II), and finally it can rotate the entire loop clockwise and forward (III). On other occasions the loop moves backwards, but with a large part to the right (IV and V).

Based on these patterns, in V1 a pattern from low voltage QS ⅋ till to RS or R only (ᒪ) may be seen

ECGs for Beginners, First Edition. Antoni Bayés de Luna.
© 2014 John Wiley & Sons, Inc. Published 2014 by John Wiley & Sons, Inc.

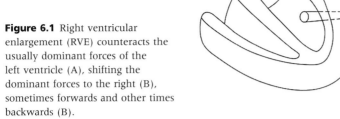

Figure 6.1 Right ventricular enlargement (RVE) counteracts the usually dominant forces of the left ventricle (A), shifting the dominant forces to the right (B), sometimes forwards and other times backwards (B).

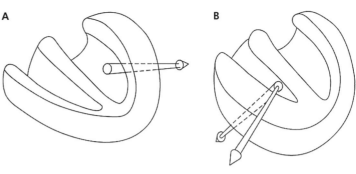

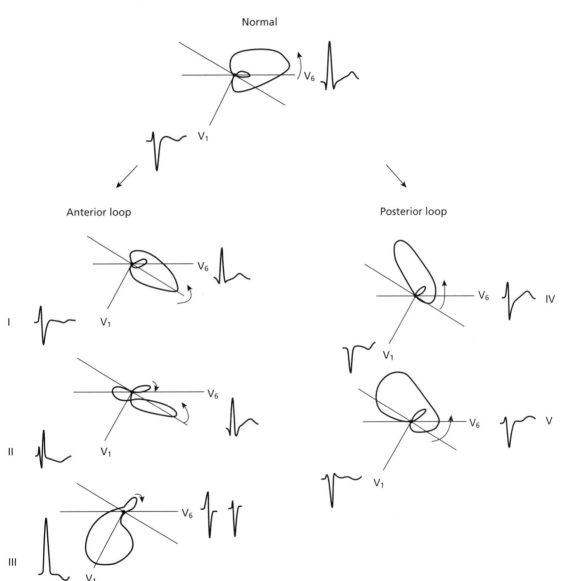

Figure 6.2 Parting from a normal loop in the horizontal plane, right ventricular enlargement always produces a rightward shift in direction, sometimes forward and other times backward. If the loop moves forward, it produces different QRS morphologies in V1 as it becomes progressively more anterior, with R gradually becoming taller and T more negative (from I to III). Often the loop begins rotating counterclockwise and ends up rotating clockwise, producing an rSr' morphology in V1 identical to that seen in partial right ventricular block. If the RVE directs the loop to the right and backward, a normal morphology (rS) or QS or rSr' can be seen in V1, always with a marked S in V6 (IV and V).

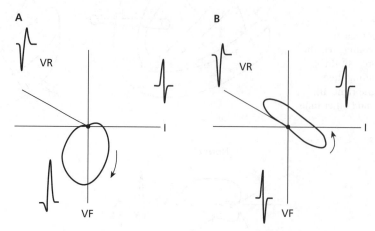

Figure 6.3 The QRS loop in the RVE may be rightwards (A) or type $S_I\ S_{II}\ S_{III}$ (B).

in V1, with always a pattern with big S (,) in V6 (Fig. 6.2).

6.2.2.2. Frontal plane

The morphology of QRS, according to the rotation and direction of the loop, presents right ÂQRS (RS in I and qR in VF) (A), or the ÂQRS is indeterminate ($S_1\ S_2\ S_3$) (B) (Fig. 6.3).

6.2.3. Diagnosis of RVE in clinical practice

The most commonly used criteria, which are very specific but not with low sensitivity, are the following:

- ÂQRS ≥110° (R < S in I).
- V1 = R/S > 1, and/or S in V1 <2 mm, and/or R ≥ 7 mm.
- V6: R/S ≤ 1 and/or S in V5–V6 > 7 mm.
- P wave of the RAE.
- It is important to make a differential diagnosis with all the processes that might originate a high R or rSr′ in V1 (Table 6.1).
- In cases of QS morphology in V1, the associated signs (S in V6, ÂQRS, P wave) facilitate the diagnosis of RVE (see before, and Fig. 6.4C).
- The signs of RVE, especially R in V1 of high voltage, may regress, at least partially, after surgery in patients with congenital heart diseases.

6.2.4. ECG morphologies in different types of RVE

6.2.4.1. Morphologies in V1 and other ECG changes according to the severity and etiology of the hypertrophy

Figure 6.4 shows examples of three groups of patients (A); valvular heart diseases (B); congenital heart diseases; and (C), cor pulmonale. In these three cases we may see patterns that present, with rs or rsr′, or even QS in patients with cor pulmonale, to only R with a strain-type pattern. In addition, we see that ÂQRS is always to the right or $S_1\ S_2\ S_3$, and that ÂP is to the right in valvular heart disease cor pulmonale, while it is somewhat to the left in congenital heart diseases (P congenitale) (Fig. 5.2C).

Figures 6.5 to 6.8 show examples of some congenital and acquired heart diseases (cor pulmonale) that present characteristic ECG patterns of RVE. Consult Sections 17.1 and 17.2 in Chapter 17, where the ECG in patients with valvular and congenital heart diseases is discussed.

6.2.4.2. ECG changes due to acute dilation of the right cavities

Acute dilation of the right cavities may be seen in patients with decompensation of chronic cor pulmonale and in patients with pulmonary embolism.

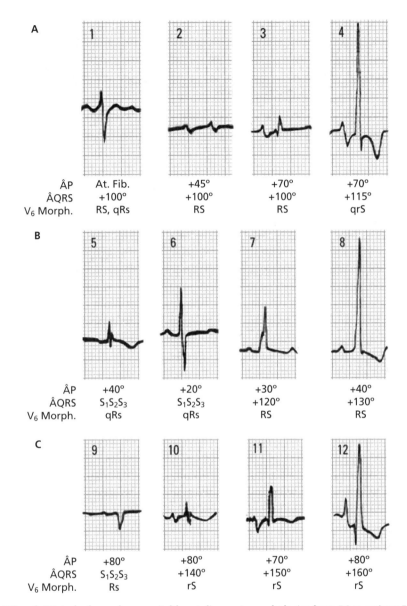

Figure 6.4 In (A) and (B) (valvular and congenital heart diseases) morphologies from RS to unique R in V1 may be seen usually in relation with the severity of the disease (loops type I to III). In (A) four cases (1 to 4) of mitral stenosis each one with more pulmonary hypertension, and in (B) four cases (5 to 8) of congenital pulmonary stenosis each one with more severe stenosis. In (C) (cases of pulmonale) different patterns of QRS in V1, from QS (number 9) to R (case 12) with strain patterns, may be seen, the latter is a case of severe subacute cor pulmonale with important pulmonary hypertension.

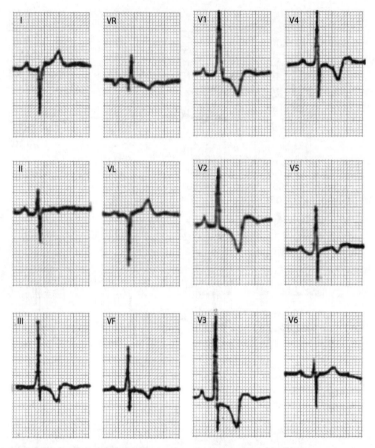

Figure 6.5 An 8-year-old patient with significant pulmonary valve stenosis with a gradient over 100 mmHg. The patient presents with a typical RVE morphology with a barrier-type systolic overload (R in V1–V2 with negative T wave). The ÂP in the ECG seems deviated leftwards. In fact the patient presents with wandering pacemaker between sinus and junctional rhythm (see strip of lead III).

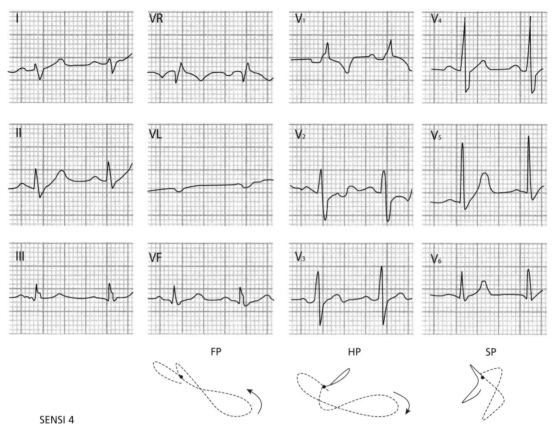

SENSI 4

Figure 6.6 Typical morphology of ostium secundum-type atrial septal defect (ASD). Observe the rSr′ morphology in V1, the right-deviated ÂQRS, and the ECG–VCG correlation.

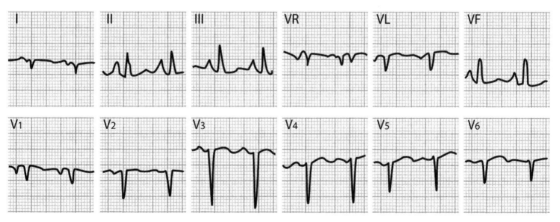

Figure 6.7 A 65-year-old patient with significant chronic obstructive pulmonary disease (COPD) and no left heart disease. There is a typical P pulmonale as well as other signs of right ventricular enlargement (RVE), with the QRS loop posterior and to the right (P negative in V1, absence of the first vector in the HP, rS in V6, ÂQRS $\geq$ 110°, etc).

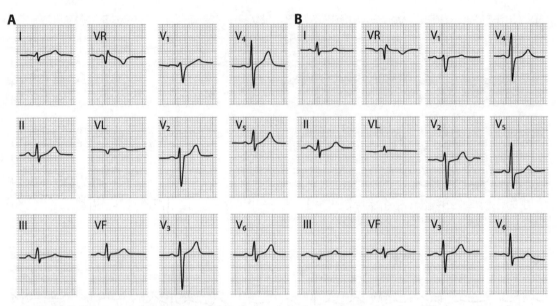

Figure 6.8 SI, SII, SIII morphology in a normal case (A) and in chronic obstructive pulmonary disease with right ventricular enlargement (RVE) (B). The ECG morphologies often do not differ. In some cases the P and T wave changes can help distinguish them. (See also Section 7.1 in Chapter 7.)

In the first group of patients, the HP may show negative, reversible T waves that may be deep, and increased S waves until V6, with ÂQRS more to the right (Fig. 6.9).

In severe cases of pulmonary embolism, evident ECG changes are often found (Chapter 17). The most noticeable changes include: (a) sinus tachycardia; (b) negative T waves in right precordial leads; and (c) appearance of advanced RBB (Fig. 15.4), or S_I Q_{III} morphology with negative T_{III} (McGinn-White sign) (Fig. 15.3). The ECG may appear normal in mild or moderate pulmonary embolism.

6.2.5. Differential diagnosis

A. Differential diagnosis of the morphology of right VE with a prominent R or r′ in V_1

Table 6.1 shows the different clinical contexts in which prominent R or r′ (R′) in V1 is observed.

B. Differential diagnosis of RVE with QS morphology in V1

These cases must be distinguished from other processes that present QS in V1, such as left branch block (LBB) and septal infarction. The presence of the associated ECG signs (S in V6, right ÂQRS or S_1 S_2 S_3, and P wave of RAE) facilitate the diagnosis of RVE (Fig. 6.3).

6.3. Left ventricular enlargement

• Left ventricular enlargement (LVE) is mainly seen in acquired heart diseases (aortic valve disease, arterial hypertension, cardiomyopathies (including ischemic cardiomyopathies, and genetically induced cardiomyopathies), and some types of congenital heart diseases (aortic stenosis, aortic coarctation, and fibroelastosis).

D

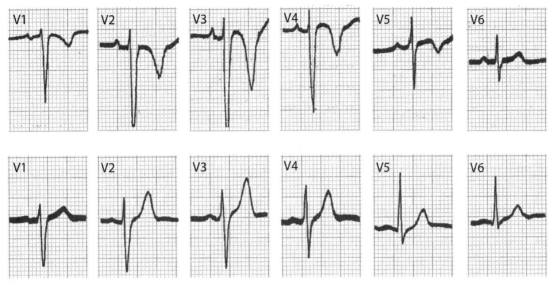

Figure 6.9 A 65-year-old patient with important chronic obstructive pulmonary disease (COPD) and no left heart disease. There is a typical P pulmonale as well as other signs of right ventricular enlargement (RVE), with the QRS loop posterior and to the right (P negative in V1, absence of the first vector in the HP, rS in V6, ÂQRS ≥ 110°, etc).

• Generally, hypertrophy predominates dilation in LVE. This is more frequent in the presence of cardiomyopathy) and in heart diseases with diastolic overload, of LV (e.g. aortic regurgitation) in VI.

E **6.3.1. Mechanisms of ECG changes**

• Figures 6.10 and 6.11 show that in LVE the vectorial forces of the free wall of LV that is the part of LV that grows the most, are directed more backwards (B), and upward and to the left (ÂQRS more or less to the left). In LVE of the hypertrophic cardiomyopathy (MH) with apical predominance the vectorial forces move less backward (Fig. 6.10C).

• The LVE is often associated with specific degrees of left branch block (LBBB).

• Repolarization changes with some ST depression, and a negative and asymmetrical T are caused more by the clinical course of the disease than the degree of overload (systolic or diastolic).

• With the passage of time, especially in severe cases, the pattern referred to as 'strain pattern' with a negative ST-T appears. These changes are in part secondary to the depolarization changes (hypertrophy). A certain degree of ischemia is often also involved, as well as the effect of certain drugs such as digitalis, for example (primary factor), originating mixed pattern (Fig. 6.13C) in which ST depression or a very negative T predominate.

6.3.2. Repercussions of the changes in the ECG

6.3.2.1. Changes in the FP and HP

Figure 6.11 shows the QRS loops in the FP and HP and the ECG morphologies in normal patients (A), patients with mild to moderate LVE (B), and those with severe LVE (C). In HM, with septal hypertrophy deep 'q' waves may be seen, and in the case of hypertrophy with apical predominance, very negative T waves may be found (D and E).

F **Table 6.1** Presence of prominent R or r′ in V₁: Differential diagnosis.

Clinical setting	R or R″(r′) morphology in V1	QRS width	P wave morphology in V1
1. No heart disease – Electrode misplacement	 2nd RIS 4th RIS	<0.12 s	P− in 2° IS P+ or ± In 4° IS
– Hypermature – Normal variant: Fewer Purkinje fibers in anteroseptal zone or extreme counter clockwise rotation	 <10 mm	<0.12 s	Normal
– Thorax abnormalities (pectus excavatum)		<0.12 s	Negative
2. Classical RBBB		From <0.12 s to >0.12 s	Normal
3. Atypical RBBB – Ebstein disease		Usually ≥0.12 s	Usually peaked and/or ±
– Arrhythmogenic RVD/C Low voltage in V1 or Σ wave		May be 0.12 s	Usually pathologic
– Brugada syndrome		Sometimes ≥0.12 s	Normal
4. Right or biventricular enlargement (athletes) or even LVH (Hypertrophic or others CM)		<0.12 s	Usually tall and peaked. Sometimes ±
5. Wolff-Parkinson-White syndrome		From <0.12 s to >0.12 s	Normal P wave with short PR
6. Lateral MI		<0.12 s	Usually normal
7. Block of middle fibers (especially if the pattern is transient (see chapter 7)?	Prominent R in V₁ or more frequently V₂	<0.12 s	Usuallly normal

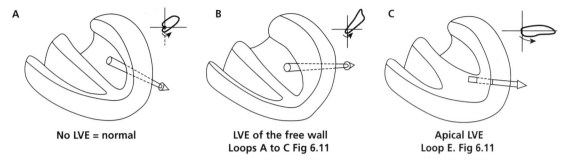

No LVE = normal

**LVE of the free wall
Loops A to C Fig 6.11**

**Apical LVE
Loop E. Fig 6.11**

Figure 6.10 See the vector and loop in normal cases (A) and in different types of LVE (B and C).

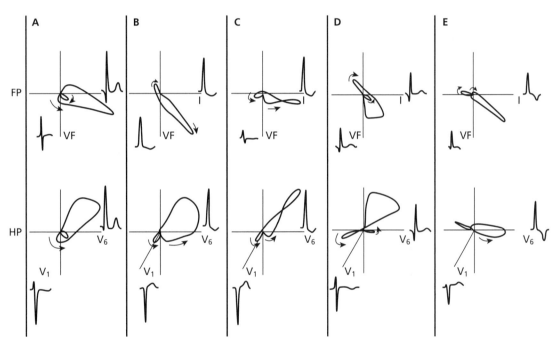

Figure 6.11 Diagram of the QRS and T loops in the frontal plane (FP) and horizontal plane (HP) in mild or moderate left ventricular enlargement (A) and severe enlargement (B and C). The D loop (or similar) is seen in some cases of hypertrophic cardiomyopathy, and the E loop is seen in cases of apical hypertrophic cardiomyopathy. Note in the five cases the typical morphology that appears in VF, I, V1, and V6 according to the loop–hemifield correlation.

G ## 6.3.3. The diagnosis of LVE in clinical practice

- **The voltage criteria, which are very specific (>90%) although with less sensitivity (20–50%) of left ventricular hypertrophy (LVH), include:**
  1. **Cornell criterion:** R VL +SV3 >24mm in men and >20mm in women.
  2. **Sokolow criterion:** SVI+RV5-6 ≥35mm.
  3. **VL criterion:** VL ≥11mm, or ≥16mm in the presence of supero-anterior hemiblock.
- **The presence of strain-type repolarization alterations and/or evidence of LAE or atrial fibrillation reinforce the diagnosis**, especially in the presence of voltage criteria.
- The associations between these criteria are the basis for **diagnostic scores**, the most well known being the **Romhilt–Estes** score (Bayés de Luna, 2012a) (Table 6.2).
- The presence of dilation of LV combined with hypertrophy is suggested by (a) the voltage of V6 is greater than or equal to that of V5; (b) IDT ≥ 0.07s; and (c) relatively low voltage in the FP compared to the HP.

Table 6.2 Romhilt-Estes score. There is left ventricular enlargement if 5 or more points are obtained. Left ventricular enlargement is probable if the sum is 4 points.

A. Criteria based on QRS modifications	
1. Voltage criteria	3 points
One of the following should be present:	
– R or S in the FP ≥ 20mm	
– S in V_1-V_2 ≥ 30mm	
– R in V_5-V_6 ≥ 30mm	
2. AQRS at −30° or more to the left	2 points
3. Intrinsicoid deflection in V_5–V_6 ≥ 0.05	1 point
4. QRS duration ≥0.09s	1 point
B. Criteria based on ST-Tchanges	
1. ST-T vector opposite to QRS (⤸) without digitalis	3 points
2. ST-T vector opposite to QRS (⤸) with digitalis	1 point
C. Criteria based on P wave abnormalities	
1. Negative terminal P mode in V_1 ≥ 1mm in depth and 0.04sec in duration	3 points

6.3.4. ECG morphologies in specific types of LVE

6.3.4.1. Small differences between the normal ECG and mild LVE
H
Occasionally, the diagnosis of LVE based on an echocardiogram may not be made by ECG, or may only be indicated by subtle ECG changes that may even be seen in healthy individuals. These changes, however, are a little different from the completely normal ECG seen in normal people. Figure 6.12 shows the rectified ST and the symmetry of the T wave in II, III, VF, and V5–V6 in cases of a patient with moderate HTA (B) compared with that of a healthy individual showing very similar QRS but with a normal ST-T (upsloping and asymmetrical) (A).

It is important to bear in mind that these subtle changes may be variants of normal patterns, especially in menopausal women and in the elderly. These cases must therefore be studied more closely because they could correspond to mild LVE or even ischemic heart disease, especially if accompanied by mild ST depression (<1mm). A good history taking and clinical examination are necessary, in addition to complementary testing (e.g. stress test, echocardiogram), before making the definitive diagnosis.

6.3.4.2. Changes during the clinical course in LVE
I
Figure 6.13 shows the clinical course of a patient with LVH evolving to strain-pattern (negative ST-T with asymmetrical branches), both in aortic stenosis (systolic overload) (A), and in aortic regurgitation (diastolic overload) (B). The latter case may present more often a small q wave. C shows the appearance of a pattern of strain with an added primary factor (digitalis and ischemia). See the rectified depression of the ST depression and the more symmetrical and deeper T wave (see above).

Figure 6.14 illustrates the ECGs of a patient with LVH, showing severe aortic regurgitation in a young person that had not been longstanding. Voltage criteria for LVE are presented, with qR in V5-6, a rectified ST segment and a symmetric and tall T

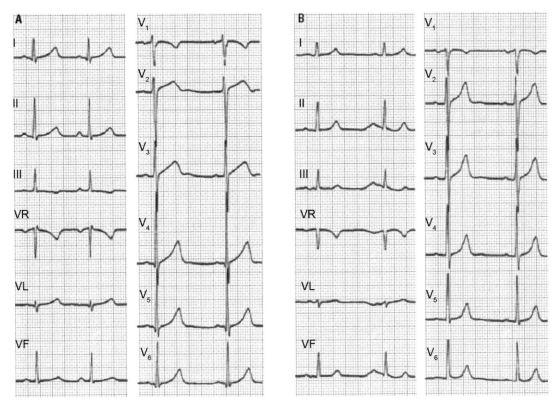

Figure 6.12 (A) ECG in a healthy, lean, adolescent (my grandson, Iker) and (B) in a patient with hypertension. Observe the mild differences in the ST segment/T wave. In (A) there is from the beginning an upsloping of the ST segment (V4–V6, I, and II). In contrast in (B) there is a rectified ST with symmetric T wave (V5, V6, I, II, VF).

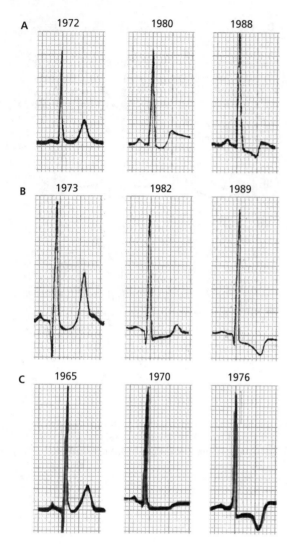

Figure 6.13 Three typical examples of morphology evolution. (A) A case of significant aortic stenoses, lacking the q wave from the first ECG, that evolves to an increase of voltage and repolarization with a 'strain pattern.' (B) Significant aortic regurgitation with a progressive decrease in the q wave with the appearance of a 'strain pattern'. (C) A patient with ischemic and hypertensive heart disease that presents a mixed pattern of LVE + ischemia, with the progression of the disease. As the ECG evolves, we can observe the changes in the ECG patterns.

wave. Figure 6.15 shows the ECG of a 45-year-old man with severe longstanding aortic stenosis presenting LVH with strain.

6.3.4.3. Regression of LVE pattern

The signs of repolarization suggesting LVH in the ECG in patients with hypertension who show LVH in the echocardiogram may regress with adequate treatment, and have a good prognosis. An example is shown in Figure 6.16. The signs of LVE may also regress after surgical correction of some valvular and congenital heart disease.

6.3.5. Differential diagnosis in LVE

1. **Advanced left bundle branch block (LBBB)**
   • In LVE the QRS never measures 120 ms or more, although many cases of severe LBBB present associated LVE.
   • LVE often shows signs that are suggestive of concomitant first-degree LBBB (missing q in V6 and I and even missing r in V1 with QRS < 120 ms).
2. **Septal infarction**
   • A missing r in V1–V2 may make the differential diagnosis difficult with septal infarction using ECG alone. Favors septal infarction negative/symmetrical T wave in V1–V2.
3. **Wolff–Parkinson–White pre-excitation type I and II**
   • This has a delta wave and PR is short.

6.4. Biventricular enlargement

(Fig. 6.17)

It is sometimes difficult to diagnose because the presence of one type of enlargement may mask the other.

Diagnostic criteria include:
1. High R in V5-6 with right ÂQRS or S1 S2 S3.
2. High R in V5-V6 with RS in V1-V2.
3. QRS with normal voltage but with considerable repolarization alterations.
4. Low-voltage QRS in V1, evident S in V2 and R or Rs in V5-6 with right ÂQRS or S_1 S_2 S_3. (Fig. 6.17).
5. The P wave may present signs of right and/or left atrial involvement (Fig. 5.4), or atrial fibrillation.

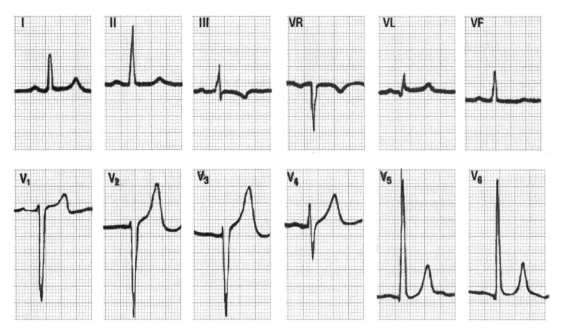

Figure 6.14 Typical ECG of a 22-year-old male with significant, although not very longstanding, aortic regurgitation. It corresponds to moderate left ventricular hypertrophy but satisfies the diagnostic criteria for LVE (Romhilt–Estes score). In effect, R in V5–V6 > 30 mm (3 points); intrinsicoid deflection time (IDT) = 0.07 s (1 point); duration of QRS = 0.10 s (1 point). Total: 5 points. Left ventricular dilation is suggested by IDT > 0.07 s and the R wave height in V6 greater than in V5.

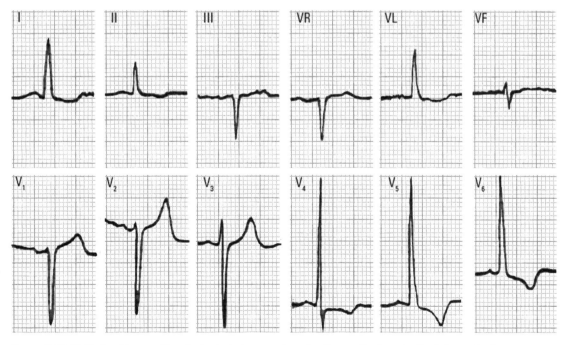

Figure 6.15 ECG of a 47-year-old male, typical of severe, longstanding aortic stenosis. The left ventricular hypertrophy pattern is typical. R in V4–V5 > 30 mm (3 points); ST–T opposite to R in V4–V6 (3 points); IDT = 0.055 s (1 point). Total: 7 points (Romhilt–Estes score).

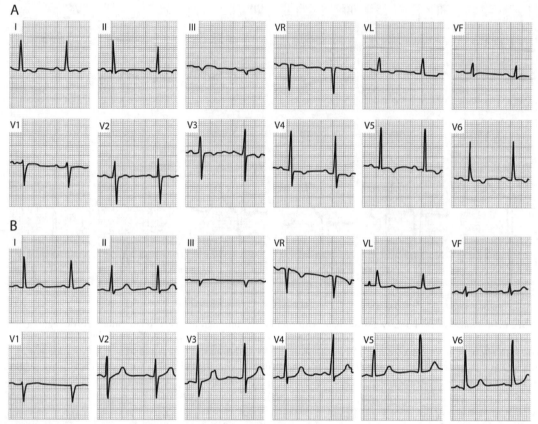

Figure 6.16 A 56-year-old male with hypertensive heart disease. ECGs before treatment (A) and seven months later (B). Observe the reduction in the left ventricular enlargement morphology.

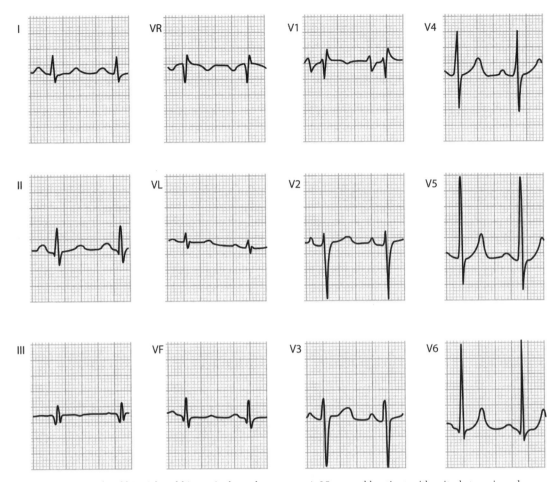

Figure 6.17 Example of biatrial and biventricular enlargement. A 35-year-old patient with mitral stenosis and regurgitation, aortic regurgitation and significant pulmonary hypertension with sinus rhythm (see text).

Self-assessment

A. List the electrophysiologic changes that explain the ECG morphologies of RVE.

B. What are the most important ECG diagnostic criteria for RVE in clinical practice?

C. List the ECG changes found in pulmonary embolism.

D. What are the criteria indicating RVE in the presence of QS in V1?

E. List the electrophysiologic changes that explain the ECG morphologies of the LVE.

F. List the causes of prominent R or rSr′ in V1 apart from RVE.

G. What are the most important diagnostic criteria for LVE in clinical practice?

H. What are the small differences between a normal ECG and that of mild LVE?

I. Name the evolutionary ECG changes that occur during the clinical course of LVE.

J. Which processes present patterns similar to those of LVE?

K. Biventricular enlargement: How is the diagnosis performed by the ECG?

CHAPTER 7
Ventricular Blocks

7.1. General concepts

• In the specific intraventricular conduction system there are four fascicles (Fig. 7.1): the right bundle branch (RBB), the left bundle branch (LBB) and its two divisions, the superoanterior (SA) and infero-posterior (IP), as well as some middle fibers that exist between two divisions and that occasionally constitute a true fascicle (see Section 7.7).

• In Chapter 5 we discussed how block in any part of the heart, whether at sinoatrial, atrial, AV junction, or ventricular level, refers to the slowing of the conduction (partial or first-degree block), or complete block of the conduction in the area in question (advanced third-degree block). When only some stimuli are blocked, either in the form of partial or advanced block we refer to it as second-degree block.

A • Block in the right and left branches may be at the proximal (trunk) or peripheral level. Here we refer mainly to the ECG criteria of proximal blocks. However. the characteristics of right and left peripheral bundle branch block, are similar to proximal ones. For details consult Bayés de Luna (2012a).

• The diagnostic criteria for bundle branch block and two divisions of LBB were established many years ago by the Mexican School (Sodi et al.) in 1967) and Rosenbaum and Elizari in 1968, respectively. Recently, some of these criteria have been questioned, especially the width of QRS for the diagnosis of advanced LBB block (LBBB) (Strauss

et al., 2011). We continue to use the classic criteria in this book.

• It is worth mentioning that block in the peripheral divisions of the RBB may originate S_I S_{II} S_{III} morphologies that are practically identical to those seen in RVE and as variants on normality (Bayés de Luna et al., 1987).

• In addition, block of the middle fibers of the LBB will be briefly discussed at the end of the chapter.

For more information regarding the diagnosis of the association of bundle branch block with ventricular enlargement, acute ischemia, or necrosis, consult Bayés de Luna (2012a).

7.2. Right bundle branch block (RBBB)

7.2.1. Advanced RBBB (third-degree)
We speak of advanced, and not of complete RBBB, and also of advanced, and not of complete LBBB (Section 7.3), because it is difficult to know whether the conduction of the stimulus through the affected branch would be possible, if transeptal depolarization from the other ventricle does not exist.

7.2.1.1 Mechanisms of ECG changes (Fig. 7.2)
The activation (depolarization + repolarization) of the right ventricle occurs transseptally producing, due to a small number of Purkinje fibers in the septum, a QRS with longer duration. The transeptal activation originates the delayed 3 and 4 vectors of

ECGs for Beginners, First Edition. Antoni Bayés de Luna.
© 2014 John Wiley & Sons, Inc. Published 2014 by John Wiley & Sons, Inc.

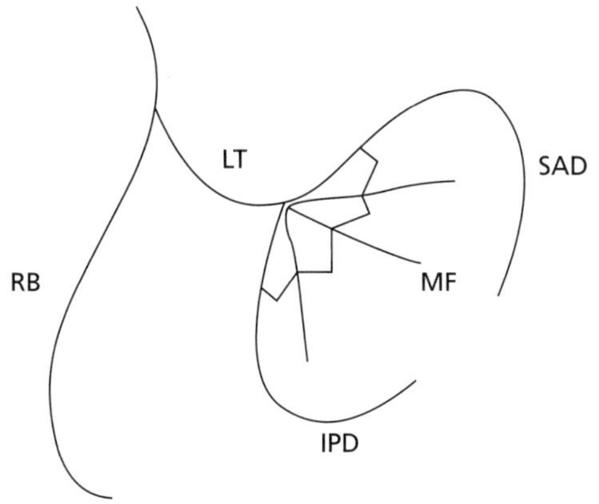

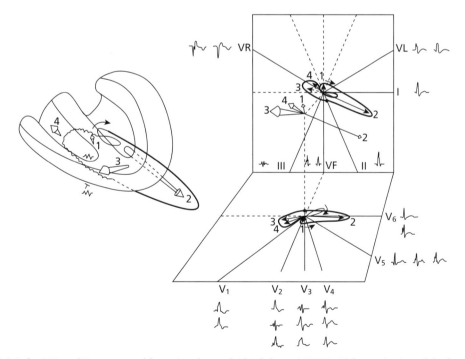

Figure 7.1 Scheme of intraventricular conduction system: RB = right bundle; LB = Leith bundle trunk; SA and IP = superoanterior and inferoposterior division; FM = middle fibers.

depolarization of the septum and RV, and the formation of a characteristic QRS loop.

Figure 7.2 shows the correlation of these vectors and the corresponding loop with the hemifield of each lead, all of which explain the morphologies observed.

Figure 7.3 shows how the morphology of ST-T changes seen in advanced RBBB are explained by septal repolarization, which dominates over that of the LV wall. The septal repolarization dipole begins in the left side of the septum, and thus the head (positivity) of the repolarization vector always faces the left side and is recorded as negative in V1 and positive in V6.

Figure 7.4 compares the QRS loop and morphologies in the FP and HP under normal conditions and in advanced RBBB.

B

Figure 7.2 Left: QRS and T vectors and loops in advanced (third-degree) RBBB. Right: projection of the loops on the two planes and the resultant morphologies most often encountered in clinical practice.

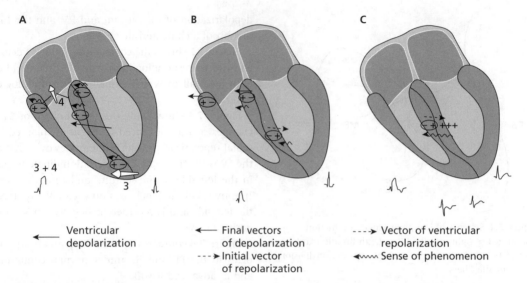

A

3 + 4

3

B

C

⟵ Ventricular
   depolarization

⟵ Final vectors
   of depolarization

--→ Initial vector
   of repolarization

--→ Vector of ventricular
   repolarization

⟞∿∿ Sense of phenomenon

Figure 7.3 Diagrams of the formation of the dipole and vector of depolarization and repolarization in advanced RBBB. The T wave is negative in V1 and positive in V6, because the vector of septal repolarization dominates and has the head (positive charge) facing the left side, although the sense of phenomenon (⟵∿∿) is going from left to right.

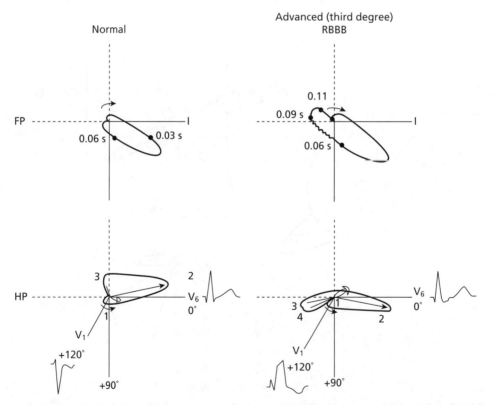

Figure 7.4 Frontal (FP) and horizontal (HP) plane loops in a normal patient and in a patient with advanced RBBB. Observe how this type of block does not modify the general loop direction in the FP, but it is somewhat more anterior in the HP.

C **7.2.1.2. Diagnostic criteria in advanced RBBB (third-degree)**

The diagnostic criteria for advanced RBBB are as follows (Sodi et al., 1967; Bayés de Luna, 2012a):

1. QRS ≥ 0.12 s with variable ÂQRS.

2. Horizontal plane: rSR' in V1 and in general V2 with slurrings in R', and in general slightly depressed ST in V1 and an asymmetrical negative T wave in V1–V2 and occasionally in V3. qRs in V5–V6 with slurrings in the 's' wave.

3. Frontal plane: QR in VR with slurrings in R, and negative T wave and qRs in I and usually VL with slurrings in S wave. ÂQRS may be located in the normal range in the absence of RBBB. More to the right or left according to the rotation of the heart and/or presence of right or left ventricular enlargement.

Figure 7.5 shows a typical example of advanced RBBB in a normal heart without rotations.

The key leads for diagnosis are V1, V6 and VR.

7.2.2. Partial RBBB (first-degree)

In this case the transseptal activation is more (B) or less (A) important (grey area) depending on the degree of stimulus delay in the right bundle branch (Fig. 7.6). Consequently, a greater or lesser part of
D the RV is depolarized with a delay (striped area).

For this reason, the ECG of first-degree RBBB is characterized by the following (Fig. 7.7):

1. QRS measures <120 ms.

2. rSr' in V1. The r' is not wide and may have a voltage more or less evident. It may be seen in the initial phases as an RS morphology, because the first part of QRS loop goes a little forwards before the last part presents the forward slurrings. This explains the RS pattern in V1 (Fig. 7.8). However, to avoid overdiagnosis, we can give the diagnosis of partial RBBB in the presence of r' in V1.

3. Terminal with 'r' that is not wide is also found in VR, and 's' in I and V6.

7.2.3. RBBB: Comparative morphologies (Fig. 7.8)

See the different morphologies in VR, V1, and V6 in the case of normal activation and in first-degree and third-degree RBBB. In V1 the morphology may be from 'rs' to 'rsR', with QRS ≥120 ms.

7.2.4. Second-degree RBBB (Fig. 7.9) **E**

In this case a pattern of transient **first- or third-degree RBBB appears in the same tracing** (see legend and Chapter 11, ventricular aberrancy).

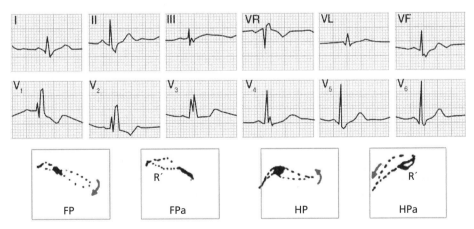

Figure 7.5 ECG and VCG of a healthy 75-year-old woman with no heart disease (M.B.V). For more than 15 years, the ECG was unchanged. This is a case of advanced RBBB in a normal heart with no apparent rotations (ÂQRS in the first half of QRS = +30° and there is a qRs morphology in V5). FPa: frontal plane amplified; HPa: horizontal amplified. See the final part of QRS depolarization that produces R' in VR and V1 (see Fig. 7.2).

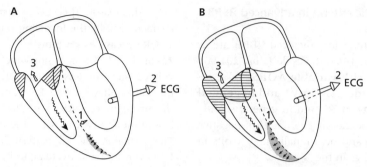

Figure 7.6 Diagram of ventricular depolarization in global but partial (first-degree) RBBB of proximal origin, less intense in (A) and more intense in (B). In this type of RBBB (see text), one part of the right septum (dotted area) depolarizes transseptally because when the impulse reaches the right septum from the left side, the impulse from the right bundle branch has still not arrived. The longer this impulse takes to reach the right septum, the larger the portion of it that depolarizes transseptally (B). This delay in the arrival of the impulse to the right ventricle means that a proportionate part of the right ventricle depolarizes later than the left ventricle (lined area), originating a final ventricular depolarization vector (3) directed upwards and to the front. It must be remembered that under normal circumstances a small portion of the right ventricle is the last to depolarize, and it produces a vector directed upward and backward. In partial RBBB, the final vector of QRS is directed upward and a little forward, and it usually falls at least a little in the positive hemifield of V1 and VR. It is also somewhat delayed. Therefore, an rSr′ or rsR′ morphology in V1 and a final r′ in VR that is wider than normal but with QRS <0.12 s is produced. However, as seen in Fig. 7.8, the first change of QRS morphology may be from rS to RS pattern (see text).

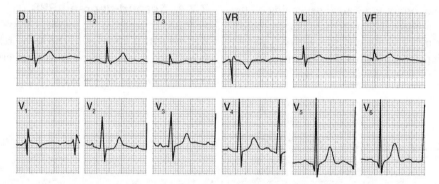

Figure 7.7 Typical example of partial RBBB. To compare with morphologies of normal conduction advanced RBBB and other morphologies of partial RBBB see Figure 7.8.

7.2.5. Differential diagnosis of RBBB morphology

• The differential diagnosis of RBBB must be made with **all processes that present a prominent R or r′ in V1**, including pre-excitation, right or biventricular enlargement, athletes, pectus excavatum, and Brugada syndrome, among others (Table 6.1 and Chapter 16).

• **A mistakenly high placement of the electrodes of V1 and V2** and other variants on the normal ECG must also be ruled out. In cases of high placement in V1–V2, the P wave is negative (Fig. 7.10). A negative P wave in V_1 with the electrode located in the correct place, is a common finding in pectus excavatum. See differential diagnosis of r′ in V1 in Table 6.1.

F

• Naturally, the differential diagnosis is more difficult in partial RBBB because the sole presence of QRS $\geq$120 ms indicates, once pre-excitation is ruled out based on normal PR, advanced RBBB.

• For more information on the diagnosis of advanced RBBB associated with necrosis, ischemic heart disease, or pre-excitation, and on the diagnosis of peripheral right bundle branch block (which as we have said may present S_I S_{II} S_{III} pattern similar to RVE and variant of normality [Fig. 6.8]), consult Bayés de Luna (2012a).

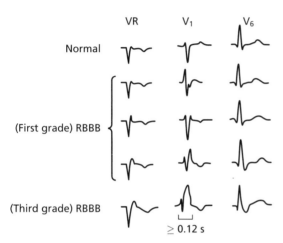

Figure 7.8 VR, V1, and V6 morphologies in a normal case and in third- and first-degree RBBB. Note that in partial (first degree) RBBB three ECG patterns corresponding to three consecutives bigger grades of first degree RBBB may be seen.

7.3. Left bundle branch block (LBBB)

7.3.1. Advanced LBBB (third-degree)

7.3.1.1. Mechanisms of ECG changes
(Fig. 7.11)

G

The activation of the entire left ventricle takes place transseptally, as also happens in advanced RBBB. This explains the slowness in forming QRS, because transseptal depolarization is slow due to the few number of Purkinje fibers that exist in the septum. Transseptal and left ventricle activation originate four vectors (Fig. 7.11) that explain the formation of a QRS loop and a wide QRS complex, the morphologies of which can be explained by the loop–hemifield correlation (Fig. 7.11).

The morphology of ST-T in the case of advanced LBBB is explained because the **repolarization of the septum dominates over that of the LV wall** (Fig. 7.12). The repolarization dipole that begins on the right side of the septum is directed from right to left, and thus the repolarization vector also moves from right to left with the head (positivity) always facing V1. As a result, the T wave is positive in V1 and negative in V6.

7.3.1.2. Diagnostic criteria for advanced LBBB (third-degree) (Fig. 7.13)

The classic diagnostic criteria (Sodi, 1967; Willems et al., 1985; Bayés de Luna, 2012a) include the following:

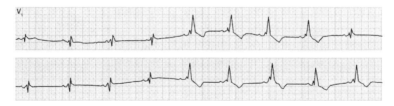

Figure 7.9 V1. Continuous recording. A 55-year-old patient with first-degree RBBB morphology (the first four complexes) who abruptly presented with advanced RBBB morphology (third-degree) for four complexes, with minimal changes in the RR interval. After five first-degree RBBB complexes, there were five advanced RBBB complexes. This is an example of second-degree RBBB (some impulses are completely blocked in the right bundle branch), although it stems from a first-degree RBBB morphology. The appearance of advanced RBBB coincides with slow decreases of heart rate (see Section 7.4).

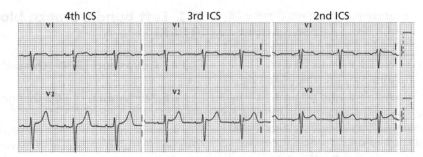

Figure 7.10 A very slim 15-year-old patient without heart disease. The rSr′ morphology is due to a misplaced V1 electrode in the second right intercostal space (see negative P wave) and disappears when the electrode is properly positioned (fourth right intercostal space).

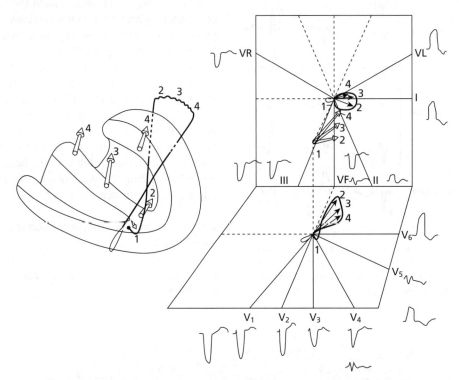

Figure 7.11 Left: QRS vectors and loops in advanced LBBB (third-degree). Right: projection of the loops on the two planes with formation of the respective loops and ECG morphologies most often seen in clinical practice.

1. QRS ≥120 ms. Recent studies suggest that in cases of heart failure, the preferred wideness of QRS for the placement of resynchronization pacemakers has to be ≥130 ms in women and ≥140 ms in men (Strauss, 2011; Gettes and Kligfield, 2012; Zareba, 2013) (see before).

2. The presence of notches or slurrings in the middle third of QRS in at least two of the following leads: V1, V2, V5, V6, I, and VL, with a prolongation at the delayed peak in R in V5-V6 to >60 ms.
3. Generally, the ST segment is slightly opposed to the QRS polarity, especially when it is ≥140 ms and

H

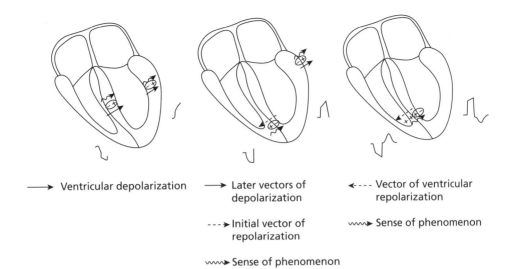

→ Ventricular depolarization

→ Later vectors of depolarization

←--- Vector of ventricular repolarization

---→ Initial vector of repolarization

∿→ Sense of phenomenon

∿→ Sense of phenomenon

Figure 7.12 Diagram of formation of dipole and the depolarization and repolarization vector in advanced LBBB. The T wave is positive in V1 and negative in V6, because it dominates the septal repolarization vector that is always from left to right (V1 faces positivity and V6 faces negativity), although the sense of phenomenon is going from right to left.

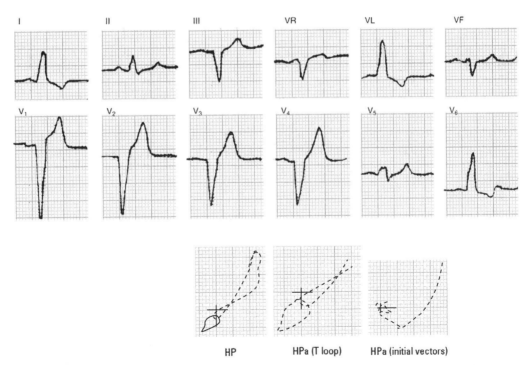

HP   HPa (T loop)   HPa (initial vectors)

Figure 7.13 ECG and VCG of a healthy 68-year-old man with advanced LBBB and no apparent heart disease. QRS >0.12 s. Its morphology is consistent with those in Figure 7.11.

it is rapidly followed by an asymmetrical T wave of opposed polarity.

4. Horizontal plane: QS or rS in V1 with small 'r' with ST slightly elevated and positive asymmetrical T wave, and unique R in V6 with negative asymmetric T wave. When the QRS is <140 ms, the T wave in V6 may be even positive.

5. Frontal plane: R exclusively in I and VL often with a negative asymmetrical T wave and slightly ST depression, and usually QS in VR with positive T wave. In cases with advanced heart failure and great dilation of right cavities, there is a delay of depolarization of RV that explains the final R in VR (QR pattern) (Van Bommel et al., 2011).

6. The ÂQRS is variable. It may be rightwards in patients with RVE and/or congestive heart failure (Fig. 7.14), and leftwards in case of associated super-oanterior hemiblock, deleted CM, etc. (Fig. 7.15).

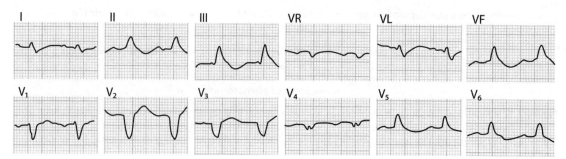

Figure 7.14 ECG of a patient with congestive heart failure and a morphology of advanced LBBB with right deviated ÂQRS, low voltage in FP and QS pattern till V4.

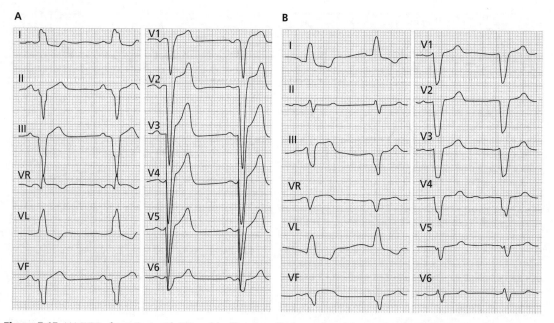

Figure 7.15 (A) ECG of a patient with idiopathic dilated cardiomyopathy with very low ejection fraction and LBBB with left ÂQRS. The ECG is similar to (B) that corresponds to an elderly patient with chronic obstructive pulmonary disease, but without evident heart failure with the same LBBB at least in the last 20 years. The only difference is that in the first case there is a QR pattern in VR that is explained by late activation of right ventricle due to its dilation (see text).

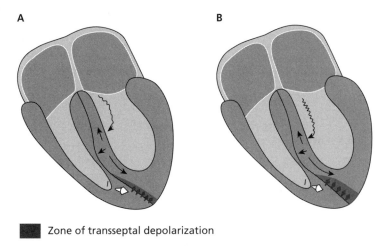

Zone of transseptal depolarization

Figure 7.16 Diagram of ventricular depolarization in first-degree LBBB. If the delay is mild (A), there is small transseptal depolarization by the right bundle branch and the only ECG repercussion is the disappearance of the first vector due to the fact that the delay in its inscription causes it to cancel out the right forces. The T wave may be positive or negative when there is associated disease. If the delay is greater (B), there is more anomalous septal depolarization, resembling more advanced LBBB, but the QRS does not reach 0.12 s in duration and the T wave is positive or negative–positive in I, VL, and/or V5 and V6 depending on the associated heart disease.

Figure 7.13 shows a typical example of advanced LBBB, and in Figures 7.14 and 7.15 two examples of advanced LBBB with associated pathology are shown (see legends). The association with IHD is briefly explained in Chapter 9 (see Section 9.6).

7.3.2. Partial left bundle branch block (first-degree)

In this case, the stimulus passes slowly down the left bundle branch. This explains that some part of the left ventricle is depolarized transseptally and some part is depolarized by a normal pathway (more in B than A in Fig. 7.16).

Because the start of septal depolarization occurs from right to left, the septal q wave is not originated and thus a unique R is seen in V6, I, and VL. Initial r is not found in V1 either, or it is very small, due to RV depolarization by the stimulus that passes down the right bundle branch.

The ECG of a .first-degree LBBB is characterized by:

1. QRS <120ms, with a unique R in I, VL, and V6.
2. Repolarization in V6 may be positive or flat/negative according to the accompanying pathology and degree of transseptal depolarization (Fig. 7.17).

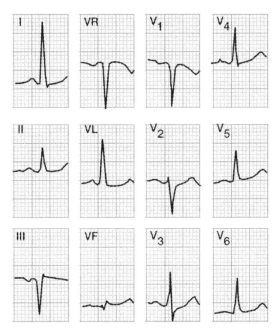

Figure 7.17 One example of partial LBBB. A 75-year-old patient without clinical heart disease.

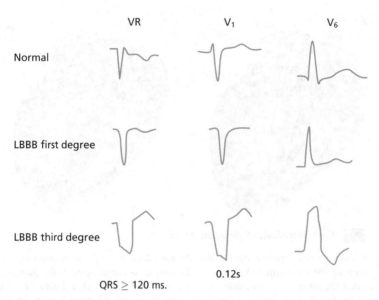

Figure 7.18 Comparative morphologies in partial (first degree) and advanced (third degree) LBBB.

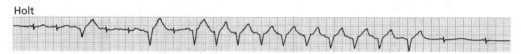

Figure 7.19 Intermittent LBBB. The third and sixth complexes manifest a LBBB morphology. The same occurs from the eighth complex to the seventeenth complex, after which rhythm becomes bradycardic and LBBB disappears (see Section 7.4).

7.3.3. Comparative morphologies

In Figure 7.18 may be seen the different morphologies in the VR, V1, and V6 in cases of normal activation and first- and third-degree LBBB.

7.3.4. Second-degree LBBB (Fig. 7.19)

As in second-degree RBBB, a pattern of transient first or third degree LBBB appears in the same tracing (see legend and Chapter 11, Ventricular Aberrancy).

7.4. Hemiblocks or fascicular blocks

See Rosenbaum et al., 1968; Elizari & Chiale, 2012.

In 1968, Rosenbaum and Elizari defined the ECG criteria of superoanterior and inferoposterior fascicular block of the left branch from a clinical and experimental point of view, calling it hemiblock. Many cases exist of superoanterior hemiblock (SAH) and few of inferoposterior hemiblocks (IPH).

7.4.1. Superoanterior hemiblock (SAH)

Figure 7.20 shows how ventricular activation occurs in a case of block in this fascicle.

The block in the superoanterior division originates a change in the start of activation that is then made through a small septal vector (**vector 1**) that moves downward, forward, and to the right, and then depolarizes the rest of the left ventricle upwards and backwards (**vector 2**).

The loop generated by this activation when projected on the positive and negative hemifields of each lead of the FP and HP explain the different QRS morphologies found in each case.

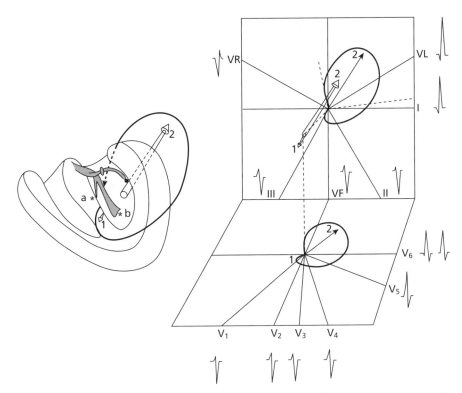

Figure 7.20 Diagram of the activation in superoanterior hemiblock. On the left are two vectors responsible for ventricular depolarization and the global QRS loop. The three stars represent the three entrances of the electric impulse in the left ventricle. On the right is the projection of the two vectors on the frontal and horizontal planes, with formation of the respective loops and the most common morphologies observed in clinical practice according to the loop–hemifield correlation. The dotted line above lead I represents what is probably the most exact situation of the positive part of lead I. As such, the entire last part of the loop would be in the positive hemifield of I, justifying the absence of S in I, which normally occurs (a line perpendicular to the true I has been added to the sketch, delimiting the positive and negative hemifields of this lead and illustrating this point).

L **7.4.1.1. Diagnostic criteria for SAH**

See Rosenbaum et al., 1968; Elizari & Chiale, 2012. The diagnosis of SAH may be made based on the presence of the following electrocardiographic criteria:

1. Leftwards ÂQRS between −45° and −75°. ÂQRS between −30° and −45° may correspond to non-advanced degrees of SAH.

2. FP morphology: qR in D1 and VL; rS in II, III, and VF, with S$_{III}$ > S$_{II}$ and R$_{II}$ > R$_{III}$, and sometimes with terminal r in VR.

3. HP morphology: S until V6 with intrinsicoid deflection time (IDT) in V6 < IDT in VL and with IDT in VL ≥50 ms. Some changes occur if the precordial electrodes are located above the normal site: in V1-V3 small q waves may appear, simulating a previous septal myocardial infarction, and in V2 an r′ wave may also appear. In V5-V6 the 'S' wave may be reduced and a small q may appear.

4. QRS duration <120 ms. However, in isolated cases the QRS may not surpass 100 ms. A QRS between 100 ms and 120 ms usually indicates associated LVE.

5. In advanced cases, mid-terminal slurrings are present in I and VL.

Figure 7.21 shows a typical example of SAH.

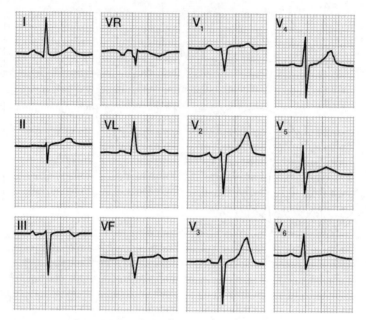

Figure 7.21 ECG–VCG of a patient with typical isolated superoanterior hemiblock. The morphology is that corresponding to Figure 7.20.

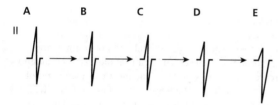

Figure 7.22 Evolution in time in a case of superoanterior hemiblock (SAH). Different drawings of QRS recording in lead II. In D and E, SAH is evident, but there must also be a certain degree of SAH in A and B, and especially in C.

7.4.1.2. Partial SAH

It is not easy to diagnose the presence of partial SAH. Leftwards ÂQRS starting at −30° may correspond to partial SAH if this pattern evolves into AQRS at −45° or more over time, as shown in Figure 7.22.

7.4.2. Inferoposterior hemiblock (IPH)

Figure 7.23 shows how ventricular activation is carried out in cases of block in this fascicle. As seen in the figure, **activation occurs inversely to that observed in SAH** (see before).

The **diagnosis of hemiblock in the inferoposterior division** (IPH), a process that is much less common than SAH because this fascicle is larger and narrower, **may only be made in the absence of RVE and very vertical heart**. According to some authors, a pathology on the left ventricle must also be present.

7.4.2.1. Diagnostic criteria for IPH

The diagnostic criteria of inferoposterior hemiblock are listed below.

1. ÂQRS greatly deviated to the right (between +90° and +140°).

2. RS or Rs in I and VL, and qR in II, III, and VF. With regard to precordial leads, the most common morphologies are seen in Figure 7.21.

3. QRS <120 ms.

4. TDI=>50 ms in VF and V6, with TDI <50 ms in VL.

5. Mid-terminal slurrings in II, III, and VF in advanced cases.

Figure 7.24 shows the appearance of an IPH morphology. Very often it appears in association with RBBB.

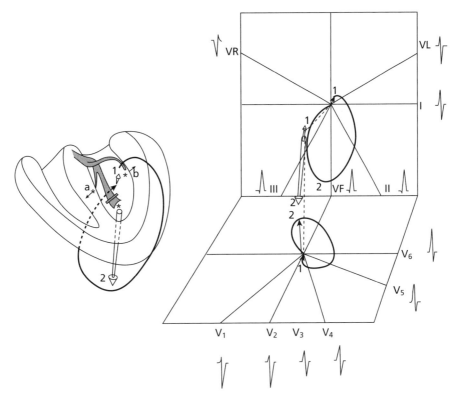

Figure 7.23 Diagram of activation in inferoposterior hemiblock. On the left are the two vectors that account for ventricular depolarization and the global QRS loop, and on the right, the projection of these vectors on the frontal and horizontal planes, with formation of the respective loops and the most common morphologies seen in practice according the loop–hemifield correlation.

In cases of IPH due to progressive conduction aberrancy of atrial extrasystoles or extrastimulus, it has been observed that cases of **partial inferoposterior hemiblock** may only be diagnosed by comparative study.

7.5. Bifascicular block

The most typical cases are due to RBBB associated with SAH or IPH.

o **A. RBBB + SAH**
See the wide QRS (>120 ms), the rsR' pattern in V1, and the very left ÂQRS with rS pattern in II, III and VF (Fig. 7.25A).

When exists an important delay of LV activation, the final vectors of activation may be directed forwards (R in V1 due to RBBB), but to the left instead of to the right. Due to this, there is no S in I and VL. Thus the HP looks like RBBB and the FP like LBBB. This type of bifascicular block is named 'masked bifascicular block' (Bayés de Luna, 2012a) (Fig. 7.25B).

B. RBBB + IPH (Fig. 7.26)
See the wide QRS (>120 ms), the rsR' pattern in V1, and the right ÂQRS with qR pattern in II, III, and VF to assure the diagnosis, the ECG has to be taken from a patient with no right heart disease or a very vertical heart.

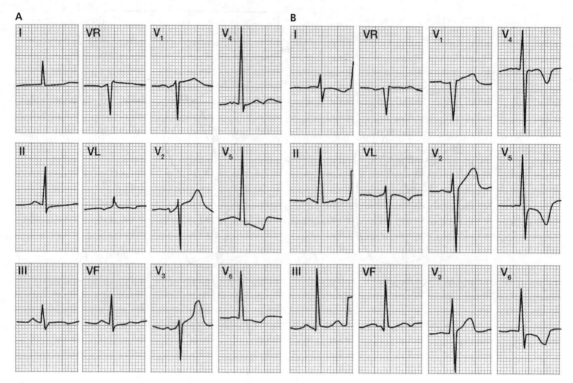

Figure 7.24 (A) ECG of a 55-year-old patient with arterial hypertension and coronary heart disease. (B) Without any clinical change, a month later the patient presented a striking ECG change: ÂQRS went from left to right, in VF Rs passed to qR with IDT = 0.06 s, and in V6 qR changed to Rs. All this may be explained by the appearance of inferoposterior hemiblock.

See Bayés de Luna (2012a) for more explanation of the clinical implications of these types of block.

7.6. Trifascicular block (Fig. 7.27)

P **In this case a block in three fascicles is present**.

The most typical case presents a morphology of **RBBB alternating with SAH and IPH**.

See (Fig. 7.27) how in the presence of a wide QRS and a pattern of RBBB in the two ECGs, an abrupt change in ÂQRS occurs in the frontal plane from −70° in A to +130° in B. These patients may present syncopes when trifascicular block coincides, because an abrupt advanced AV block occurs (Rosembaum–Elizari syndrome). These situations require the urgent implantation of a pacemaker.

The presence of **LBBB alternating with RBB + SAH** has the same clinical considerations as the previous case.

The cases of bifascicular block with a long PR interval may be explained by first degree block in the His bundle. Therefore they cannot be considered due to trifascicular block.

7.7. Block in the middle fibers of the left branch

Q

The presence of block in the middle fibers (MF), also known as the septal fascicle (SF), probably originate some ECG changes. At present the following two criteria are the most used to describe this type of block: **(1) lack of septal q** (lack of q in

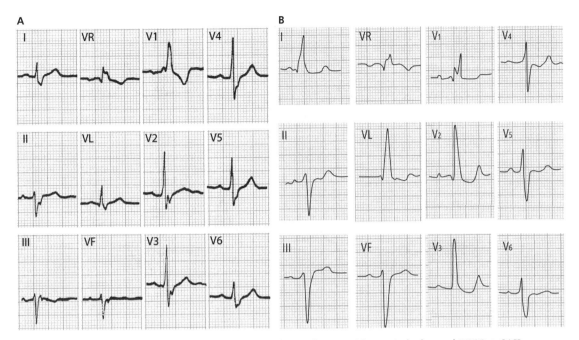

Figure 7.25 (A) A 70-year-old patient with no apparent heart disease with a typical advanced RBBB + SAH morphology. (B) An example of masked bifascicular block (see text).

leads V5-v6 and I) and **(2) the presence of a prominent R in V1-V2**. The Brazilian school supports more this last criterion.

The presence of these patterns (missing septal q wave in I, V5-V6, or presence of R/S in V₁–V₂) if transient, confirm that they are due to some type of intraventricular conduction disturbance, although the location of the conduction delay is not certain. The lack of septal q wave in V6, I, may be also explained by first-degree LBBB, and the presence of RS in V1-V2 may occur in case of MF/SF block or partial right bundle branch block (Fig. 7.8) or both. Many other processes may also present prominent R or r' in V1 (see Table 6.1) (Bayés de Luna et al., 2012d).

Self-assessment

A. What types of block exist at the ventricular level?

B. How is the activation modified in advanced RBBB?

C. What are the diagnostic criteria for advanced RBBB?

D. What are the diagnostic criteria for partial RBBB?

E. What are the diagnostic criteria for second-degree RBBB?

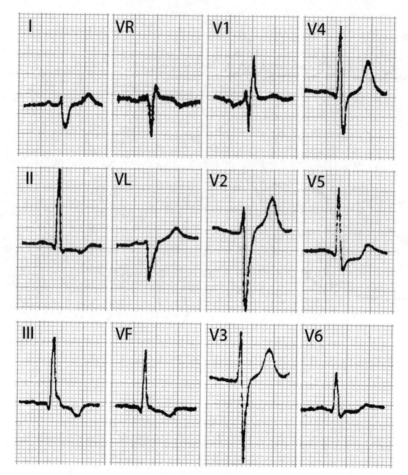

Figure 7.26 A 76-year-old patient with ischemic heart disease and arterial hypertension, and with no right heart disease or vertical heart, who presented with a morphology typical of advanced RBBB + IPH (see text). The ST segment is depressed in the left precordial leads because of the underlying disease.

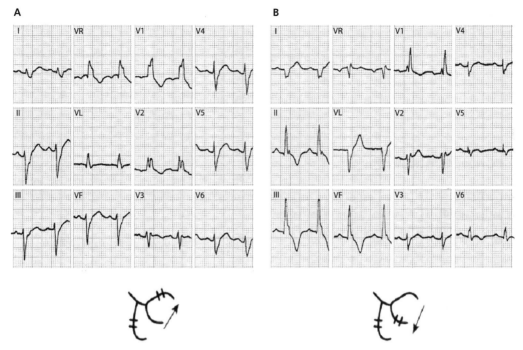

Figure 7.27 Typical example of trifascicular block. (A) RBBB + SAH. (B) The next day the frontal ÂQRS passed from −60° to +130°, indicating the appearance of an inferoposterior hemiblock substituting the superoanterior hemiblock.

F. Do you remember the differential diagnosis of RBBB?

G. How is the activation of advanced LBBB modified?

H. What are the diagnostic criteria for advanced LBBB?

I. What are the diagnostic criteria for first-degree LBBB?

J. What are the diagnostic criteria for second-degree LBBB?

K. Describe the activation in superoanterior hemiblock.

L. What are the diagnostic criteria for superoanterior hemiblock?

M. What produces activation in inferoposterior hemiblock?

N. What are the diagnostic criteria for inferoposterior hemiblock?

O. List the most common types of bifascicular block.

P. List the most common types of trifascicular block.

Q. Can block of the middle fibers of left branch be diagnosed on the ECG?

CHAPTER 8
Ventricular Preexcitation

8.1. Concepts and types

A • **Ventricular preexcitation occurs when the electrical stimulus reaches the ventricles before the normal activation through the specific conduction system (SCS).** In fact, this phenomenon is not really a preexcitation, but rather early ventricular excitation.

• Early ventricular excitation, mistakenly known as preexcitation, was described by Wolff, Parkinson, and White in young persons presenting paroxysmal arrhythmias, and is known as **Wolff–Parkinson–White (WPW) syndrome**. Early excitation occurs because of the existence of **short muscular bundles with accelerated conduction** (accessory pathway), known as **Kent bundles**, that connect the atria to the ventricles. These bundles may involve conduction that is anterograde, retrograde, or both. The degree of anomalous activation is variable (Fig. 8.1).

• Rarely, early excitation takes place through long bundles that connect the right atrium with the fascicles or muscular mass of the right ventricle and present **anterograde decremental conduction only**. This is known as **atypical** preexcitation and includes the phenomenon previously known as Mahaim preexcitation.

• Also the preexcitation may be due to the existence of an atrial-hisian bundle, which carries the stimulus from the atrium to the ventricle faster, or may be due simply to accelerated AV conduction. This is known as **short PR-type preexcitation**, or **Lown–Gannon–Levine syndrome**.

• The presence of preexcitation, especially WPW syndrome, favors the appearance of potentially dangerous supraventricular arrhythmias (see later).

8.2. WPW-type preexcitation

8.2.1. Electrocardiographic characteristics (Fig. 8.2)

B

(A) Short PR interval
This is due to early ventricular excitation through an accessory pathway, that occurs before the normal excitation arrives through the SCS.

(B) QRS morphology
The QRS is usually wide (≥ 0.11 s) and its morphology depends on the location of the accessory pathway. However, in all the cases as the location in the ventricular muscle of the accessory pathway takes place in an area with few Purkinje fibers, some initial slurrings in the QRS complex, known as **delta wave**, are present. Later, the stimulus arrives through the normal pathway, and the ventricles are activated through two fronts, configuring a true fusion complex that presents a greater or lesser degree of preexcitation depending on the quantity of preexcited ventricular mass (Fig. 8.1).

Figure 8.2 shows various degrees of **WPW-type preexcitation** (above right). See how from A to C an increasing degree of delta wave. D is a case of atrial fibrillation with a second complex presenting the maximum degree of preexcitation. In the

ECGs for Beginners, First Edition. Antoni Bayés de Luna.
© 2014 John Wiley & Sons, Inc. Published 2014 by John Wiley & Sons, Inc.

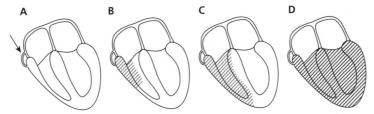

Figure 8.1 The accessory bundle is indicated with an arrow. Ventricular depolarization is realized by two routes: normal (through the SCS and abnormal (through the accessory bundle). The zone depolarized by the abnormal route is shaded in B and C; the resulting complex is a fusion complex, since part of the ventricles are depolarized by the normal route (unshaded area) and part by the abnormal route (shaded area). In A, the complete depolarization is effected in the normal route and in D, entirely by the abnormal route (maximum preexcitation).

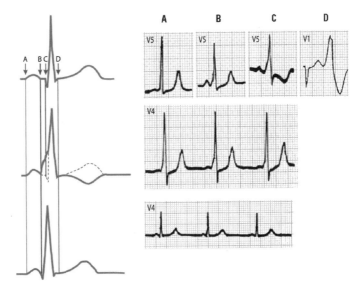

Figure 8.2 Left top panel: Diagram of the P–QRS relationship in normal cases. (AB) P wave; (BC) PR segment; (CD) QRS. Middle panel: WPW-type preexcitation (the broken line represents the QRS complex if no preexcitation occurred). AD distance is the same as under normal conditions, with a wide QRS complex in detriment to the PR segment (BC distance), which partially or totally coincides with the delta wave. Lower panel: in cases of short PR segment, the QRS complex is shifted forward because the PR segment is shortened or may even disappear. Top right: Four examples of delta wave (arrow) by increasing order of relevance. (D) Atrial fibrillation patient in whom the first QRS is conducted over the normal pathway, while the second QRS is conducted over the accessory pathway with maximum preexcitation. Middle panel: example of four complexes with preexcitation, with an average-sized delta wave. Lower panel: four complexes in a case of short PR preexcitation.

middle part of the figure, four successive complexes are seen in a case of moderate preexcitation. With a clear short PR and an exclusive short PR-type preexcitation below. On the upper left, normal ventricular activation is shown. In the middle, WPW preexcitation shows short PR and a delta wave with an earlier QRS complex seen in points, but with the same final QRS resembling that found in normal patients. This is because ventricular activation is a fusion complex between the first preexcited part and the second part activated by a normal pathway.

C **8.2.2. Types of WPW-type preexcitation**

WPW-type preexcitation may be classified into four types according to the accessory pathway location. Figure 8.3 shows this organization and the repercussions of the anomalous pathway location on ECG morphology. We must always remember that in WPW preexcitation ventricular activation is shared by the accessory pathway and the normal pathway (Figs 8.1–8.3). Figures 8.4 and 8.5 show examples of the four types of preexcitation with evident delta waves.

Many algorithms have been described based on the location of the delta wave in certain leads. These algorithms can be used to locate the accessory pathway quite precisely (Bayés de Luna, 2012a). However, the predicted location must always be confirmed before performing ablation of the pathway.

Sometimes preexcitation is intermittent and occasionally may appear **progressively** (concertina effect). Figure 8.6 shows a case of sudden intermittent preexcitation and Figure 8.7 shows how preexcitation disappears progressively (concertina effect).

8.2.3. Confirming or ruling out preexcitation

D • **The injection of adenosine**, a selective blocker of the AV node, can confirm (if the ECG pattern appears clearly), or rule out (if the ECG pattern does not modify) the preexcitation.
• **The presence of q in V6** practically rules out preexcitation.

8.2.4. WPW-type preexcitation and arrhythmias

WPW preexcitation may be related to certain types of arrhythmia.

E **A. Reentrant paroxysmal tachycardias of the AV junction with an accessory pathway (JRT-AP; also named AVRT, see Chapter 11.)**
• The accessory bundle may participate in the **reentrant circuit** of a paroxysmal tachycardia of the AV junction, with retrograde conduction through the accessory pathway and anterograde conduction through the SCS. The atria are activated through the accessory pathway after anterograde activation of the ventricles through the normal pathway, and thus P′ is located after a narrow QRS. This differentiates these tachycardias from those in which the re-entrant circuit is found exclusively in the AV junction (JRT-E) (see Chapter 10).
• Figure 8.8 shows in the first two complexes (A) the activation through the accessory pathway (∼∼∼➔) and later (B), after an atrial extrasystole (P′), the activation blocked in the accessory pathway and carried anterograde in through the AV junction of the SCS with a narrow QRS (1), originating a re-entrant tachycardia with retrograde atrial activation through the accessory pathway (P′ located after QRS) (P′R > RP′). The subsequent QRS complexes are also narrow (3) (**orthodromic tachycardia**) (see Chapter 11).
• In rare cases of reentrant tachycardia, the anterograde conduction to the ventricles is made through one accessory pathway (Kent bundle or a long anomalous pathway in atypical preexcitation with retrograde conduction (see Fig. 8.3). This is known as **antidromic tachycardia**.
• ECGs can generally be used to identify these two types of antidromic tachycardias that present a similar morphology to that of LBBB (QS in V1 and R in V6). Antidromic tachycardia through the Kent bundle presents a LBBB-like morphology with transition to R in precordial leads before V4 and the antidromic tachycardia through a long atriofascicular pathway of atypical preexcitation presents a LBBB-like morphology with a transition to R in precordial leads in V4 or later (see Bayés de Luna, 2011 and 2012a). For the differential diagnosis of antidromic tachycardia with ventricular tachycardia. See Section 12.2.3.2 in Chapter 12 (Steurer et al., 1994).

B. WPW preexcitation and atrial fibrillation or flutter
• Patients with WPW more frequently present episodes of atrial fibrillation (AF) or flutter (AFL). Usually this is explained because a ventricular extrasystole (VE) carried quickly and retrogradely through the accessory pathway encounters atria

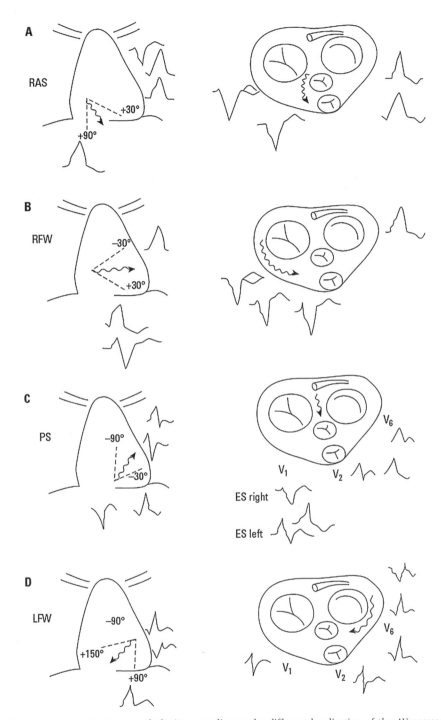

Figure 8.3 WPW-type preexcitation morphologies according to the different localization of the AV accessory pathway: (A) Right anteroseptal area (RAS); (B) right ventricular free wall (RFW); (C) inferoseptal area (IS); and (D) left ventricular free wall (LFW). ES = early stimulation.

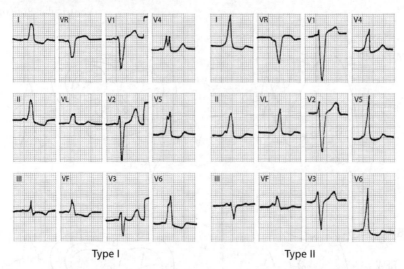

Type I   Type II

Figure 8.4 Left: ECG of WPW preexcitation type I in a 28-year-old patient. Right: ECG of WPW preexcitation type II. The most important difference is the ÂQRS direction; in type I around +50° and type II around +15°: see Fig. 8.3). These cases mimic LBBB pattern, case A with a less advanced pattern.

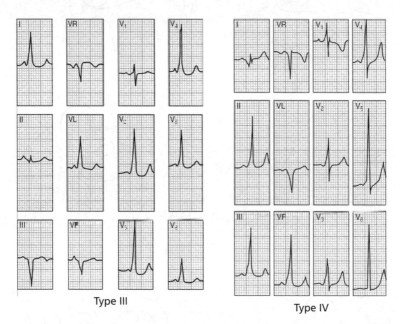

Type III   Type IV

Figure 8.5 Left: A WPW patient with the accessory pathway located in the inferoseptal heart wall (type III WPW). This case may be mistaken for an inferior infarction, right ventricular hypertrophy, or right bundle branch block (RBBB). Right: One case of a WPW patient with the accessory pathway located in the left ventricular free wall (type IV WPW). This case may be mistaken for a lateral infarction, right ventricular hypertrophy, or right bundle branch block.

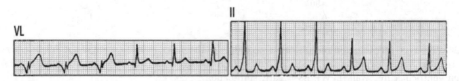

Figure 8.6 Intermittent type IV preexcitation: the pattern with preexcitation is similar to Q wave MI (see VL).

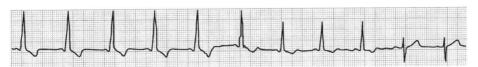

Figure 8.7 Concertina effect. The five first complexes are identical and show short PR and preexcitation. In the next four complexes, preexcitation decreases with a shorter PR = 0.12 s. The three last complexes do not show any preexcitation and the PR = 0.16 s.

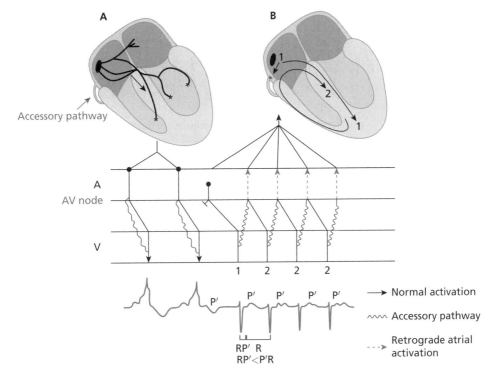

Figure 8.8 Scheme of a heart with a right accessory AV pathway, which leads to faster than normal AV conduction (short PR) and early activation of part of the ventricles and appearance of abnormal QRS morphology (delta wave) (A). All this may be observed in the first two P-QRS complexes of the scheme. The QRS is a fusion complex due to initial depolarization through the accessory AV pathway (curved tracing) and the rest of depolarization through the normal AV pathway (rectilinear tracing). The third P wave is premature (atrial ectopic P') that finds the accessory AV pathway in the refractory period. Due to this, the impulse is only conducted by normal AV conduction (rectilinear tracing in AV node) usually with a longer than normal P'R interval, because the AV node is in a relative refractory period. This stimulus produces a normal QRS complex (1), due to the fact that the accessory AV pathway is already out of the refractory period. Then it is conducted retrogradely to the atria, through the accessory pathway generating an evident P' after the QRS complex (RP' < P'R). In the case of junctional reciprocal tachycardia with circuit exclusively in the AV junction (JRT-E), the P' is within the QRS complex or can be seen in its final part, modifying the QRS morphology (Fig. 11.7). After that the impulse re-enters and is conducted down to the ventricles via normal AV conduction (2). Due to this macroreentry circuit, the reciprocating tachycardia is maintained. The conduction in this circuit is retrograde via accessory AV pathway (curved tracing) and anterograde via the normal AV conduction (rectilinear tracing). The RP' interval is smaller than the P'R interval, which is typical of junctional reciprocating tachycardia that involves an accessory AV pathway (WPW). (See Plate 8.8.)

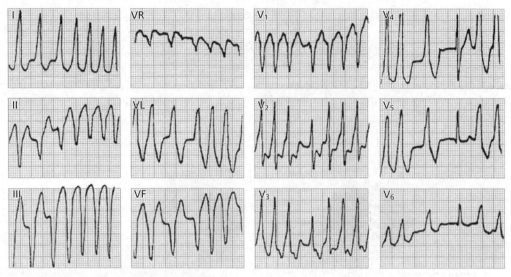

Figure 8.9 Twelve-lead ECG of a Wolff–Parkinson–White (WPW) syndrome in atrial fibrillation. Note the great degree of aberrancy of the complexes, that makes necessitates differential diagnosis with ventricular tachycardia (VT); this may be very difficult especially in the presence of a regular ventricular conduction (atrial flutter) (see Fig. 8.10B). In this example the diagnosis of WPW syndrome with atrial fibrillation and not of VT is supported by: (i) the presence of delta waves in some leads (V2, V3) and the presence of different morphologies of QRS, with more or less degrees of aberrancy, as the expression of different degrees of conduction over the accessory pathway; (ii) irregular RR; (iii) narrow QRS, which may or may not be premature (see asterisk). In ventricular tachycardia, narrow QRS complexes are always premature (captures) (Fig. 12.11); and (iv) awareness of the existence of this arrhythmia.

that are vulnerable because they are outside the refractory period, which is generally shorter, and may trigger AF or AFL.

• Occasionally, a supraventricular paroxysmal tachycardia may also trigger AF or AFL for a similar reason.

F • The differential diagnosis between AF of WPW syndrome and ventricular tachycardia is relatively easy, even though QRS is wide in both scenarios. The diagnostic criteria are exposed in the legend of Figure 8.9. However, the differential diagnosis is more difficult when AFL, rather than AF, is present (Fig. 8.10).

C. Atrial fibrillation in WPW syndrome and sudden death

G • Sudden death (SD) in WPW may appear **in the presence of very fast AF when the RR is very short, allowing the supraventricular stimulus to fall into the vulnerable stage** in the ventricles (Fig. 8.11). This usually does not occur if preexcitation disappears at high heart rate during a stress

test, and if the refractory period of the accessory pathway is long.

8.2.5. Differential diagnosis in WPW-type preexcitation

• **WPW types I and II** = LBBB.   H
• **WPW type III** = inferior infarction, right ventricular enlargement (VE), and RBBB.
• **WPW type IV** = lateral infarction, right VE, and RBBB.

The key in every case is to measure the PR interval and to detect any delta waves.

8.3. Atypical preexcitation

• The accessory bundle is long, with slow con-   I
duction and goes from the right atrium to the right ventricle (atriofascicular or atrioventricular bundle).
• The ECG is often almost normal, or with only small degrees of preexcitation in the form of small

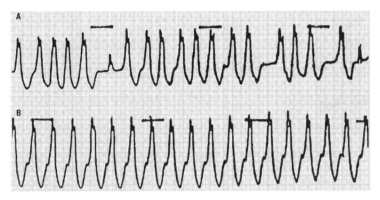

Figure 8.10 A 50-year-old patient with type IV Wolff–Parkinson–White (WPW) atrial fibrillation (top) and atrial flutter (bottom) episodes simulating a ventricular tachycardia (A). The isolated, wide R morphology, with a notch in the descending arm does not correspond to a right bundle branch block (RBBB) aberrancy. Furthermore, the following facts are in favor of a WPW syndrome with atrial fibrillation and not of ventricular tachycardia (in addition to other clinical features and the prior awareness of the WPW syndrome diagnosis): (i) The wide complexes show a very irregular rate and morphology (varying wideness) because of the presence of different degrees of preexcitation. (ii) The two narrow complexes – 6 and the last one in A – are late and premature, respectively. In sustained ventricular tachycardia, QRS are more regular and if captures occur (narrow complexes), they are always premature (see Fig. 12.11). (B) In the WPW syndrome with atrial flutter (in this case 2 × 1, 150 bpm) differential diagnosis with sustained ventricular tachycardia through the ECG is even more difficult. It is important to obtain the clinical history and to follow the criteria of differential diagnosis between VT and supraventricular tachycardia with aberrancy, especially those described by Steurer (Chapter 12).

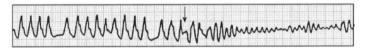

Figure 8.11 Patient with WPW syndrome presenting with a very fast atrial fibrillation triggering a ventricular fibrillation (VF). See especially the short RR interval previous to PVC that triggers VF (see arrow). This was treated with electrical cardioversion.

initial slurrings of R wave in I and V6, and often with rS in lead III that mimick partial LBBB (accessory pathway in RV).

• It may originate tachycardias with wide QRS usually of LBBB type, because the anterograde conduction is made through one long right accessory bundle (see Figure 8.2.4.A and Bayés de Luna 2011, and 2012a).

8.4. Short PR-type preexcitation

J • In this case early excitation is produced by an accelerated AV conduction, or by the existence of an atrial hisian bundle that avoids slow conduction through the AV node.

• Figure 8.2 (bottom) shows a case of short PR-type preexcitation in which the end of QRS complex occurs earlier because the entire activation, which starts early, occurs through the SCS.

• Figure 8.12 shows a typical example of short PR-type preexcitation. It is important to remember that these patients are also at risk for potentially serious arrhythmias, especially in cases of rapid AF.

Self-assessment

A. What is ventricular preexcitation and how many types exist?

B. What are the ECG characteristics of WPW-type preexcitation?

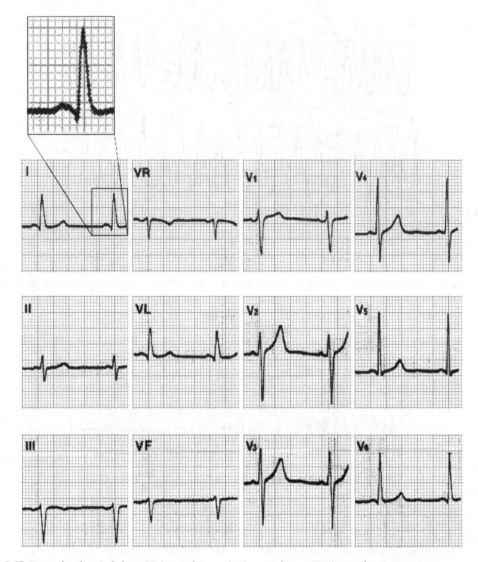

Figure 8.12 Example of typical short PR interval preexcitation syndrome (PR interval = 0.10 sec).

C. How many types of WPW-type preexcitation exist?

D. How can preexcitation be confirmed or ruled out?

E. What are the most common arrhythmias associated with WPW-type preexcitation?

F. How is the differential diagnosis made between atrial fibrillation with WPW syndrome and VT?

G. When can a patient with WPW be at risk for SD?

H. How is the differential diagnosis of WPW-type preexcitation made?

I. What is atypical preexcitation?

J. What is short PR-type preexcitation?

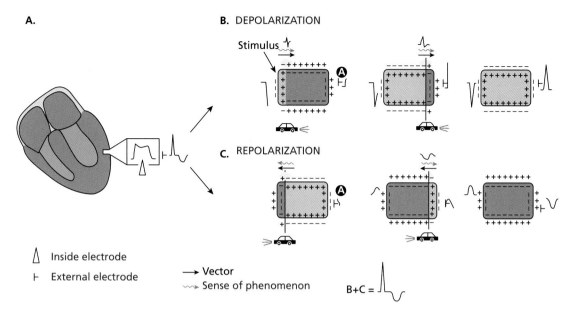

Plate 2.1 (A) An electrode located in a wedge section of myocardial tissue records TAP curve similar to the TAP recorded when a microelectrode is located inside the cell (Fig. 1.6). When one electrode is placed outside a curve, the so-called 'cellular electrogram' is recorded. (B and C) Diagram showing how the curve of the cellular electrogram originates, based on the dipole theory (B depolarization and C repolarization).

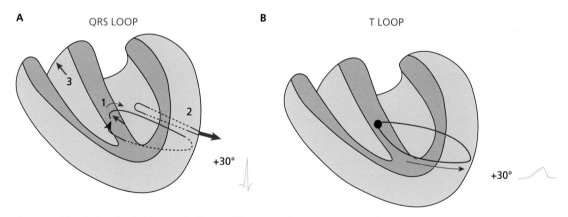

Plate 2.9 QRS (A) and T (B) loops of a heart without rotations (see Chapter 4).

ECGs for Beginners, First Edition. Antoni Bayés de Luna.
© 2014 John Wiley & Sons, Inc. Published 2014 by John Wiley & Sons, Inc.

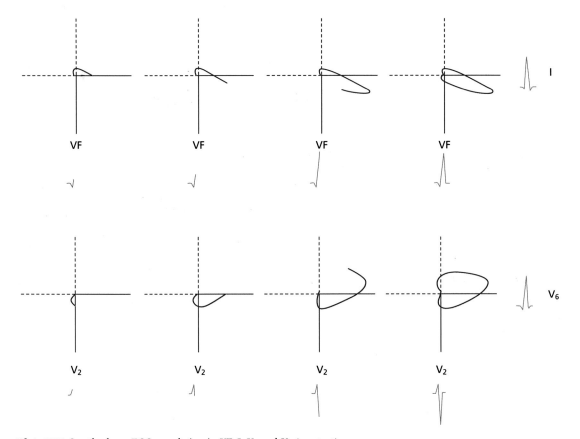

Plate 2.23 See the loop–ECG correlation in VF, I, V$_2$ and V$_6$ (see text).

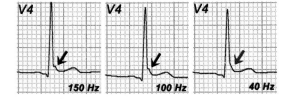

Plate 3.7 Forty-year-old patient with ECG morphology typical for early repolarization. Observe how a low-pass filter (40 Hz) can make the typical J curve disappear.

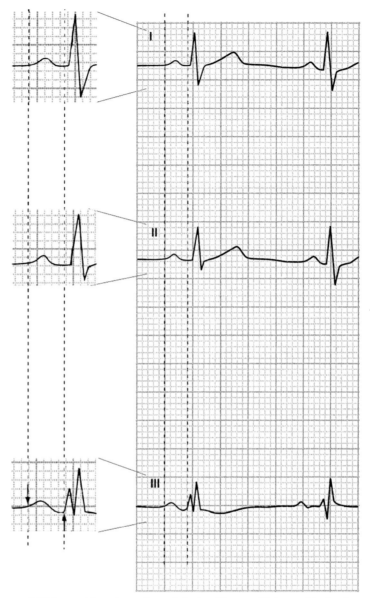

Plate 4.3 Measurement of PR interval in a three-channel device: The true PR interval is the distance between the first inscription of P wave and QRS complex in any lead. In this case (see solid lines) this happens in lead III but not in I and II.

A

B

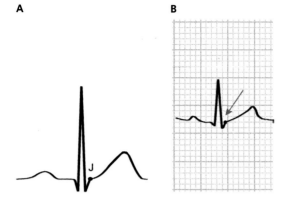

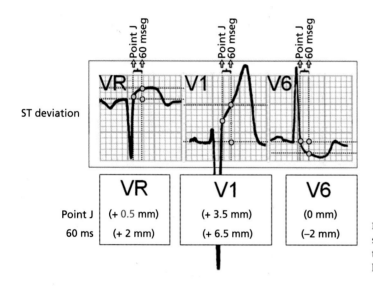

Plate 4.8 (A) Drawing showing the location of the J point. (B) The J point (arrow) in an ECG tracing.

ST deviation

	VR	V1	V6
Point J	(+ 0.5 mm)	(+ 3.5 mm)	(0 mm)
60 ms	(+ 2 mm)	(+ 6.5 mm)	(–2 mm)

Plate 4.9 Method of measuring the ST shifts. The figure shows the results with the measurements at J point, and 60 ms later.

A

B

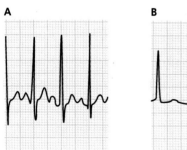

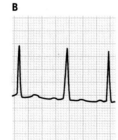

Plate 4.11 (A) Heart rate during sympathetic overdrive, and (B) after beta blockers in a case of physiological stress (parachuting). (Holter recording.)

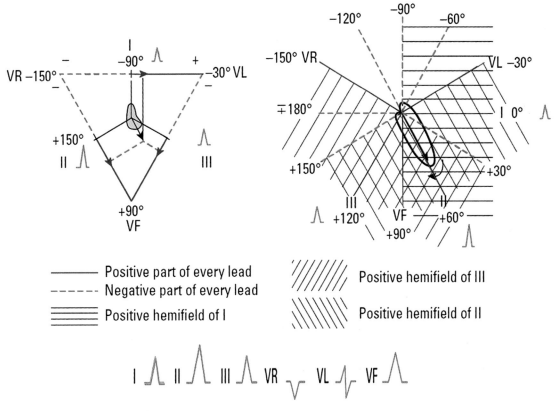

Plate 4.14 Calculation of the ÂQRS: when this is situated at +60°, the projection on I, II, and III and the situation in the positive and negative hemifields of these leads originate in I, II, and III, the morphology shown at the left of the figure.

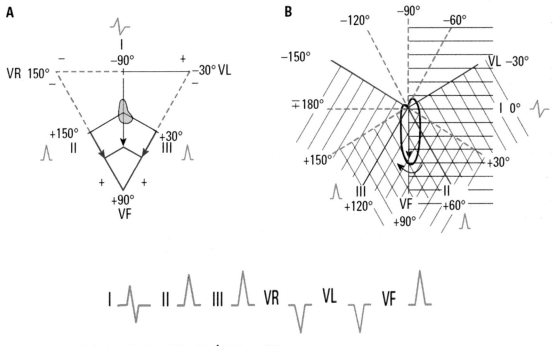

Plate 4.15 Morphologies of I, II and III with ÂQRS at +90°.

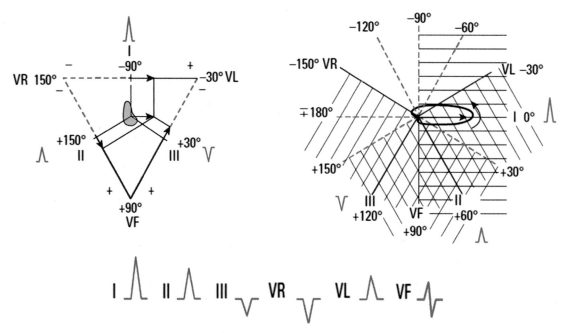

Plate 4.16 Morphologies of I, II and III with ÂQRS at 0°.

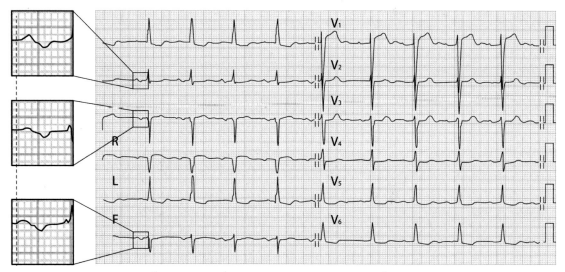

Plate 5.7 Typical ECG of advanced interatrial block (P ± in II, III, and VF and duration > 120 ms) in a patient with ischemic cardiomyopathy. When amplified we can see the beginning of P in the three leads.

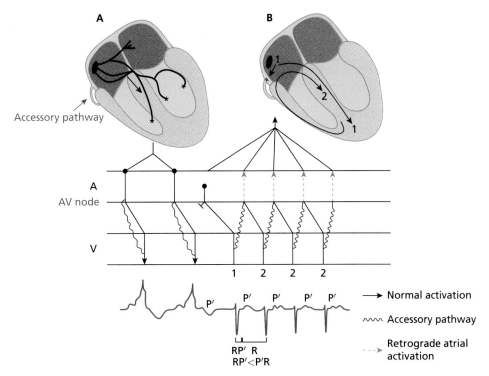

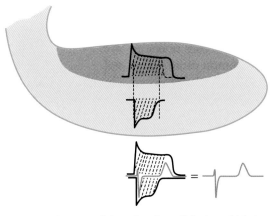

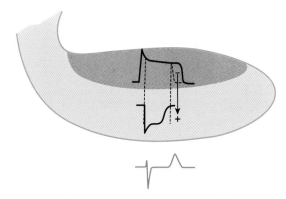

Plate 8.8 Scheme of a heart with a right accessory AV pathway, which leads to faster than normal AV conduction (short PR) and early activation of part of the ventricles and appearance of abnormal QRS morphology (delta wave) (A). All this may be observed in the first two P-QRS complexes of the scheme. The QRS is a fusion complex due to initial depolarization through the accessory AV pathway (curved tracing) and the rest of depolarization through the normal AV pathway (rectilinear tracing). The third P wave is premature (atrial ectopic P′) that finds the accessory AV pathway in the refractory period. Due to this, the impulse is only conducted by normal AV conduction (rectilinear tracing in AV node) usually with a longer than normal P′R interval, because the AV node is in a relative refractory period. This stimulus produces a normal QRS complex (1), due to the fact that the accessory AV pathway is already out of the refractory period. Then it is conducted retrogradely to the atria, through the accessory pathway generating an evident P′ after the QRS complex (RP′ < P′R). In the case of junctional reciprocal tachycardia with circuit exclusively in the AV junction (JRT-E), the P′ is within the QRS complex or can be seen in its final part, modifying the QRS morphology (Fig. 11.7). After that the impulse re-enters and is conducted down to the ventricles via normal AV conduction (2). Due to this macroreentry circuit, the reciprocating tachycardia is maintained. The conduction in this circuit is retrograde via accessory AV pathway (curved tracing) and anterograde via the normal AV conduction (rectilinear tracing). The RP′ interval is smaller than the P′R interval, which is typical of junctional reciprocating tachycardia that involves an accessory AV pathway (WPW).

Plate 9.2 The sum of the subendocardial TAP, which is lengthened but maintains the same form as that of the subepicardium, and the subepicardial TAP explains how the ST segment remains isoelectric, the T wave is wider or higher, and the QT somewhat longer.

Plate 9.3 The formation of the subendocardial vector of ischemia in the second part of repolarization, which moves from the endocardium (the area not yet repolarized) with negative charges toward the epicardium (already repolarized) explains the higher and wider T wave.

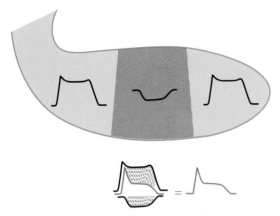

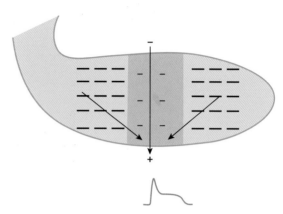

Plate 9.4 The TAP in the transmural zone affected by severe ischemia presents a slower descent and an inverted polarity (Ashman phenomenon). The sum of this TAP with the TAPs in neighboring areas explains the ECG morphology with ST elevation.

Plate 9.5 The vector of severe transmural ischemia (historically called the subepicardial injury vector) is directed from the subendocardium to the subepicardium and recorded as ST elevation. This is due to the lesser negative charge in the affected transmural zone compared to the rest of the myocardium and thus functions as relatively positive.

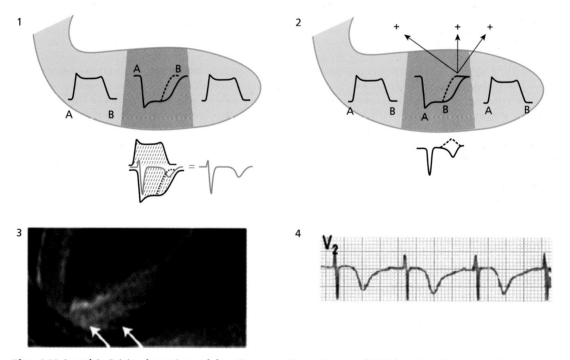

Plate 9.18 1. and 2. Origin of negative and deep T wave. 1. Due to increased TAP duration of transmural area affected, the sum of this TAP of this area with the TAP neighboring areas, that is shorter, explain the negative T wave. 2. The explanation based on the vector of ischemia theory. 3. Transmural involvement (CMR) in a case of negative T wave after aborted (Migliore et al., 2011). See the transmural edema. 4. Deep and negative T wave in V2 in a case of transient LAD occlusion (negative T wave of reperfusion-edema).

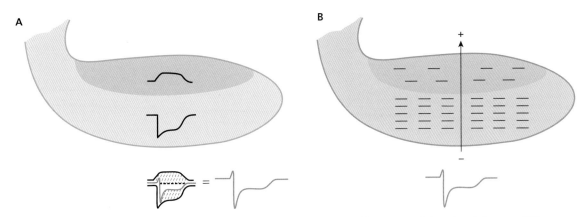

Plate 9.21 (A) The sum of the TAP in the subendocardium (TAP with smaller area) and the TAP of the rest of VI (normal) explains the ST depression. (B) The area with severe endocardial ischemia presents less negative charges than the rest of VI and is thus relatively positive. For this reason the severe ischemic vector (injury vector) points to the subendocardium and is recorded as negative from the end of QRS in the elevations of the ECG.

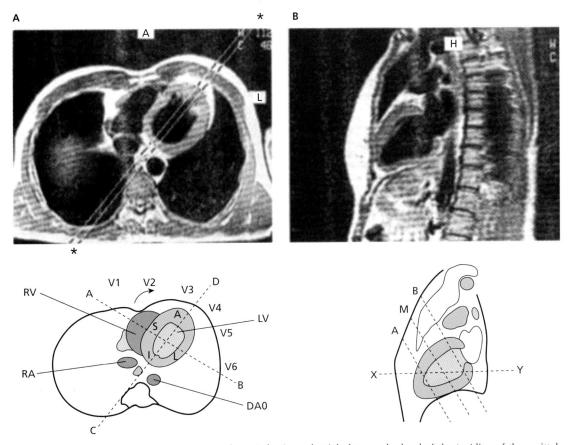

Plate 9.32 Magnetic resonance imaging. **(A)** Thoracic horizontal axial plane at the level of the 'xy' line of the sagittal plane of right side of the figure. The four walls can be adequately observed: anterior (A), septal (S), lateral (L), and inferior (I), with the inferobasal portion of the wall (segment 4 of Cerqueria statement) that bends upwards in this case. **(B)** Sagittal plane following the line seen in (A) (asterisk). B, M, and A, basal, middle, and apical plane. DAo = descending aorta; RA = right atrium; RV = right ventricle. An R wave (mirror pattern of Q wave in back leads) is not originated in V1, in the case of infarction of the basal area of inferior wall, because this basal zone always depolarizes after the first 40 ms, and then the QRS pattern has already started the recording. Furthermore although a necrosis vector (NV) could be generated this would face V3–V4 and not V1 (see in A the asterisk and the line C D).

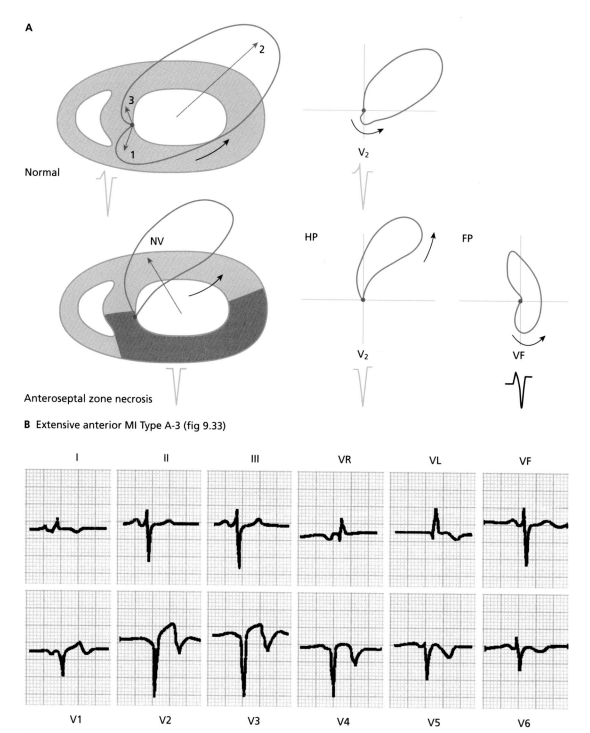

A

Normal

Anteroseptal zone necrosis

NV

HP

FP

V_2

V_2

VF

B Extensive anterior MI Type A-3 (fig 9.33)

| I | II | III | VR | VL | VF |

| V1 | V2 | V3 | V4 | V5 | V6 |

Plate 9.34 (A) A comparison of normal activation and in case of in extensive anterior infarction (Q beyond V2 and in I and VL) (type A.3 in Fig. 9.33). The direction of the infarction vector in the FP and HP explains the morphologies in precordial leads and in lead 1 and VL. (B) Example of infarction in this zone. QS until V4 and qr in D1 and VL.

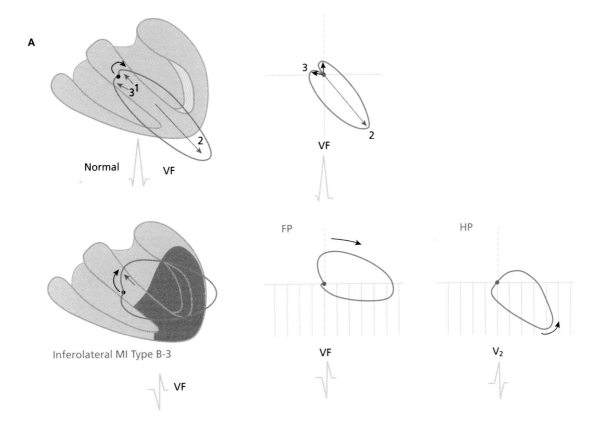

A

Normal   VF

VF

3

2

Inferolateral MI Type B-3

VF

FP

VF

HP

V₂

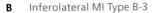

B   Inferolateral MI Type B-3

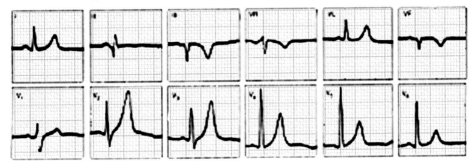

Plate 9.38 (A) A comparison of normal activation with the activation in a case of infarction of the inferolateral zone (type B-3 in Fig. 9.33). The inferior infarction vector moves upward and in the FP the loop–hemifield correlation explains the appearance of the Q wave in inferior leads. The involvement of the lateral wall originates an anteriorization of the loop in the HP, explaining the prominent R wave in V1. (B) An example of Q infarction in the inferolateral zone in II, III, and VF and RS in V1 (type B-3).

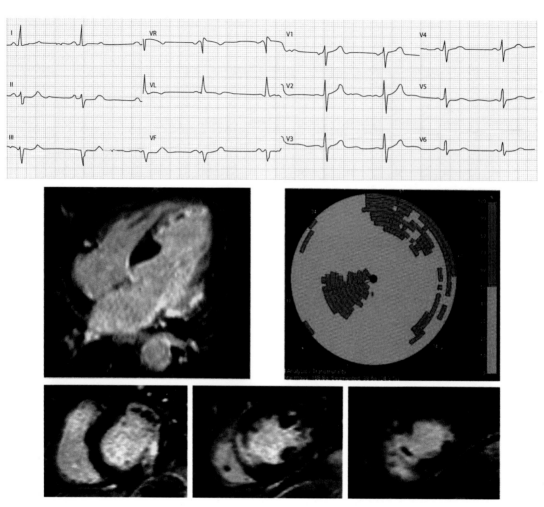

Plate 9.43 Patient with septal and lateral infarctions clearly visible with CE-CMR using MRI. The ECG is practically normal because the two vectors of necrosis cancel each other and thus the Q wave is not visible.

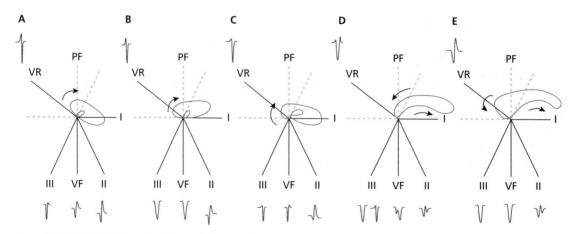

Plate 9.51 (A–E) ECG loops in different inferior infarctions associated in D and E with SAH. In these last two cases (D and E), the final part falls in the negative hemifield of II because of the special rotation of the QRS loop due to SAH and this explains the terminal 'r' inVR (D and E). Thus, the QS (qs) morphology without a terminal r in II, III, and VF (although qrs morphology may be seen) and with terminal 'r' in VR suggests associated SAH. In the absence of SAH, even if the entire VCG loop falls above 'X' axis (lead I) (B), there will always be a terminal r, at times small, at least in lead II, but never a terminal r in VR (A-C).

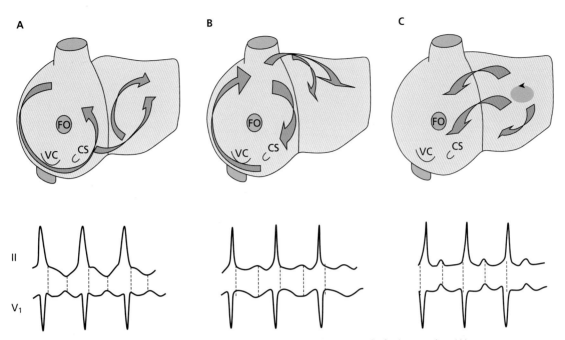

Plate 10.8 Circuits explaining the presence of common flutter with counterclockwise rotation (A); non-common (reverse) flutter with clockwise rotation (B); and one case of atypical flutter arising in the left atrium (C).

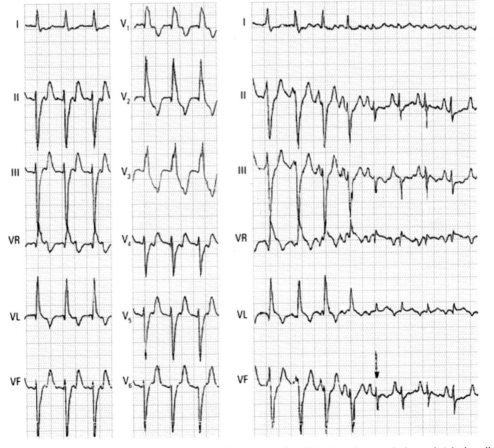

Plate 12.4 An example of verapamil-sensitive ventricular tachycardia (VT). Note the morphology of right bundle branch block + superoanterior hemiblock (RBBB + SAH), but with qR morphology in V1. In the right panel it can be appreciated how the sinus tachycardia exceeds the VT rate during exercise testing.

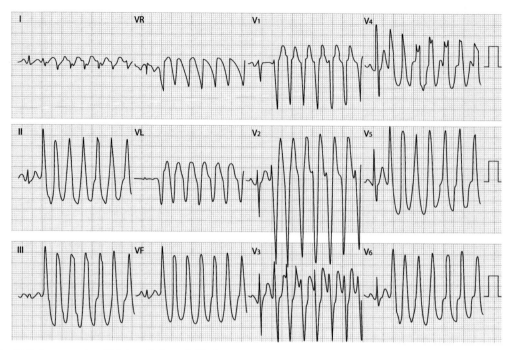

Plate 12.5 An example of left bundle branch block (LBBB)-type ventricular tachycardia (VT) with rightwards QRS occurring as repetitive runs during exercise testing in an individual without heart disease.

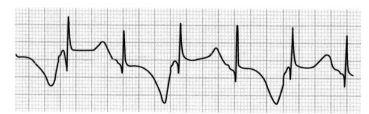

Plate 16.2 Repolarization alternans in a congenital long QT syndrome.

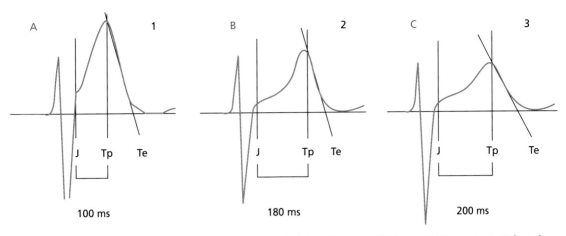

Plate 16.3 Symptomatic short QT pattern (A), asymptomatic (B), and normal QT (control) (C) (see text) (Adapted with permission from Anttonen et al., 2009).

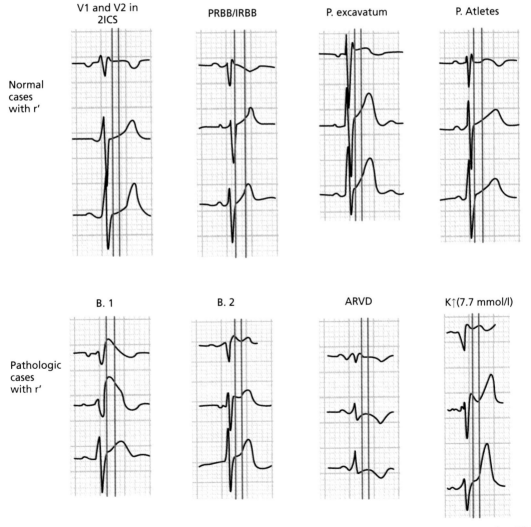

Plate 16.6 This figure shows clearly (first vertical line) the difference in the duration of QRS in V1 compared to V3 in Brugada patterns 1 and 2 ARVD and hyperkalemia (lower row). However, in four variants of normality (upper row) the duration of QRS in V1-V3 is the same. The second vertical line measured 80 ms later, clearly shows that in the two Brugada patterns the ST segment is downsloping (ratio ST↑ at J point / ST↑ 80 ms later > 1) (Corrado index), but it is upsloping in at least V2 in normal variants (upper row) (ratio <1) (see text and Fig. 17.10).

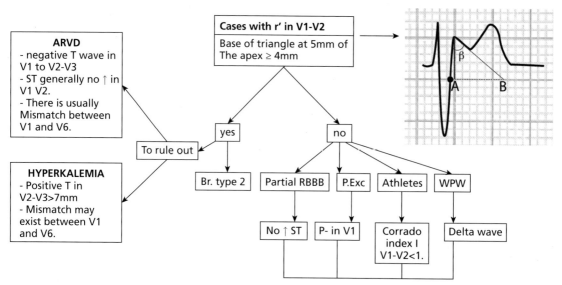

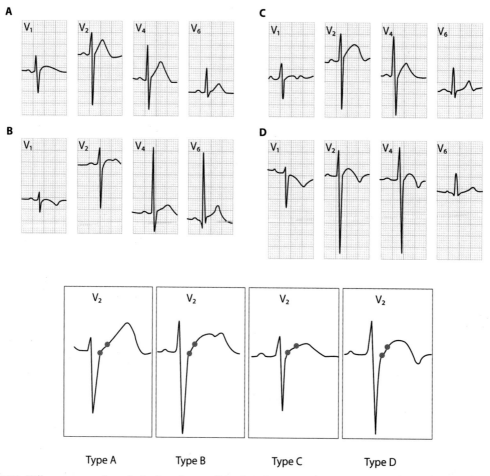

Plate 16.7 Flow chart for performing differential diagnosis of patients with r' in V1-V2 based on the measurement of the base of triangle of r'. If AB ≥ 4 mm, this is very suggestive of Brugada type 2 (see text and Baranchuk et al., 2014).

Plate 17.11 Different types of repolarization abnormalities found in athletes. These are usually benign, but it is essential to perform an echocardiogram to rule out hypertrophic cardiomyopathy. Below may be seen (·) the placement in V2 of the two lines (separated by 80 ms) to measure the Corrado index. In all cases the index ST elevation at J point/ ST elevation 80 ms later in <1 in athletes, and in Brugada syndrome is >1 (see Fig. 16.6 and Section 16.2.3.2 in Chapter 16).

CHAPTER 9
Myocardial Ischemia and Necrosis

9.1. Introduction

• Table 9.1 shows the various clinical presentations with ECG abnormalities due to myocardial ischemia and/or necrosis.

• These ECG disturbances occur mainly in the T wave, ST segment, and the QRS complex.

• Myocardial ischemia can also alter the P wave and other ECG parameters, such as the PR and QT intervals. In fact, the first disturbance due to ischemia is a delay in repolarization in the ischemic tissue, which can originate a lengthening of the QT interval. However, this is usually very difficult to recognize because we do not have the baseline value.

• This ischemia can provoke all types of arrhythmias and is the main cause of SD. We will review these types of arrhythmia at the end of the chapter. In addition, some of these aspects will be briefly discussed in the section on arrhythmias (Chapters 11–13).

A • Ischemia may originate ECG abnormalities due to reduced coronary blood flow or increased blood demand. **We discuss especially the ECG abnormalities caused by reduced blood flow** due to coronary occlusion produced by atherothrombosis in patients with a narrow QRS. **In the acute phase, this includes acute coronary syndrome** (ACS), of which there are two types depending on the presence of ST elevation, **and in the chronic phase it includes infarction with or without a Q wave**.

B • ECG abnormalities due to increased blood demand usually present clinically as exercise angina or its equivalent (Table 9.1).

• We will briefly mention ECG abnormalities in patients with wide QRS and other confusing factors (left ventricular hypertrophy), as well as ACS not due to atherothrombosis.

• For more information especially on these aspects, we will refer first and mainly to cases with narrow QRS (Bayés de Luna, 2012a).

9.2. ACS with ST elevation (STEACS)

This is caused by total occlusion, or in the hyperacute phase sometimes subtotal occlusion of a coronary artery due to atherothrombosis with **transmural involvement**. This process must be treated immediately with percutaneous coronary intervention (PCI). If this is not possible, fribrinolysis should be used to avoid extensive infarction.

This clinical syndrome due to acute ischemia, with occluded-near occluded artery with transmural involvement that presents an ST elevation in its evolving phase as a more clear ECG manifestation, is named ST elevation ACS **(STEACS)**. However, it has to be understood that in the evolving process of STEACS, other ECG patterns may be present at different moments of evolution. We call them **atypical patterns**, which may be confused with ECG patterns of no ST elevation ACS **(NSTEACS)**.

ECGs for Beginners, First Edition. Antoni Bayés de Luna.
© 2014 John Wiley & Sons, Inc. Published 2014 by John Wiley & Sons, Inc.

It is important to know this for the better management of each case (see atypical patterns of STEACS).

C **9.2.1. Evolutive ECG abnormalities**
The successive degrees of ischemia that appear after total occlusion of a coronary artery in ACS-STE are accompanied of different ECG patterns (Fig. 9.1). First, in the hyperacute phase occlusion originates

Table 9.1 Clinical settings due to myocardial ischemia and ECG abnormalities

---

1. **Reduced blood flow**
   Acute coronary syndrome – myocardial infarction (ACS-MI)
   (a) Due to atherothrombosis
      • Acute ischemia: with narrow QRS due to total or near total occlusion of the artery and transmural involvement (ACS with ST elevation [STEACS]) and with arterial subocclusion and non transmural involvement (ACS without ST elevation [NSTEACS])
      • Necrosis: chronic MI with narrow QRS
      • Ischemia and necrosis in patients with wide QRS or other confounding factors (LVH)
   (b) Myocardial ischemia, sometimes true ACS, not due to atherothrombosis: Coronary spasm, Takotsubo syndrome, X syndrome, myocardial bridging, coronary dissection, congenital heart diseases, toxins, etc.
2. **Increased demand**
   Exercise angina or its equivalent due to atherothrombosis, psychological stress, tachyarrhythmia, pulmonary hypertension, chronic anemia, etc.

---

a predominantly subendocardial ischemia: a high, and sharp T wave (B). Next, the ischemia, which is now more severe, becomes transmural: ST elevation (C). Finally, if the occlusion is not successfully treated or spontaneously resolved, a necrosis pattern may appear: necrosis Q wave and negative T wave (D).

9.2.2. Electrophysiological mechanisms of typical ECG patterns during the acute phase of STEACS

9.2.2.1. Origin of the high, wide T wave
The initial changes in the T wave into wider, more symmetrical morphology, and a generally higher and more peaked wave in the hyperacute phase of STEACS, are due to subendocardial ischemia (A). **This may be explained by two mechanisms:** (1) the sum of TAP of the subendocardium and subepicardium and (2) the formation of a vector of subendocardial ischemia that moves away from the ischemic zone.

A. TAP sum (Fig. 9.2)
The high, peaked T wave are explained by changes that occur in the second part of repolarization. This occurs because the TAP in the subendocardial zone, which is the first to suffer ischemia because it is more poorly perfused than the subepicardial zone (e.g. terminal perfusion, etc.), is prolonged more than the TAP in normal circumstances (see the normal endocardial TAP, pointed in B and C).

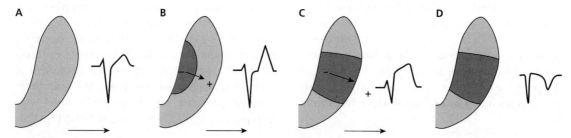

Figure 9.1 The ECG morphology explains the different degrees of ischemia that appear sequentially following total coronary occlusion. (A) ECG with no previous ischemia. (B) Predominating ischemia in the subendocardial area (T wave is symmetrical and often higher than normal with a longer QT interval). (C) If ischemia is severe and become transmural, ST elevation appears. (D) If ischemia persists, transmural necrosis appears and is expressed as the Q wave of necrosis and a negative T wave with left intraventricular patterns: (window effect of Wilson).

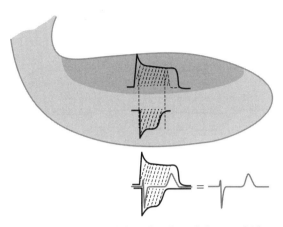

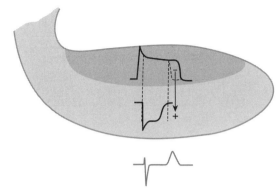

Figure 9.2 The sum of the subendocardial TAP, which is lengthened but maintains the same form as that of the subepicardium, and the subepicardial TAP explains how the ST segment remains isoelectric, the T wave is wider or higher, and the QT somewhat longer. (See Plate 9.2.)

Figure 9.3 The formation of the subendocardial vector of ischemia in the second part of repolarization, which moves from the endocardium (the area not yet repolarized) with negative charges toward the epicardium (already repolarized) explains the higher and wider T wave. (See Plate 9.3.)

However, it conserves the same morphology if the ischemia is not very severe or was already previously present in the subendocardial zone. Consequently, the sum of the two TAPs, one positive and longer (subendocardial) and the other negative and shorter (subepicardial) explain, according to Ashman (Fig. 2.4), the presence of a higher, wider T wave and/or symmetrical T wave. This is because the area it encompasses is greater, but without apparent changes in the ST segment, because the morphologies of the two TAPs in the initial phase (as we have just explained) are usually the same (Fig. 9.2A).

However, when the subendocardial ischemia is more severe but still is not transmural, the shape of subendocardial TAP is different (lower area) and the sum of both TAP may then originate an ECG pattern with high T wave and some degrees of ST depression (see Fig. 9.2B) (Birnbaum et al., 2012; Bayés de Luna, 2012a).

B. Ischemic vector (Fig. 9.3)
Because repolarization is longer in the ischemic subendocardium, subepicardial repolarization finishes beforehand. In this ischemic subendocardial zone with remaining negative charges that are not

repolarized, an ischemia **vector is generated** that moves to the already-repolarized area of the subepicardium. The head of this vector faces the subepicardium which is already repolarized (+), while the subendocardium still presents negative changes as the TAP of the subendocardium is not yet complete. This bigger area of subendocardial TAP which is still not repolarized explains the increase in voltage in the T wave, without, in general, (see before) changes in the first part of repolarization (ST segment).

In addition, due to lengthening repolarization, the QT interval is also longer, but this parameter is more difficult to evaluate because we do not generally know its value before the appearance of ischemia.

9.2.2.2. Origin of ST elevation   E
Ischemia quickly becomes transmural and the ECG shows a change typical of STEACS, ST elevation, often known as the pattern of subepicardial injury, but this is wrongly named, because this pattern appears when **acute ischemia is of a higher degree (what was termed injury) and become transmural**.

This transmural severe acute ischemia in the surface ECG (ST elevation) appears only during

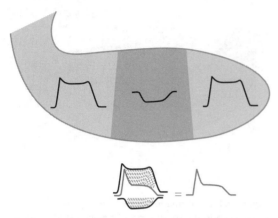

Figure 9.4 The TAP in the transmural zone affected by severe ischemia presents a slower descent and an inverted polarity (Ashman phenomenon). The sum of this TAP with the TAPs in neighboring areas explains the ECG morphology with ST elevation. (See Plate 9.4.)

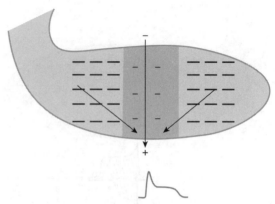

Figure 9.5 The vector of severe transmural ischemia (historically called the subepicardial injury vector) is directed from the subendocardium to the subepicardium and recorded as ST elevation. This is due to the lesser negative charge in the affected transmural zone compared to the rest of the myocardium and thus functions as relatively positive. (See Plate 9.5.)

systole, already at the end of QRS, because the ECG recording devices are designed based on the isoelectric line being stable during diastole.

The mechanisms that explain the appearance of ST elevation are as follows:

A. Sum of TAP in the transmurally affected zone with TAP in neighboring areas (Fig. 9.4)

The transmurally affected area presents a TAP with a shorter and slower phase 1, and a smaller area because it presents a degree of depolarization in the diastole and thus its DTP is closer to zero, explaining the formation of what we call a 'poor quality' TAP. The sum of this abnormal TAP, which, according to Ashman (1941) is negatively recorded because the exploratory electrode located in this area faces the most negative areas of the neighboring zones, with a normal TAP in the healthy neighboring zones, explains the ST elevation pattern.

B. Formation of the severe transmural ischemic vector (classically named injury vector) (Fig. 9.5)

The transmural zone with severe ischemia presents fewer negative charges than the rest of LV and

therefore are relatively positive. Consequently the flow of the current generated between the two zones which comes from the most negative part to the least negative part (the ischemic one proportionally positive) originates a vector, of severe transmural isquemia called the **injury vector**, which is directed to the subepicardium. An electrode placed in the subepicardium records this in the form of ST elevation already from the end of QRS (end of depolarization). On the contrary, the ischemic vector of subendocardial ischemia (peaked T wave) is recorded only in the second part of repolarization (see before).

9.2.3. Electrocardiographic diagnosis

9.2.3.1. Diagnostic ECG criteria in STEACS

The key ECG criteria are represented by ST elevation, and hence the name ACS with ST elevation (STEACS)*.

---

*Frequently is used the term STEMI (STE-Myocardial infarction) because often STEACS evolves to STEMI. **F**

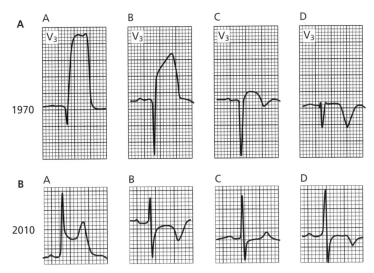

Figure 9.6 (A) Course of a patient who suffered an extensive anterior myocardial infarction in the 1970s who in 1 month (A to D) presented a typical pattern of the Q wave of necrosis with a deep negative T wave. **(B)** Course of STEACS today. After 2 hours of pain (A) the patient underwent emergency PCI successfully (B). Note the negative T wave. A few hours later the pain returned and the T wave pseudonormalized (C). A reocclusion of stent was suspected. The patient underwent a second PCI that reopened the artery and showed improvement, presenting a new negative T wave in the ECG.

9.2.3.1.1. ST elevation due to ischemia

A. Typical pattern. New elevation of the ST segment in at least two continuous leads at the level of the J point and ≥1 mm in all leads except V2–V3, where the new elevation must be >2 mm in men (>2.5 mm in younger than 40 years) and ≥1.5 mm in women (Thygessen, 2012). **The elevation and depression in the ST segment** (see later) may also be measured several ms (20, 40, 60, etc) from the J point. In these cases the value of an abnormal shift is different. The elevation is measured from the level above the PR segment and depression from the lower level. If the PR segment is down-sloping, it is measured from the start of QRS (Fig. 4.12). Figure 4.9 shows an example of how the ST shifts in STEACS are measured (Bayés & Fiol-Sala, 2008).

B. Evolution of ST elevation in STEACS. Before the current treatment (PCI) or, when not possible, fibrinolysis, the evolution of STEACS almost always evolves to Q-wave MI with negative T wave (intraventricular pattern due to electrical window) effect (see Figs 9.30 and 9.31), with a considerable loss of myocardial mass that may be expressed by a reduction in the ejection fraction (EF) from 10 to more than 20 points.

Figure 9.6A shows a typical example of this in a patient with proximal left anterior descending coronary artery (LAD) occlusion who suffered acute infarction in the 1970s. See the evolution over a 1-month period in which a necrosis Q wave and a negative T wave appear. This negative T wave is not indicative of subepicardial ischemia, but rather is a postischemic pattern (electric window effect) (see before) (see Figs 9.30 and 9.31).

Today this situation is very different. In the ECG in Figure 9.6B, we see a patient with a similar previous STEACS (A) in whom an emergency PCI was performed to avoid infarction. See the negative T wave of reperfusion (post-ischemic T wave) (B). A few hours later the patient presented once again with pain, and the ECG pseudonormalized (C), suggesting the stent thrombosis. A new PCI allowed the artery to be opened and the infarction was

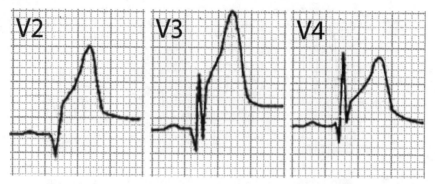

Figure 9.7 The S wave is carried upward due to the maximum degree of ischemia on the anteroseptal zone caused by LAD occlusion.

avoided (aborted infarction) (D), with a negative T wave appearing once again. The entire process took place in less than 24 hours.

Although this clinical course is seen in countries that have ideal conditions for optimal treatment of ACS, there are still many parts of the world, especially in developing or undeveloped countries, where neither emergency PCI nor even sometimes fibrinolysis can be used to treat STEACS.

Persistent ST elevation (for days), which rarely occurs with today's treatment, is a sign of poor prognosis and can be a marker for cardiac rupture or ventricular aneurysm.

C. The importance of ST to evaluate the degree of ischemia. ST elevation allows the severity of ischemia to be quantified. According to the Birnbaum–Sclarovsky grading system (1993), severity increases proportionally as ST elevation pulls the S upward. See a typical example of maximum grade ischemia in Figure 9.7.

D. The importance of ST to evaluate the extension of ischemic area. Even with limitations, it may be assumed that the spread of ischemia is considerable if the sum of the shifts in ST (elevation and depression) is ≥15 mm (Hatheway et al., 1998).

9.2.3.1.2. Other electrocardiographic patterns that may be seen in STEACS that are useful in the diagnosis and prognostic evaluation

We refer to the presence of mirror pattern and atypical electrocardiographic patterns.

A. Mirror patterns

In the acute phase of STEACS mirror patterns may appear (ST depression) in opposite leads.

The correlation of the leads with ST elevation and mirror patterns allow, in cases of LAD occlusion (ST elevation in precordial leads), the site of occlusion to be located (Fig. 9.8). In cases of ST elevation in II, III and VF (right coronary [RC] or circumflex [CX] occlusion), this correlation allows the occluded artery to be identified (Fig. 9.11).

Locating the site of occlusion in LAD. (Figs 9.8–9.10): In ACS due to LAD occlusion and ST elevation in precordial leads, the mirror pattern allows the site of occlusion to be located (Figs 9.8–9.10). If the occlusion is high, proximal to the first diagonal (D_1), and the LAD is long, wrapping the apex which is something that frequently occurs, the vector of severe transmural ischemia (injury vector) moves upward (↑ of ST in V2-V4-5) and from II, III, and VF we see its tail. Thus, an ST depression is recorded in the inferior leads (Fig. 9.10A). If the occlusion is also proximal to the first septal (S_1), ST would also be elevated in V_1 (Bayés & Fiol-Sala, 2008).

However, if the occlusion is distal to the first diagonal (Figs 9.8 and 9.9), the vector of severe ischemia (injury vector) would also be directed forward but downward instead of upward, and thus II, III, and VF would record an isoelectric or positive ST segment (Fig. 9.10B).

It is important to remember the rare cases of total occlusion of the left main trunk (LMT) that arrives alive to the hospital, present STEACS resembling

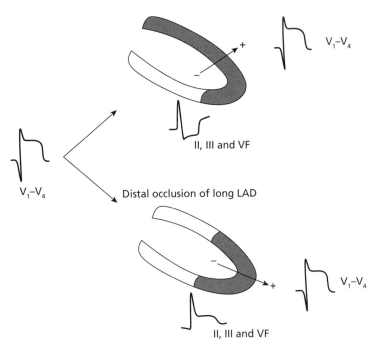

Proximal occlusion of long LAD

V_1–V_4

II, III and VF

V_1–V_4

Distal occlusion of long LAD

V_1–V_4

II, III and VF

Figure 9.8 In cases of ST elevation in precordial leads due to LAD occlusion (STEACS) if the occlusion is proximal (above D1) the injury vector moves forward but upward and ST depression is seen in II, III, and VF. If the occlusion is distal (below D1), the injury vector moves forward but downward, with isoelectric and somewhat elevated ST in II, III, and VF (see Fig. 9.10).

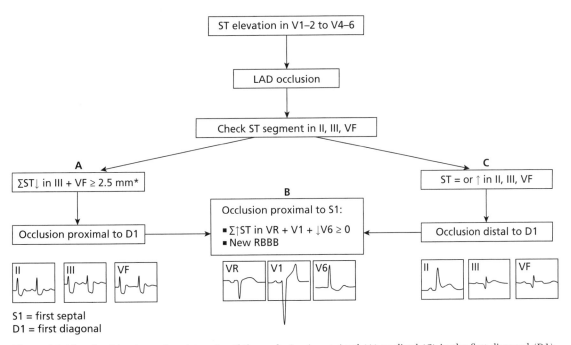

ST elevation in V1–2 to V4–6

LAD occlusion

Check ST segment in II, III, VF

A
ΣST↓ in III + VF ≥ 2.5 mm*

Occlusion proximal to D1

B
Occlusion proximal to S1:
- Σ↑ST in VR + V1 + ↓V6 ≥ 0
- New RBBB

C
ST = or ↑ in II, III, VF

Occlusion distal to D1

II   III   VF

VR   V1   V6

II   III   VF

S1 = first septal
D1 = first diagonal

Figure 9.9 The algorithm is used to determine if the occlusion is proximal (A) or distal (C) in the first diagonal (D1) in cases of ST elevation in precordial leads. If a complete RBB appears or the sum of the ST elevation in millimeters in VR+V1 and the ST depression in V6 totals ≥0, the occlusion is probably located above the first septal (S1) (B).

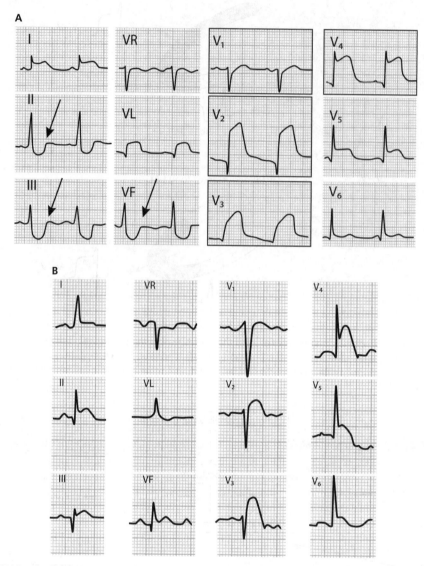

Figure 9.10 (A) An STEACS due to LAD occlusion proximal to D1 and distal to S1. The ECG shows ST elevation in V2-V5, I, and VL (not in V1 or VR) with a clear ST depression in inferior leads. (B) An STEACS due to LAD occlusion distal to D1 and S1. Note the ST segment elevation in V2-V5-V6 with some ST segment elevation in II, III, and VF (II>III) and ST depression in VR.

proximal LAD occlusion to D1 and S1. Very frequently in these cases RBBB+LAH appear, that sometimes may make it difficult to evaluate the ECG changes.

The hemodynamic presentation in total occlusion of LMT is much serious that in LAD proximal occlusion. Approximately 50% of patients die from cardiogenic shock (Fiol et al., 2012). Later on we will see that in most cases LMT involvement is shown by subocclusion, not total occlusion, originating NSTEACS, with a depression of ST in seven or more leads.

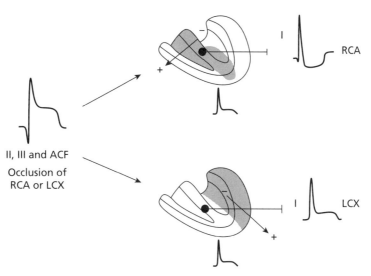

Figure 9.11 In ST elevation in II, III, and VF if there is ST depression in I, RC occlusion is most probable because the injury lesion in the affected zone (top) moves away from D1, while if ST is elevated in I CX occlusion occurs because the injury vector moves to the left. In doubtful cases (isoelectric ST) the algorithm in Figure 9.12 may be useful especially in the absence of very dominant RC or CX artery.

In conclusion, the algorithm of Figure 9.9 can be used to locate the site of occlusion in the LAD in the case of STEACS (Fiol et al., 2009). We must look at (1) the appearance of ST in II, III, and VF to determine if the occlusion is proximal or distal to D1 and (2) whether occlusion is proximal to the first septal (S1) (Fig. 9.9B). Figure 9.10 shows the ECG in two cases of LAD occlusion, one proximal and one distal to D1.

CX occlusion versus RC occlusion in the case of ST elevation in II, III, and VF (Fig. 9.11–13): In ACS with ST elevation in II, III, and VF the occluded artery is RC at the proximal or distal level if a depression in the ST segment is seen in lead I. This occurs because the severe ischemia vector (injury vector) is directed more toward the right since the affected area in RC occlusion is located more in this zone (Figs 9.11 and 9.13A and B). By contrast, if occlusion is in the CX artery, the severe ischemia vector (injury vector) is directed more to the left because it is the most affected area and then in lead I we may see ST elevation (Figs 9.11 and 9.13C).

In case of doubt or when the ST is isoelectric, we may use other criteria to identify the culprit artery (Fig. 9.12) (Fiol-Sala et al., 2004). This figure shows the successive steps that allow the location of the involved artery with high SP and SE, in case of STEACS with ST elevation in II, III and VF.

B. Atypical patterns of STEACS
In addition to typical patterns of ST elevation, there are some ECG patterns seen in the evolving course of an STEACS considered atypical and that we discuss below (De Winter et al., 2008; Nikus et al., 2010; Bayés de Luna, 2012; Birnbaum et al., 2012).
• **STE equivalent** (Figs 9.14 and 9.15): Is a mirror image of true STEACS. It corresponds to a mirror pattern of severe transmural lateral ischemia due to occlusion in CX, that originates an ST elevation in the back leads but are recorded in V1–V2 as mirror pattern (ST depression in V1–V2). Often they are considered to be a true ST depression and they are incorrectly diagnosed as NSTEACS. The presence of sometimes very small ST elevations in inferior and/or lateral leads and in V7–V9 (Fig. 9.15), and above all to know that this pattern exists, is useful to make the correct diagnosis.
• In the hyperacute phase a final positive T wave is not present at the end of the ST depression

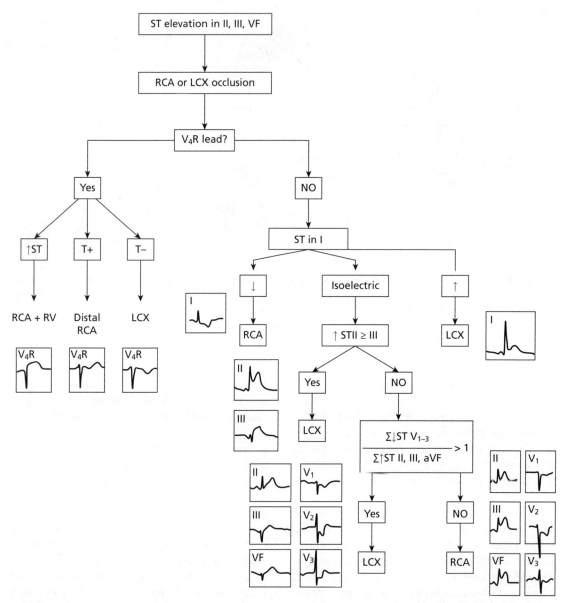

Figure 9.12 An algorithm used to determine whether occlusion is CX or RC in ACS-STE with ST elevation in II, III, and VF. First, the ECG is examined to see if the V4R lead is recorded. If so, the morphology of this lead indicated the site of occlusion (Wellens, 1999). However, V4R is often not recorded. In our experience, by following the steps shown on the right, the correct diagnosis may be reached with high specificity and sensitivity. It starts with the first criterion already outlined in the previous figure. In cases of doubt (isoelectric ST), the two following criteria are used. (1) ST elevation in II ≥III indicates that the affected artery is CX. If this is not the case, (2) we examine whether the ↓ST V1 V3 / ↑STII,III,VF relationship >1. If so, the affected artery is the CX, and if not, the affected artery is the RC.

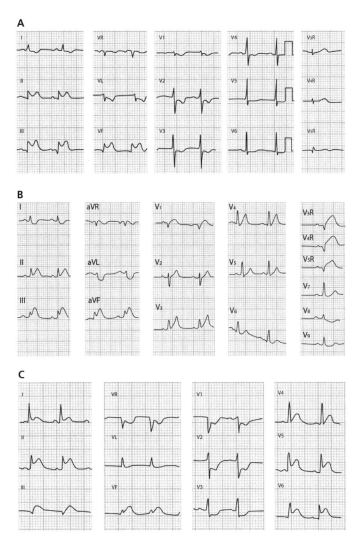

Figure 9.13 (A) Typical ECG in STEACS due to RC occlusion distal to the RV branches. (B) Typical ECG in case of STEACS due to proximal RCA occlusion with right ventricular involvement. Observe the ST segment elevation in II, III, and VF with III > II, ST segment depression in I and isoelectric or elevated in V1–V3 as well as in V3R–V4R leads with positive T wave. (C) Typical ECG in case of LCX occlusion. See the ST elevation in lead I, ST↑ II>III, and ST↓ V1-V3 > I / ST↑II, III,VF > 1.

(Fig. 9.14). However, a positive T wave usually appears after a few hours coinciding with a decrease in the ST depression. This **change of pattern** corresponds to the mirror image that appears in the back leads; less ST elevation and the appearance of a negative T (Fig. 9.15). Also often, a high R of lateral infarction appears in V1 that is the mirror pattern of Q in back lead. These considerations are

important in making the differential diagnosis with the pattern of severe subocclusion in the proximal LAD (Figs 9.15 and 9.23A).

• **Peaked, symmetric and tall T wave** (Fig. 9.16) may appear in the hyperacute phase of STEACS and is caused by the isolated initial subendocardial ischemia that is present in this phase in STEACS. It occurs usually in case of LAD occlusion,

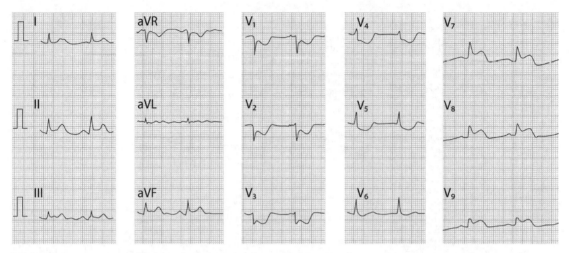

Figure 9.14 Mirror image of severe lateral ischemia. An example of total CX occlusion with ST depression from V1 to V3–V4 without a final positive T wave and very few changes in II, III, and VF. Note, however, the ST elevation in V7–V9.

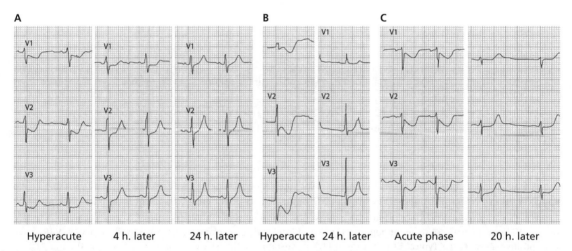

Figure 9.15 (A & B)Two examples of ACS with ST depression in V1–V3 due to LCX occlusion evolving to lateral MI (ST elevation equivalent). In the hyperacute phase the terminal part of ST is not followed by positive T wave. However, after some hours the ST is less negative and is followed by positive T wave. A tall T wave is also seen corresponding to mirror pattern of lateral MI.

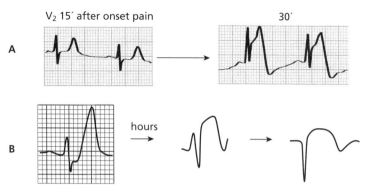

Figure 9.16 (A) High, peaked T wave in the hyperacute phase of STEACS due to LAD occlusion. Note the clear ST elevation appearing after 30 min. (B) In this case the tall T wave with ST depression remains some hours before it evolves to a Q-wave MI when the artery is completely occluded and a transmural involvement exists.

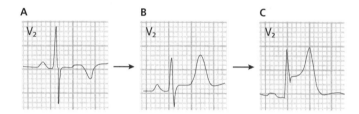

Figure 9.17 (A) Deep inverted T wave. An STEACS without pain. The artery is now partially open and the ACS does not evolve to Q wave infarction and the STE become negative T wave (reperfusion pattern). With a new episode of angina, there is again an occlusion of the artery (LAD), and the ECG pseudonormalices the negative T wave (B), and after an ST elevation appears (C).

(V_1 to V_2–V_3), but rarely may be seen in cases of LC or CX occlusion.

The presence and duration depends on when the first ECG is taken. It is generally brief (Fig. 9.16A) and usually is recorded during this first ECG because already an ST elevation is present. There are times, however, that the duration is longer and it may rarely ($\approx$2% of LAD occlusion cases) be accompanied by a generally small ST depression, especially if subendocardial ischemia was already present previously (De Winter, 2009) (see before and Fig. 9.16B).

• **Deep inverted T wave** (Fig. 9.17). This is a pattern often seen in STEACS if the artery, usually LAD, opens spontaneously or under treatment (PCI or fibrinolysis) before the ST elevation pattern evolves to Q-wave MI. Therefore, a deep negative T wave from V1-V2 to V4-V5 may appear, generally

with some lengthening of QT, indicating that the artery is more or less open (T wave of reperfusion), although it may close again (Fig. 9.17). In these cases it is necessary to carry out PCI as an urgent, but not emergent, procedure. At this time the negative T wave pattern indicates that there is no active ischemia (no pain). Therefore, this is mainly a reperfusion pattern as seen following fibrinolysis or PCI, or coronary spasm. However, without treatment the process can resume (Fig. 9.17), presenting pseudonormalization or even if angina persists, an ST elevation.

This post-ischemic T wave that appears in the clinical course of STEACS or coronary spasm (see later) occurs because a slower repolarization persists in the affected transmural zone when compared to neighboring areas due to a slowing in the ionic exchange during repolarization (Fig. 9.18). This

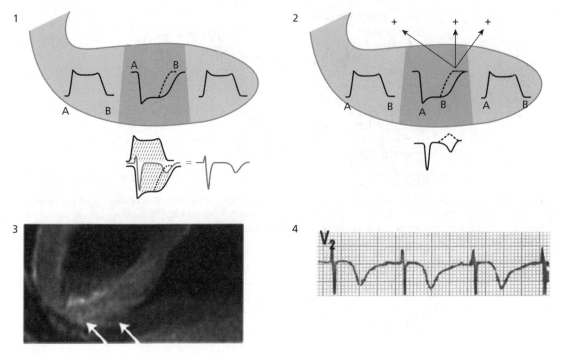

Figure 9.18 1. and 2. Origin of negative and deep T wave. 1. Due to increased TAP duration of transmural area affected, the sum of this TAP of this area with the TAP neighboring areas, that is shorter, explain the negative T wave. 2. The explanation based on the vector of ischemia theory. 3. Transmural involvement (CMR) in a case of negative T wave after aborted (Migliore et al., 2011). See the transmural edema. 4. Deep and negative T wave in V2 in a case of transient LAD occlusion (negative T wave of reperfusion-edema). (See Plate 9.18.)

may be explained (A) (Fig. 9.18-1) by the sum of the longest TAP in the affected transmural zone and the shortest TAP of the neighboring areas, and (B) because a vector is generated in the affected transmural zone in the second part of repolarization (not yet completely repolarized and with a longer TAP) that goes from this to the neighboring areas (vector of ischemia) (Fig. 9.18-2). MRI in small series of these cases has shown transmural edema with the negative T wave disappearing conjointly with the edema (Migliore et al., 2011) (Fig. 9.18-3).

Later in this chapter, we will explain the basis for other negative T waves that appear during the clinical course of ischemic heart disease (e.g. NSTEACS, Q wave infarction) (see Figures 9.25, 9.34, 9.38).

• **Other patterns**. On rare occasions, a negative U wave may be seen when a negative T wave is pseudonormalized or a residual negative U wave may remain in an aborted STEACS.

9.2.4. Differential diagnosis

9.2.4.1. Differential diagnosis of the high, peaked T wave of subendocardial ischemia

We must remember that the high, peaked T wave in subendocardial ischemia is generally transitory, although some cases of LAD occlusion with persistently high T wave have been described, sometimes with a slight ST depression, that appears in the hyperacute phase of an STEACS (see before and Bayés de Luna, 2012a).

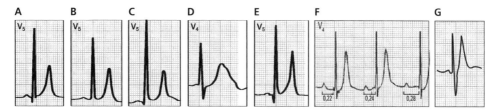

Figure 9.19 Some of the morphologies of the high, peaked T wave in situations other than ischemia. (A) High, peaked T wave in a case of variant of normality (vagal overdrive). (B) Alcoholism. (C) LVH. (D) Cerebrovascular accident. (E) Hyperkalemia. (F) Congenital AV block. (G) Short QT syndrome.

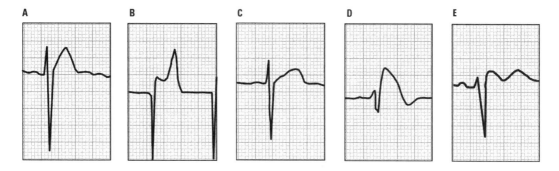

Figure 9.20 The most frequent causes of ST elevation other than ischemia. (A) Pericarditis (see Chapter 15). (B) Hyperkalemia. (C) Athletes. (D) Type 1 Brugada pattern with coved pattern. (E) Type 2 Brugada pattern (saddle back type). See differential diagnosis with variants of normality such as pectus excavatum and athletes in Chapter 16.

In the chronic phase of lateral infarction RS is sometimes seen in V1–V2 with a high T wave as a mirror pattern of Q and negative T wave that are recorded in direct lateral leads (see Fig. 9.38).

Figure 9.19 shows examples of non-transitory high, peaked T waves which are not due to subendocardial ischemia.

K **9.2.4.2. Differential diagnosis in ischemic ST elevation**

ST elevation can also be seen in certain clinical situations other than the acute phase of STEACS, including normal variants, hyperkalemia, Brugada pattern, etc. (Fig. 9.20). We should remember that in patients with STEACS, if ST persists in the subacute phase, it is a risk marker for cardiac rupture. On the other hand a persistent ST elevation that remains in the chronic phase post-MI, obliges us to rule out ventricular aneurysm (see Fig. 9.45).

9.3. Acute coronary syndrome without ST elevation (NSTEACS)

This syndrome includes the cases **of subtotal thrombotic occlusion of one coronary artery without transmural involvement**. Only in more serious cases is this indicated an emergent PCI. The myocardial area most affected by hypoperfusion is the subendocardium, although ischemia may often reach patching parts of the rest of the ventricular wall. L

ST depression is the most frequent ECG change in the acute phase, starting the depression already at the end of QRS. When the clinical situation improves usually the ECG changes to a flat/mildly negative T wave, or even a normal ECG may be recorded. If angina again appears, the ECG may change from flat/negative T wave to ST depression.

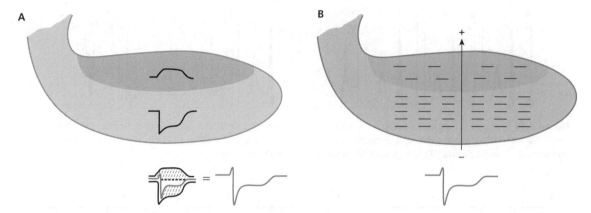

Figure 9.21 (A) The sum of the TAP in the subendocardium (TAP with smaller area) and the TAP of the rest of VI (normal) explains the ST depression. (B) The area with severe endocardial ischemia presents less negative charges than the rest of VI and is thus relatively positive. For this reason the severe ischemic vector (injury vector) points to the subendocardium and is recorded as negative from the end of QRS in the elevations of the ECG. (See Plate 9.21.)

If a patient with suspected NSTEACS arrives at the hospital, already without pain, the first ECG may present a flat or mildly negative T wave, or the ECG is normal or unchanged. The negative T wave is formed in the second part of repolarization.

Patients showing ST depression have a poorer prognosis, especially when ST shows a clear depression in various leads (see later).

We remember that in the evolving phase of STEACS, ST depression may be seen with a tall T wave, or deep negative T wave. The first may occur in the early phase of STEACS before the artery is completely occluded (Fig. 9.16B). The deep negative T wave occurs when an STEACS, usually with treatment, does not evolve to Q-wave MI (pattern C) (see before atypical patterns of STEACS). Also sometimes a clear STEACS with ST elevation become a NSTEACS (ST depression) after treatment that partially opens the artery.

M 9.3.2. Electrophysiologic mechanisms that explain the patterns of ST depression and flat negative T wave

9.3.2.1. Origin of ST depression
A. Sum of the TAPs (Fig. 9.21A)
The subendocardium presents an important change in the TAP, with a slower ascent and smaller area with varying length (often longer), due to severe hypoperfusion in a zone that is already poorly perfused. The sum of the TAP of the subendocardium and the remaining areas of LV explains ST depression, sometimes with a final positive T wave.

B. Vector of severe subendocardial ischemia (injury vector) (Fig. 9.21B)
Another way to explain ST depression, when severe ischemia occurs in an already poorly perfused area such as the subendocardium, is the presence of a **vector** of severe ischemia known as an **injury vector**. An injury vector moves from the most perfused area, the subepicardial zone with the most negative charges, to the least perfused area, the subendocardial zone, which is only partially depolarized and thus presents fewer negative charges and is relatively positive compared to the subepicardium (B). The vector points toward the subendocardium and an ST depression is recorded on the surface of the body.

9.3.2.2. Origin of flat or negative T wave in NSTEACS
The pattern reflects a certain degree of improvement in the subendocardial ischemia in the affected zone in patients who generally no longer present

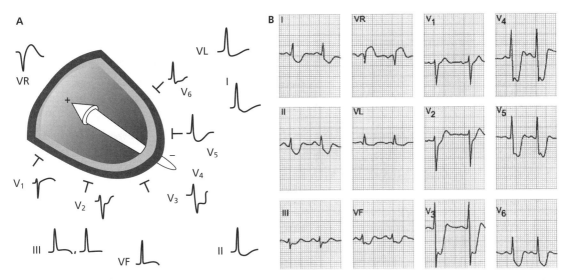

Figure 9.22 (A) 68-year-old patient with NSTEACS due to subocclusion of the left main trunk. The injury vector is directed upward, backward and to the right, explaining the ECG morphology. (B) ECG with ST depression in more than seven leads with maximum expression in V3–V5 and without a positive T wave at the end of ST. Note the ST elevation in VR >1 mm.

symptoms. Although there is not a clear electro-physiological explanation for this pattern, probably the TAP duration in the ventricular wall is similar, and this may explain why the T wave becomes flat or only slightly negative.

As previously explained, when a flat or negative T wave exists in NSTEACS it is never deeply negative and generally does not appear during an angina crisis (see Fig. 9.25). In the opposite situation, during angina if previous ECG shows a negative T wave, this may evolve into ST depression (see Fig. 9.26). This represents another argument in favor of the belief that a negative T wave is not induced by acute ongoing ischemia.

9.3.3. Electrocardiographic diagnosis

N **9.3.3.1. ECG diagnostic criteria for NSTEACS**
9.3.3.1.1. ST depression due to ischemia
• **ST depression**, with sometimes a mirror pattern of ST elevation in one or two leads, generally VR and V1, **is the most characteristic ECG pattern in NSTEACS**.

• ST depression is considered to be indicative of ischemia when the ST depression is new, at J point measures ≥0.5 mm, and is horizontal or descending for at least 80 ms in two contiguous leads (Thygessen, 2012). Many studies have described that this measurement may be performed later than the J point (20, 40 or 60 m). However, then the measurement of abnormal ST is different (Fig. 4.9).

• **NSTEACS with ST depression may be categorized into two groups:**

A. Extensive involvement (circumferential) **O**
(See Figs. 9.22 and 9.23; Nikus et al., 2010; Kosuge et al., 2011.)
1. This is usually due to subocclusion of the main trunk (LMT) or two or three proximal vessels. Less frequently it is due to proximal LAD severe subocclusion, and rarely to proximal occlusion of the dominant LCX artery.
2. In all cases, ST depression exists in ≥7 leads (for some authors in ≥8 leads). When the subocclusion occurs in the left main trunk (Fig. 9.22) the ST depression in precordial leads does not present a final positive T wave, or it is only minimal. The

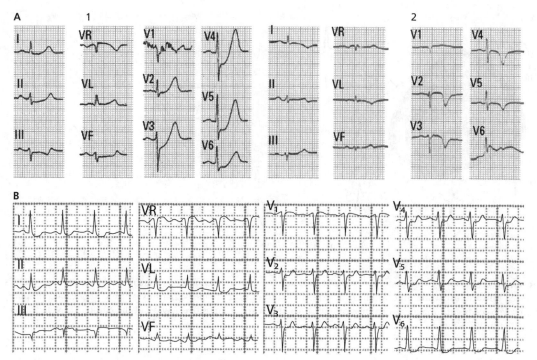

Figure 9.23 (A) Patient with critical proximal LAD subocclusion. The ECG shows ST depression in eight leads with elevation in VR of approximately 1 mm. Note the clear ST depression in V3–V5, followed by a high T wave. Note on the right how the patient finally presents a Q wave MI accompanied by a symmetrical deep negative T wave. The patient that presented NSTEACS, evolves to STEACS when the artery was occluded and then presented a Q wave MI. (B) During non-ST segment elevation ACS (NSTEACS) diffuse and mild ST segment depression is seen in many leads, especially in I, V5, and V6 with small ST segment elevation in III, VR, and V1. The coronary angiography shows three-vessel disease with important proximal obstruction in the left anterior descending (LAD) and left circumflex artery (LCX).

final positive T wave is usually more evident if the subocclusion is in the proximal LAD or in two to three vessels (Fig. 9.23).

3. In all cases ST elevation in VR exists and often in V1; this is more evident in LMT/2–3 vessel disease.

4. Differentiating between subocclusion in 2–3 vessels and in proximal LAD (Fig. 9.23) is difficult in the ECG, because in both cases there is ST depression in the right or middle precordial leads. In our experience, patients with subocclusion in 2–3 vessels present more ST elevation in VR than in the isolated subocclusion of proximal LAD, and the final T wave in mid-precordial leads is less evident (Fig. 9.23A and B). Cases of severe subocclusion of the proximal LAD may evolve more

often to Q-wave myocardial infarction if not treated in time (Fig. 9.23A), and are equivalents of atypical pattern B2 of STEACS (Fig. 9.16B).

5. The differential diagnosis between critical proximal LAD subocclusion and CX occlusion is not easy, especially after the hyperacute phase. In both cases (see before) an ST depression in V1–V3 may be seen, but in LCX occlusion the T wave is usually negative in the hyperacute phase, although in the follow-up a final positive T wave appears as a mirror pattern of evolving lateral MI (Fig. 9.15B). In the critical subocclusion of the LAD the final T wave is positive already in the early phase. This is relevant to evaluating the degree of urgency in performing PCI.

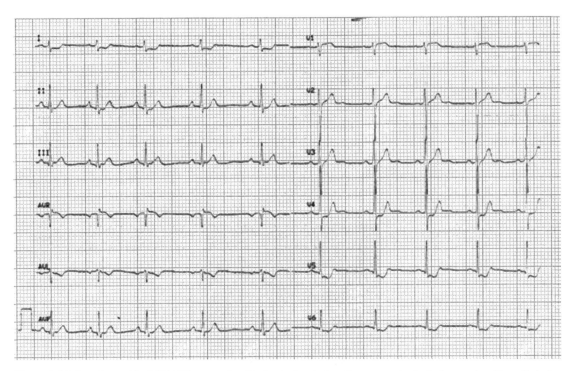

Figure 9.24 A patient with NSTEACS presenting ST depression in less than seven leads during angina. The affected artery is always difficult to identify, but often is the RC, when ST elevation is seen in lead I.

As a summary: If the final positive T wave appears late in the evolving phase of an ACS when the ST depression is not very evident, much probably the occluded artery is the LCX. In case of subocclusion of LAD, the final positive T wave already is present from the first moment, and often evolves to complete occlusion (STEACS and Q wave MI) (compare Figs 9.15 and 9.23A).

B. Regional involvement (Fig. 9.24)
1. Usually there are 1-2 vessels involved.
2. The most ECG criteria are the following:
   • **ST depression** in less than seven leads.
   • **ST elevation in VR, if present, is usually <1 mm**
3. **The ST depression may be seen (Pride et al., 2010):**
   • **V1 to V4**. In 80% of cases, it is explained by LAD subocclusion. In these cases there is usually,

as has been explained in the case of circumferential involvement (Fig. 9.23), a final positive T wave, and in V1 there is nearly no ST depression. There may be slight depression in some leads of the FP. The regional involvement in the case of proximal LAD subocclusion is more frequent than the circumferential involvement already discussed (Fig. 9.23A).

• It should be emphasized that in 20% of patients the presence of ST depression in V1–V4 is due to total CX occlusion, in which case the ECG pattern is equivalent to STEACS (atypical pattern A) (Pride et al., 2010). In this case, the acute phase of ST depression generally occurs without a final positive T wave, at least in V1 and V2, and almost always a slight ST elevation in inferior or lateral leads (Fig. 9.13A) (see before). We have already commented on the differential diagnosis between LCX occlusion

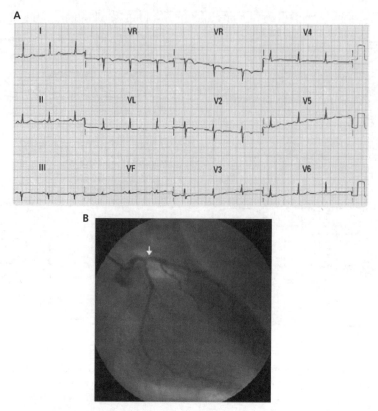

Figure 9.25 (A) ECG with flat or negative T wave in V1-V4. Despite the cessation of angina and the unremarkable ECG, the artery may be very occluded (B) yet sufficiently open to avoid active ongoing ischemia (without angina).

(STEACS) and LAD subocclusion (NSTEACS) that often evolves to STEACS (see before).

• **In II, III, and VF**. Very infrequent. Due to RC/CX subocclusion.

• **In V3-V5-6** and some FP leads. Frequently there is 2–3 vessel disease, but it is very difficult to identify the culprit artery, although if ST depression is present in lead I, more frequently the RCA is affected (Fig. 9.24).

P **9.3.3.1.2. Flat or negative T wave**
(Figs 9.25 and 9.26)

In NSTEACS, a flat or slightly negative T wave may also be observed, although not generally ≥2 mm:

• **The flat or slightly negative T wave** in NSTEACS usually **appears after the resolution phase of angina**. During angina the negative T wave either is not modified, or it is converts into a more or less evident ST depression (Fig. 9.26).

• The symmetrical flat or negative T wave is shallow (<2.5 and usually <1.5 mm) and in general appears in leads with a tall R. However, it may also be seen in V1–V3 and other leads with rS (Figs 9.25 and 9.26).

• In our opinion, the presence of a **negative T wave with the nadir measuring ≥1 mm in two contiguous leads with R or R/S ≥1, does not correspond to acute ischemia**, as described by Thygessen (2012). However, it may appear immediately after acute ischemia, as occurs with deep negative T waves that appear just after aborted STEACS (post-fibrinolysis, post-PCI) or after coronary spasm.

Without pain   With pain

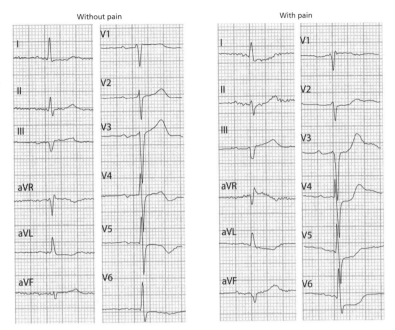

Figure 9.26 Patient with 3-vessel disease and LMT subocclusion. When recorded without pain, the ECG shows a negative T wave in V4-V6 of 2 mm. With pain, ST depression, which encompasses the T wave, clearly appears or increases in these leads and in FP leads.

• We must also remember that a deep negative T wave following a Q wave infarction does not correspond to acute ischemia (electric window effect) (Fig. 9.30A).

The negative T wave of ischemic origin may be due to a different post-ischemic mechanism:
(a) After Q-wave MI. Intraventricular pattern (window effect of Wilson).
(b) Post-reperfusion (aborted SCAEST, coronary spasm). The artery is open.
(c) Evolutive phase of NSTEACS. Never appears during angina crisis.

9.3.3.1.3. Changes in the U wave (Fig. 9.27)
Occasionally during the course of ACS, generally without ST elevation, when the patient does not feel pain (B), a U wave with a different polarity than the T wave is seen. Sometimes the voltage of the T and U waves is very small, as seen in Fig. 9.27, but the difference is clear when comparing the tracing with that of a normal ECG (A).

9.3.3.1.4. The ECG may remain normal or unmodified (≈5–10%)
In general the prognosis is these cases is good.

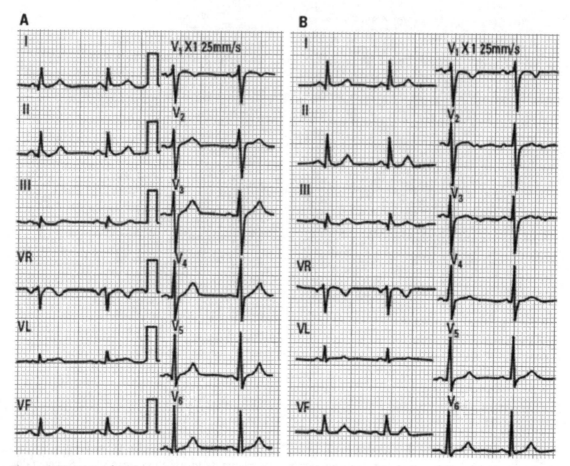

Figure 9.27 (A) Basal ECG of a 52-year-old man was normal and similar to previous ones. (B) Some hours after precordial pain, the ECG shows a negative T wave in V1 and a flat T wave in V2 and V3 with a slightly negative U wave. This suggests ischemic heart disease without acute ongoing ischemia, that was confirmed by coronarography (severe LAD occlusion).

9.3.4 In Table 9.2 the most important global characteristics of both STEACS and NSTEACS are shown.

Table 9.2 Summary of ECG, clinical, angiographic, and pathologic findings in ST elevation acute coronary syndrome (STEACS) and non-ST elevation acute coronary syndrome(NSTEACS)

ECG	Clinical	Angiographic	Pathology	Treatment
ACS with narrow QRS **STEACS (30% of total)** • Tall T wave • ST elevation • Evolving MI • Atypical patterns (Table 9.3)	Rest pain or equivalents	• Total or nearly occluded artery by fresh thrombus • TIMI 0/1 flow	• Usually ruptured plaque. After some time of subendo-cardial involvement there is a transmural homogeneous involvement	• Emergent PCI • Medical treatment (see guidelines scientific societies) • Fibrinolysis if PCI is not feasible
NSTEACS (50% of total)ᵃ (During pain) • ST depression (70%) • Flat/negative T wave ($\approx$15%) • U changes (<1%) • Normal or unchanged ($\approx$15%) • Sometimes in absence of pain the ECG is normal/nearly normal	With or without permanent rest pain	• Patent artery in >70% cases. • Non-occluded thrombus ($\approx$50%) • Acute total occlusion in10–20% case but with collaterals/ preconditioning	• Usually ulcerated plaque • Predominant subendocardial involvement • Usually non-transmural homogeneous involvement or, if exists (10-20% cases)is in general in the 'mute' (basal) areas	• Antithrombotic and antiplatelet agents (see guidelines scientific societies) • Non-emergent PCI except in a high-risk group. However often PCI is urgent (see Table 9.3)

ᵃThe rest (20%) are cases of ACS with confounding factors (see text).
ACS: acute coronary syndrome; STEACS: ST elevation acute coronary syndrome; NSTEACS; non-ST elevation acute myocardial infarction;PCI percutaneous coronary intervention.

9.3.5. Differential diagnosis

Q **9.3.5.1. ST depression**

ST depression may be seen under various circumstances other than ischemic heart disease. Often it appears as a secondary change to a depolarization disorder such as branch block or ventricular enlargement with a strain pattern.

As a primary change, or in other words, changes not due to disturbances in depolarization (enlargement or block), it may be seen due to the administration of many drugs, electrolytic disorders, and also some cardiomyopathies and other heart condi-

tions. Figure 9.28 shows examples of these situations. Additionally, Chapters 6 and 7 in particular outline these processes.

9.3.5.2 Differential diagnosis of negative T wave

R

Determining whether the T wave is of ischemic origin using the ECG alone is not easy. Given that ischemic heart disease (IHD) generally affects a certain area of the heart specifically, the negative T wave related to it is more localized and often deeper than the negative T wave due to factors affecting

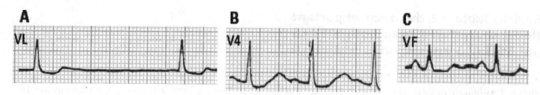

Figure 9.28 (A) ST depression due to digitalis effect. (B) ST depression due to hypokalemia in a patient taking high doses of diuretics. (C) ST depression in a patient with mitral prolapse.

the entire heart, such as myocarditis, pericarditis, toxic or drugs effect.

The most frequent cases of negative T waves not related with ischemic heart disease cardiopathy are linked to pericarditis in the chronic phase (Fig. 15.1), myocarditis, and some cardiomyopathies (Fig. 17.6A).

Figure 9.29 shows some examples of negative or flat T wave which are not due to IHD or myopericarditis.

9.4. More frequent pitfalls in the ECG interpretation of ACS

Table 9.3 summarizes the most frequent pitfalls that are performed in patients with ACS, due to lack of knowledge of ECG changes that occur in the presence of ACS. It is important to carefully study this table in order to avoid mistakes.

9.5. Necrosis pattern

9.5.1. Q wave of necrosis

9.5.1.1. Concept
- STEACS usually evolves, without swift and adequate treatment, to myocardial infarction. The typical ECG pattern includes the presence of a pathologic Q wave (see Section 9.5.1.2). Historically, a Q wave of necrosis was considered to represent a transmural infarction. Today, thanks to MRI correlation we know that this is not always the case. Transmural infarctions can occur without Q (see Section 9.5.2), and Q waves can appear without transmural involvement (Moon et al., 2004).

9.5.1.2. Electrophysiological mechanisms
The Q wave of necrosis can be explained by two theories as outlined below.

1. Electric window theory (Figs 9.30A and 9.31A).

The electrode facing the necrotic area records the left intraventricular pattern of negative QS with negative T wave. In cases in which necrosis does not reach the subepicardial zone, QRS may have a QR-type morphology (Fig. 9.31B). However, if subepicardial zone without necrosis is hypokinetic/akinetic a QS pattern with negative T wave may also be present.

2. Vector of necrosis theory (Figs 9.30B and 9.30C).

In the necrotic zone as shown in Figure 9.30C, electrical forces are not generated due to the loss of myocardial mass. This originates a vector that moves away from this area (Figs 9.30C and 9.31). Thus, an epicardial electrode faces the tail of this vector and records negativity.

9.5.1.3. Diagnosis of the Q wave of necrosis
The ECG characteristics that define a Q wave or its equivalent (R in V1) as being due to myocardial necrosis are outlined below (Thygesen et al., 2012):
- Any Q wave in V2–V3 $\geq$0.02 s or a QS complex in leads V2 and V3.
- Q wave $\geq$0.03 s and $\geq$0.1 mV in depth, or a QS complex in leads I, II, VL, VF, or V4–V6 in two of any leads in the group of continuous leads (I, VL, V6; V4–V6; II, III, and VF).
- R wave $\geq$0.04 s in V1 and R/S $\geq$1 with a concordant positive T wave in the absence of a conduction defect, RVE, or pre-excitation. We have reported that is very suggestive of lateral scar in post-MI patients the presence of tiny 's' wave in V1 with a ratio r/s $\geq$0.5 (Bayés de Luna, 2008).

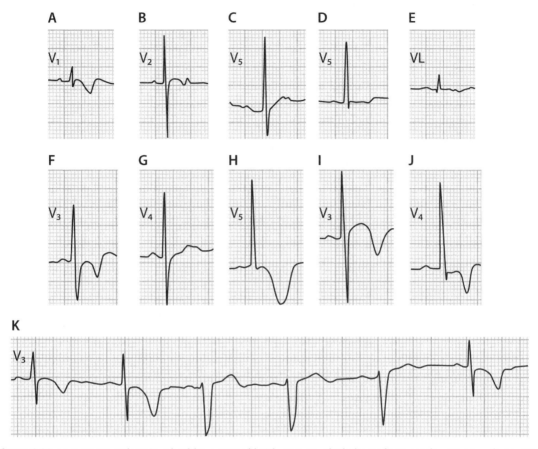

Figure 9.29 (A & B) V1 and V2 in a healthy 1-year-old girl. (C & D) Alcoholic cardiomyopathy. (E) Myxedema. (F) A negative T wave following paroxysmal tachycardia in a patient with cardiomyopathy in the initial phase. (G) Bimodal T wave with long QT often seen following long-term treatment with amiodarone. (H) A negative T wave with a very wide base sometimes seen in patients with cerebrovascular accident. (I) A negative T wave preceded by ST elevation in an apparently healthy tennis player Hypertrophic CM has to be rule not. (J) A very negative T wave in a patient with apical cardiomyopathy. (K) A negative T wave in complexes with normal ventricular activation in a patient with intermittent LBBB without apparent heart disease.

U **9.5.1.4. Locating the Q wave of necrosis**

Until recently, it was accepted for more than 30 years (Surawicz et al., 1978) that the location of necrosis according to the lead in the Q wave of necrosis existed as follows:

• Septal infarction: V1-V2; anterior infarction: V3-V4; lateral infarction: V5, V6, I, and VL (VL high lateral infarction); inferior infarction: II, III, and VF; posterior infarction: R/S >1 in V1 (mirror image of the Q wave recorded in posterior leads).

• However, the following has now been shown using correlations with delayed enhancement MRI (gadolinium) (Bayés de Luna et al., 2006 a,b; Van der Weg et al., 2009; Rovai et al., 2007):

(a) There are seven ECG patterns that correspond to the necrotic areas as demonstrated by real time CE-MRI (Fig. 9.33). The location of necrosis and its correlation with the ECG leads may be seen in the figure. According to this classification, four types of infarction are due to LAD

Table 9.3 More common pitfalls in the ECG interpretation: see ECG pattern, type of ACS and involved artery, zone involved, and recommended management

ECG patterns • and pitfalls –	Type of ACS and involved artery	Zone and characteristics of involvement	Management. Emergent (1) or urgent (2) PCI, associated to medical treatment
A • ST depression in V1–V4: in the acute phase, prominent ST depression in V1 without significant terminal positive T wave in V1-V2 (Fig. 9.14). – Consider it to be a NSTEACS	– Probably, it is true STEACS (STEACS equivalent) mirror pattern due to LCX occlusion (rarely distal RCA). – Patients have ongoing active symptoms	Transmural lateral involvement	Emergent PCI (1)
B • Leads V1-V4: isoelectric ST segment with tall, wide, positive T wave. Often a transient pattern (Figs 9.16 A) – Consider that the ECG is normal	– Hyperacute phase of STEACS. Patient with angina – Repeat ECG in few minutes – Evolving to LAD total occlusion	Subendocardial involvement evolving to transmural involvement	Probably emergent PCI (1)
C • Leads V1-V4: ST↓ plus tall positive T wave that evolves to Q wave MI. The change occurs in hours (Fig.9.16 B and 9.23 A) – Consider that the PCI is not emergent	– NSTEACS evolving to STE ACS usually in hours – Usually LAD subocclusion evolving to total occlusion – Patients have ongoing symptoms	Nontransmural involved wall evolving to transmural involvement	Emergent PCI (1)
D • Leads V1–V3: NSTEACS with isoelectric ST segment with mild negative T wave in V1–V3 (Fig. 9.25) – Consider that the problem is over	– Resolution phase (spontaneous, drugs, PCI) of NSTEACS. LAD Subocclusion that may be important – Patients usually have resolution of symptoms	No transmural involvement	Most probably urgent PCI (2)
E • Leads V1 to V4–V5: isoelectric ST segment with deep symmetrical negative T wave (Fig. 9.17). Not angina at this moment. – Consider it to be NSTEACS	– Resolution phase (spontaneous, drugs, PCI) of STEACS due to LAD subocclusion (or occlusion with collaterals) – Patients usually have resolution of symptoms	At least in some cases, transmural edema that disappears if pattern normalizes	Urgent PCI (2)
F • ST ↑ in I and VL, without evident ST ↓ in V1-V6 (Fig.9.37) – Consider it is LCX occlusion	More frequently occlusion of first diagonal usually angina	Transmural involvement mid/low anterolateral wall	Emergent PCI (1)
G • ST depression in ≥ 7 leads+ST elevation in VR–V1, and without evident final positive T wave in V1–V2 (Fig. 9.22). – Do not consider it to be LMT subocclusion	NSTEACS due to LMT subocclusion or 3 vessel disease	Without transmural involvement	Urgent or Emergent PCI according hemodynamic state (1,2)
H • ST elevation in I, VL, V2 to V3-6 No ST elevation aVR and V1 Frequent RBBB +superoanterior hemiblock. – Do not recognize that it corresponds to a complete LMT occlusion.	STEACS due to LMT total occlusion	Transmural involvement	Emergent PCI (1)

RBBB indicates right bundle-block branch. LMT = left main trunk.

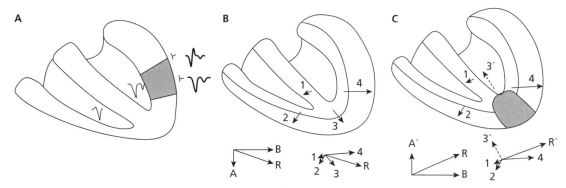

Figure 9.30 (A) The appearance of a Q wave of necrosis when a homogenously affected transmural infarction exists in left the ventricle (LV), may explain why the necrotic tissue, which cannot be activated, acts as an electric window and allows the LV intracavitary QRS in (QS complex with negative T wave) to be recorded from the outside. The QS complex explains why the vectors with normal activation, 1, 2, and 3, move away from the infarction zone. In fact, (B), under normal conditions, the QRS vector (R) is formed by the sum of the different ventricular vectors 1 + 2 + 3 + 4. (C) If there is a necrotic area (infarction) the infarction vector has the same magnitude as the previous vector but moves in the opposite direction (3′ in C). This change of direction in the initial electrical depolarization forces one part of the heart, the necrotic area (infarction), and also indicates a global change of direction in the R vector, which converts to R′.

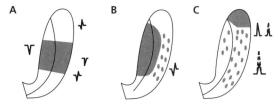

Figure 9.31 The theory of the Wilson's electric window (A) explains how a clinical transmural infarction originates a QS morphology, while in an infarction affecting the subendocardium and part of the subepicardium (B) produces a QR morphology that is not transmural. Finally (C), an infarction that affects the basal areas, or part of the myocardial wall, in patches without areas of necrosis allows the formation of early depolarization vectors that are recorded as R waves with notches, slurrings or low voltage (fragmented QRS).

occlusion at different levels (**anteroseptal zone**) and three types are due to RC or CX occlusion (**inferolateral zone**).

(b) The classic posterior wall (segment 4 in the Cerqueira classification [2002]) does not exist because this segment does not curve upward, or it only does so to a very small degree (Bayés & Fiol-Sala, 2008) (Fig. 9.32). It may still not reg-

ister in these cases as an R wave in V1, because it cannot originate a Q wave in the back. In this area, depolarization occurs after the first 40 ms, by which time QRS has already started and in any case produces a fragmented QRS. Furthermore, although a necrosis vector originates, it is directed toward V3 and not V1 (Fig. 9.32).

(c) The prominent R in V1 corresponds to a lateral infarction and not to a previous posterior infarction (currently segment 4-inferobasal in the Cerqueira classification) (see Figs 9.40 and 9.41).

(d) The Q wave in VL as an isolated manifestation, or accompanied by a small q in I, is generally due to infarction in the anteromedial zone (occlusion of the first degree diagonal) and not to infarction in the lateral-basal zone (left CX occlusion–high lateral infarction) (Fig. 9.37).

9.5.1.4.1. Q infarction in the anteroseptal zone

This zone encompasses four types of infarction (Fig. 9.33): septal (A-1), anterior apical (A-2); extensive anterior (A-3); and anterior middle (A-4).

Figure 9.34 shows the ventricular activation in Q infarction due to proximal LAD occlusion

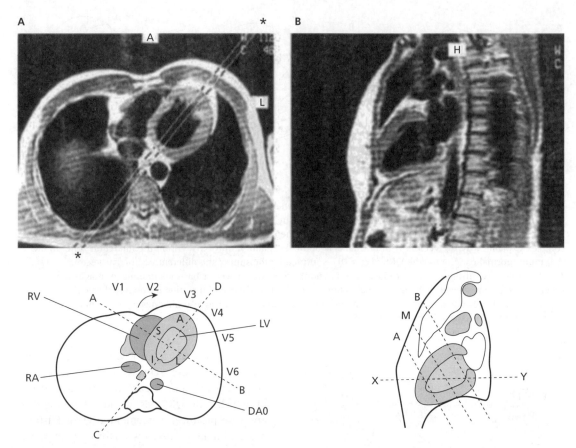

Figure 9.32 Magnetic resonance imaging. **(A)** Thoracic horizontal axial plane at the level of the 'xy' line of the sagittal plane of right side of the figure. The four walls can be adequately observed: anterior (A), septal (S), lateral (L), and inferior (I), with the inferobasal portion of the wall (segment 4 of Cerqueria statement) that bends upwards in this case. **(B)** Sagittal plane following the line seen in (A) (asterisk). B, M, and A, basal, middle, and apical plane. DAo = descending aorta; RA = right atrium; RV = right ventricle. An R wave (mirror pattern of Q wave in back leads) is not originated in V1, in the case of infarction of the basal area of inferior wall, because this basal zone always depolarizes after the first 40 ms, and then the QRS pattern has already started the recording. Furthermore although a necrosis vector (NV) could be generated this would face V3–V4 and not V1 (see in A the asterisk and the line C D). (See Plate 9.32.)

	Name	Type	ECG pattern	Infarction area (CE-CMR)	Most probable place of occlusion
Anteroseptal, zone	Septal	A1	Q in V1–V2 SE: 100% SP: 97%	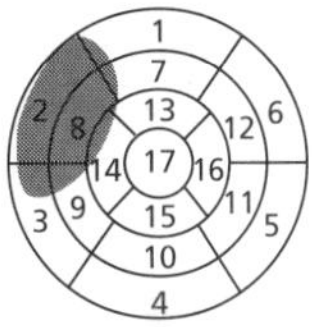	LAD 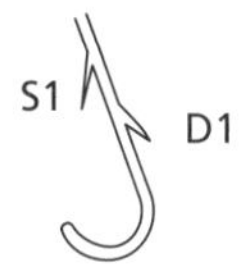
	Apical–anterior	A2	Q in V1–V2 to V3–V6 SE: 85% SP: 98%	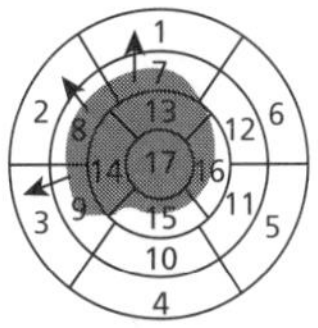	LAD 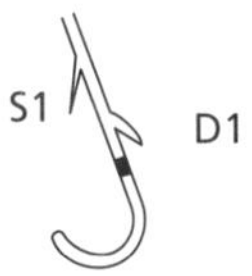
	Extensive anterior	A3	Q in V1–V2 to V4–V6, I and aVL SE: 83% SP: 100%	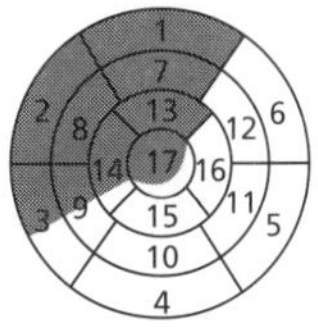	LAD 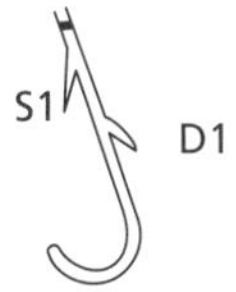
	Mid–anterior	A4	Q(qs or qr) in aVL (I) and sometimes in V2–V3 SE: 67% SP: 100%	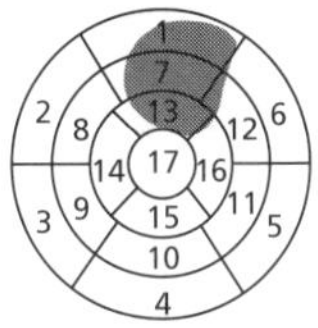	LAD 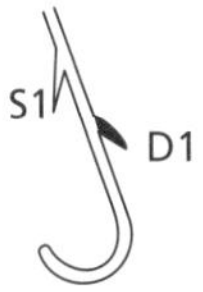
Inferolateral, zone	Lateral	B1	RS in V1–V2 and/or q wave in leads I, aVL, V6 and/or diminished R wave in V6 SE: 67% SP: 99%	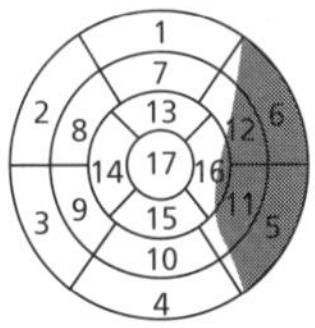	LCX 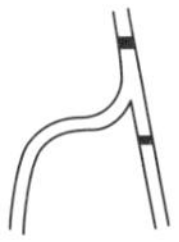
	Inferior	B2	Q in II, III, aVF SE: 88% SP: 97%	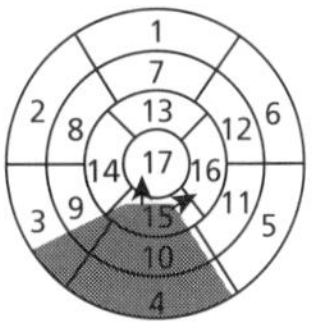	RCA LCX 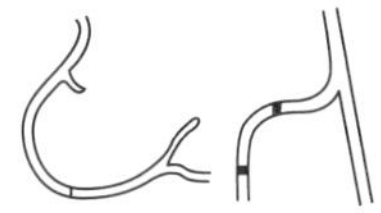
	Inferolateral	B3	Q in II, III, Vf (B2) and Q in I, VL, V5–V6 and/or RS in V1 (B1) SE: 73% SP: 98%	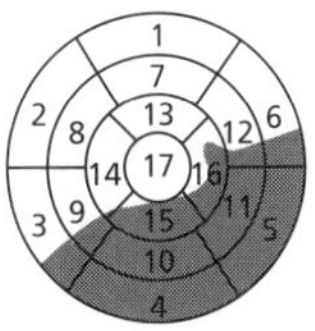	RCA LCX 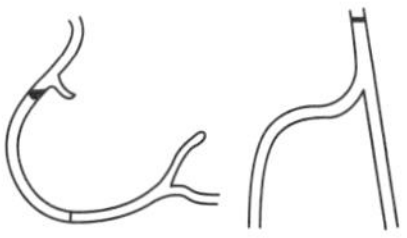

Figure 9.33 The segments affected by necrosis in the presence of Q infarction do not always present transmural involvement, although the preserved zones are generally hypokinetic. The sensitivity of these correlations is generally not very high, and thus there can be cases of infarction in an area without a characteristic ECG pattern. However, specificity in terms of the ECG pattern corresponding to the zone affected by necrosis using MRI, is almost 100%.

A

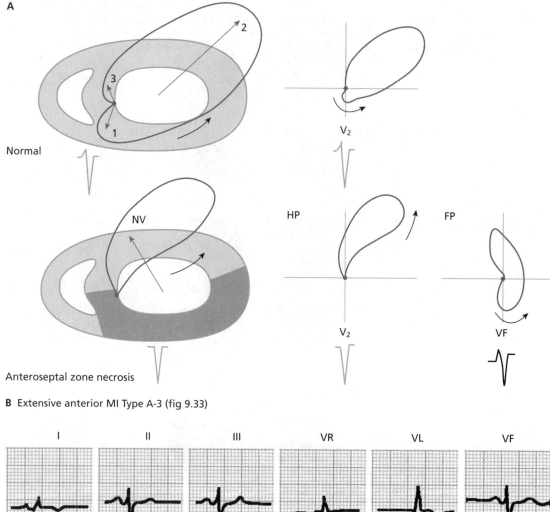

Normal

Anteroseptal zone necrosis

B Extensive anterior MI Type A-3 (fig 9.33)

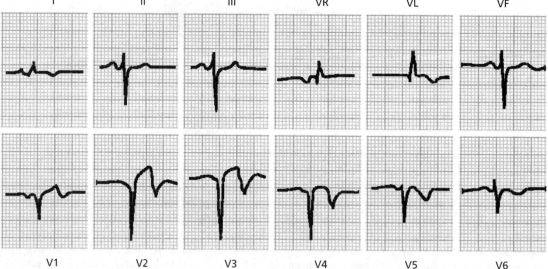

Figure 9.34 (A) A comparison of normal activation and in case of in extensive anterior infarction (Q beyond V2 and in I and VL) (type A.3 in Fig. 9.33). The direction of the infarction vector in the FP and HP explains the morphologies in precordial leads and in lead 1 and VL. (B) Example of infarction in this zone. QS until V4 and qr in D1 and VL. (See Plate 9.34.)

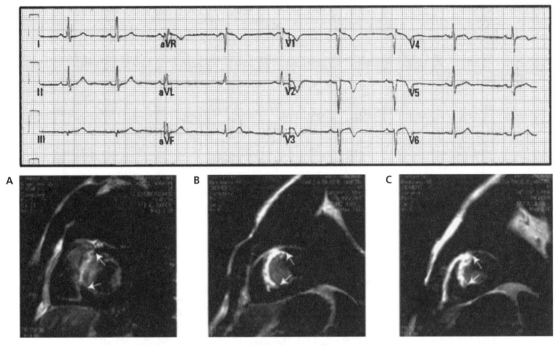

Figure 9.35 Example of septal infarction (type A-1), ECG criteria (Q in V1-V2 with rS in V3). MRI: The septal infarction is extensive and affects most of the interventricular septum at all levels (basal [A], middle [B], and apical [C]) in the transversal plane. There is a small extension toward the anterior wall at the middle and apical levels (arrows).

(**type A-3 extensive anterior infarction**) in comparison with a normal ECG. The vector of necrosis moves away from the posterior aspect towards the right and thus the precordial leads record a Q wave from V1 to V4-V5 and in VL with a minimal r in V1. This also explains the Q wave due to the electric window phenomenon previously described.

Figures 9.35 and 9.36 show two examples: one of **septal infarction (A-1)** and **antero-apical infarction (A-2)** along with their MRI correlations.

Figure 9.37 shows a case of **infarction due to first diagonal occlusion (type A-4 anterior middle infarction)**. The presence of Q (QR) in VL generally corresponds, in our experience, to first diagonal infarction, but it may also be found in some cases of CX occlusion. In the acute phase in CX occlusion, however, an evident ST depression

is observed from V1 to V3, a pattern that does not occur in first diagonal occlusion (Fig. 9.37A), or the ST depression is much less evident and is followed by a positive T wave. Furthermore, in cases of CX occlusion there is often in the subacute or chronic phase high R in V_1 (lateral infarction) (Figs 9.39 and 9.40).

In conclusion, when the most evident ECG sign presented by a postinfarction patient is Q in VL, it is generally due to infarction caused by first diagonal occlusion (A-4) and not to high lateral infarction (B-1).

9.5.1.4.2. Q wave in infarction in the inferolateral zone

This zone encompasses three types of infarction (Fig. 9.33): lateral (B1); inferior (B-2); and inferolateral (B-3).

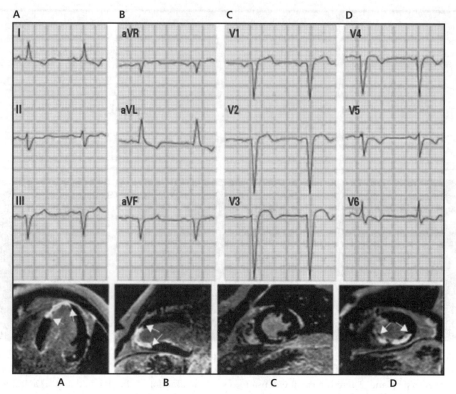

Figure 9.36 Example of an apical-anterior infarction (Type A-2) (Q wave beyond V2 but without Q in I and VL). MRI showing septal and apical involvement in the HP (A). The saggital plane (B) shows greater inferior involvement than the anterior plane, and in the middle and lower transversal sections (C and D, especially in D) septal and inferior involvement is seen.

Figure 9.38 shows activation in inferolateral Q infarction due to occlusion of very long RC artery (type B-3 inferolateral infarction). The vector of necrosis moves upwards, forwards, and somewhat to the right. This explains the presence of the Q wave in II, III and VF as well as the RS morphology in V1.

Figure 9.39 shows a clear example of inferior isolated infarction (type B-2) with only q in the inferior wall and without high R in V1, despite the fact that the infarction encompasses segment 4 (previously-named posterior wall).

Lastly, the most important conclusion to make thanks to the Q wave–MRI correlation is that **the prominent R wave in V1 is not due to poste-rior infarction as previously believed** (segment 4 in the Cerqueira classification) (Fig. 1.1), **but rather to lateral infarction** (segments 5, 6, 11, and 12) (Figs 1.1 and 9.33). Figure 9.40 shows different patterns of lateral (A to C) (type B-1) and inferobasal (old posterior) infarction (D) (segment 4) (type B-2). As shown in the figure, the inferobasal infarction does not originate a high R wave in V1.

We must remember that the pattern of a high R wave in V1 as an expression of lateral infarction is very specific and indicates that the infarction is most likely located in this area (in our experience 100% of the time). However, there are many lateral infarctions without high R in V1, mainly because

A

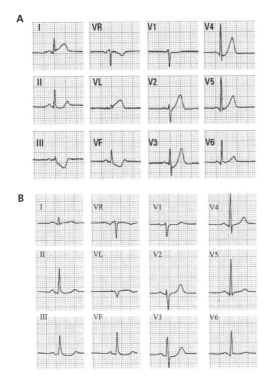

Figure 9.37 Example of mid-anterior MI (Type A-4) due to occlusion of the first diagonal. The upper part (A) is shown in the acute phase and the lower part (B) shows the infarction already established (q in VL and low R in I).

the infarction is located in the more basal parts of the lateral wall (relatively low sensitivity). In patients with STEACS who have had a lateral infarction in V1 the following morphologies as already shown may be observed (Fig. 9.40A-C): Single R wave (A); R/S ≥1 with an evident S wave; and R wave >3 mm (B); and R/S >0.5 with small S wave and R wave <3 mm (C). R/S ≥1 is 100% specific to lateral infarction.

Figure 9.41 shows the difference between the old classification (left) and the current classification (right) with respect to the types of infarction in the inferolateral zone in cases of Q-wave MI.

9.5.1.5. The evolution of the Q wave of necrosis

Generally, the Q wave does not disappear, but it may occur due to the presence of collateral circulation, especially in inferior infarctions (Fig. 9.42).

The Q wave of necrosis may also disappear with the appearance of bundle branch block especially LBBB, or infarction in the opposite zone (Fig. 9.43).

9.5.1.6. Differential diagnosis of the Q wave of necrosis: pathologic Q wave not due to myocardial infarction

W

It is well-known that pathologic Q waves not due to necrosis are frequent. Table 9.4 shows the most frequent cases: during an acute process, transitory patterns, and as a chronic pattern.

9.5.2. Fragmented QRS

X

• **When necrosis affects areas of delayed depolarization, even if transmural, Q waves are not originated** because when the stimulus reaches the necrotic area the formation of QRS is already started and thus the start of the R wave is not seen in many leads. **In this case, the necrosis is shown by an amputation of R or by slurrings in the middle of QRS** (Das et al., 2006) (Figs. 9.31C and 9.44).

9.5.3. Suspected ventricular aneurysm

Occasionally, in a chronic patient a certain degree of ST elevation may be seen, with or without fragmented QRS, suggesting the presence of a ventricular aneurysm (Fig. 9.45) secondary to ischemic heart disease with old necrosis. It is not a very sensitive sign.

9.5.4. Infarction without the Q wave

(Table 9.5)

This type of infarction occurs quite frequently, especially in cases of NSTEACS, but also with new treatments in the case of STEACS; it either does not originate infarction or this is no Q wave MI.

Table 9.5 contains a list of the different myocardial infarctions that may occur without the Q wave of necrosis. Some of these

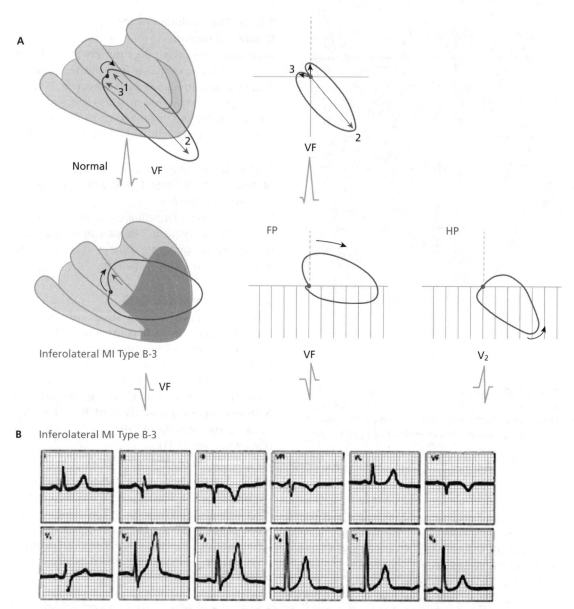

Figure 9.38 (A) A comparison of normal activation with the activation in a case of infarction of the inferolateral zone (type B-3 in Fig. 9.33). The inferior infarction vector moves upward and in the FP the loop–hemifield correlation explains the appearance of the Q wave in inferior leads. The involvement of the lateral wall originates an anteriorization of the loop in the HP, explaining the prominent R wave in V1. (B) An example of Q infarction in the inferolateral zone in II, III, and VF and RS in V1 (type B-3). (See Plate 9.38.)

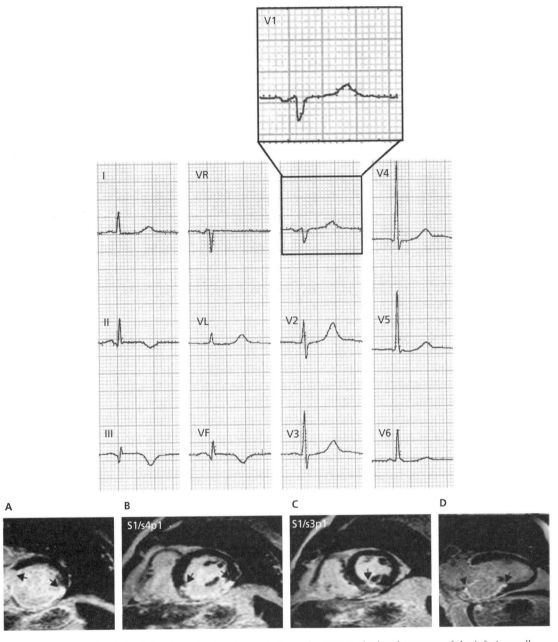

Figure 9.39 Isolated inferior infarction with involvement shown by MRI in the basal segment of the inferior wall (former posterior wall (Type B-2) (A, B & C) Transversal basal CORTES, middle and inferior sections. (D) Lateral section. Segment 4 (former posterior wall) (A & D) is involved without high R in V1 (r = 1 mm).

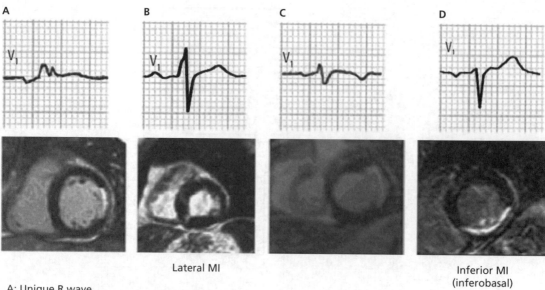

Lateral MI

Inferior MI
(inferobasal)

A: Unique R wave

B: R/S = 1 with large S wave and R wave > 3 mm

C: R/S > 0.5 with small S wave and R wave < 3 mm

Figure 9.40 The lateral wall shown by MRI shows a transversal section that is always facing the septum. The inferior wall is always located between the lateral and septal walls. Three cases of lateral infarction (Type B-1) are shown (A, B & C) with clear gadolinium enhancement (white area) and present three distinct patterns of dominant R or RS. However, (D) presents r in V1 measuring 1 mm and the necrotic zone corresponds to segment 4 of the inferior wall (inferobasal segment, or former posterior wall).

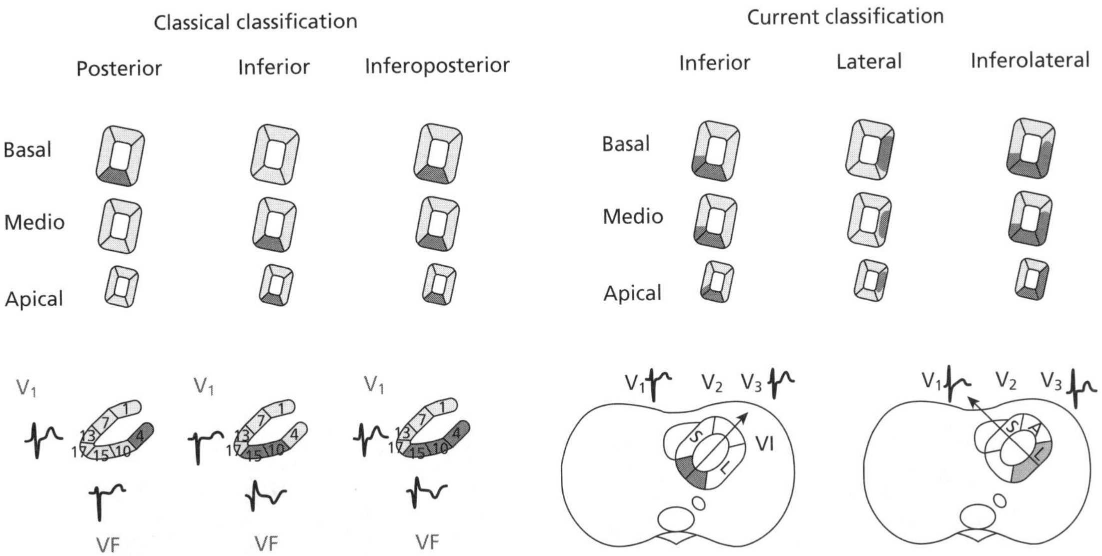

Classical classification | Current classification

Posterior · Inferior · Inferoposterior | Inferior · Lateral · Inferolateral

Basal · Medio · Apical | Basal · Medio · Apical

V₁ ... VF

Figure 9.41 Left, the area implicated in inferior, posterior, and inferoposterior infarction with the classical ECG patterns in the chronic phase according to historical classification. Right, the new concept outlined in this book. The concept of posterior wall or posterior infarction is no longer used, the RS pattern in V1 is explained by lateral infarction, and infarction of the inferobasal segment in the inferior wall (former posterior wall) does not generate a Q wave because it is an area of delayed depolarization. Thus, infarction in the inferolateral zone is of three types: inferior (Q in II, III, and VF), lateral (RS in V1 and/or pathologic Q wave in lateral leads), and inferolateral (both patterns) (see Figs 9.33, 9.39 and 9.40).

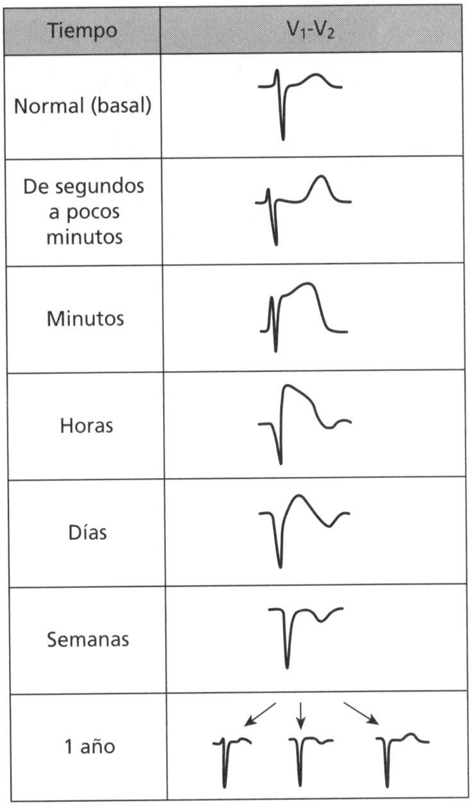

Tiempo	V₁-V₂
Normal (basal)	
De segundos a pocos minutos	
Minutos	
Horas	
Días	
Semanas	
1 año	

Figure 9.42 Sequential ECG changes in a patient with anterior infarction with Q wave (rectified ST and positive, peaked T wave are recorded in V1-V2 at the start). Note the different evolutive ECG patterns without modern treatment during the first year. <Spanish to be translated on Fig. 9.42>

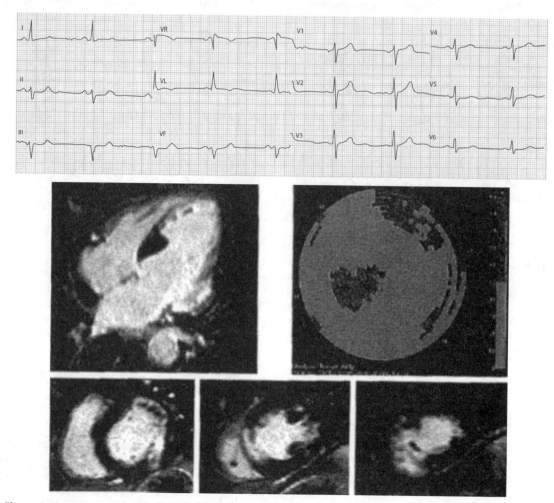

Figure 9.43 Patient with septal and lateral infarctions clearly visible with CE-CMR using MRI. The ECG is practically normal because the two vectors of necrosis cancel each other and thus the Q wave is not visible. (See Plate 9.43.)

Table 9.4 Q waves not due to ischemic heart disease

---

1. **During an acute process**
   - Myocarditis
   - Takotsubo (Fig. 9.54)
   - Pulmonary embolism
   - Miscellaneous: toxic agents, etc.
2. **Chronic phase**
   - Variants on normality (positional Q in III) (Fig. 4.26)
   - RVE and/or LVE (Chapter 6)
   - Left bundle branch block (Chapter 7)
   - Infiltrative processes (amyloidosis, sarcoidosis, cardiomyopathy) etc. (Chapters 9 and 16)
   - WPW-type pre-excitation (Chapter 8)
   - Miscellaneous: Pheochromocytoma, congenital heart diseases, etc (see Bayés de Luna, 2012a).

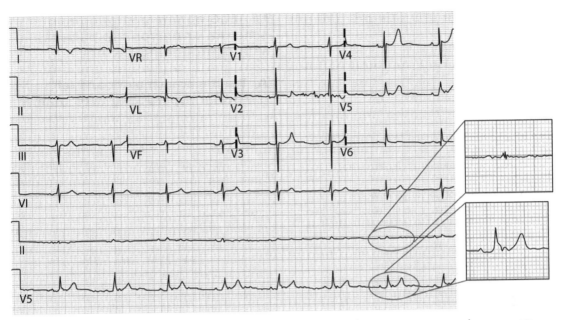

Figure 9.44 ECG in a patient with two MIs in the inferolateral zone in whom two aortocoronary bypasses were implanted. An important aneurysm exists in the left ventricle. Note the presence of RS in V1, the Q wave in lateral leads, and the anomalous morphology (fragmented QRS) in various leads (amplified leads II and V5).

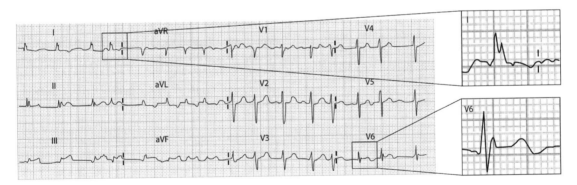

Figure 9.45 An ECG of a 65-year-old woman with atrial fibrillation who presented with two previous infarctions due to CD and CX occlusion showing a typical fragmented QRS (above). In addition, ST elevation in the chronic postinfarction phase (V6 below) is suggestive of ventricular aneurysm as shown by echocardiography.

underlying infarctions, however, do present this Q wave on occasion.

Figure 9.47 summarizes all the possible evolutions of two types of ACS (STEMI and NSTEMI) (see legend).

Y **Table 9.5** Myocardial infarctions (MI) without Q wave

– **Non Q-wave MI:** ST depression with enzymatic elevation.
– **Infarction in areas that do not generate Q**
 • atrial zones: infarction is never exclusively atrial. Generally associated with extensive inferolateral infarction
 • right ventricle: generally associated with inferior infarction due to proximal RC occlusion
 • basal zones in VI: generally without Q wave but often with **fractionated QRS** (Fig. 9.44).
– **Microinfarctions** (necrosettes). They do not alter the ECG. Enzymatic MI.
– **Q-wave MI that disappears** with time (Fig. 9.42)
– **Aborted Q-wave MI** (Fig. 9.6)
– **Masked Q-wave MI** (see Section 9.6)
 • Presence of two or more infarctions (Fig. 9.43)
 • ranch block
 • Pacemaker
 • WPW syndrome

Non Q-wave MI is characterized by an STEACS with some ST depression along with enzymatic elevation. It may evolve to normal ST with positive T wave (Fig. 9.46). Often there is a residual repolarization disturbance (ST depression <1 mm and/or flat or slightly negative T wave).

9.6. ECG abnormalities due to ischemia or necrosis in patients with confounding factors

ZA

(A) Bundle branch block and left ventricular hypertrophy with strain

It is always easier to identify ischemia and necrosis in RBBB and LVH than in LBBB.

1. STEACS: Often it is easy to observe ST elevation in the acute phase (A), even in LBB (Fig. 9.48A) (Sgarbossa criteria) (1996), which normalizes in the chronic phase (Fig. 9.48B).

2. NSTEACS: This is more difficult to observe, but often a mixed pattern of repolarization due to the basal ECG and ischemia may be seen. Figure 9.49 shows a case of LVH with strain.

3. Q-wave MI: Generally, there are no problems in presence of RBB. The Q wave is easily seen. In LBBB, however, the block usually hides the Q wave of necrosis. In the following example with MRI correlation in a patient with extensive infarction, the Q wave and slurrings in QRS are nevertheless well seen (Fig. 9.50).

4. LVH with strain pattern:
In the acute phase, ST depression due to associated ischemia may be modified (mixed pattern).
Meanwhile, in LVH with strain, the septal q wave disappears, originating QS in V1. This pattern may be confused with septal infarction. The extension of the QS morphology to V2 and the primary disturbance of repolarization (negative T wave) suggests necrosis.

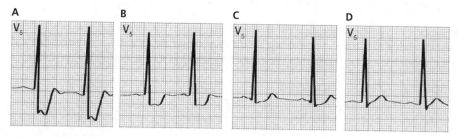

Figure 9.46 Course of an infarction without Q wave and with an important ST depression at the start, which normalized in a few weeks (A–D).

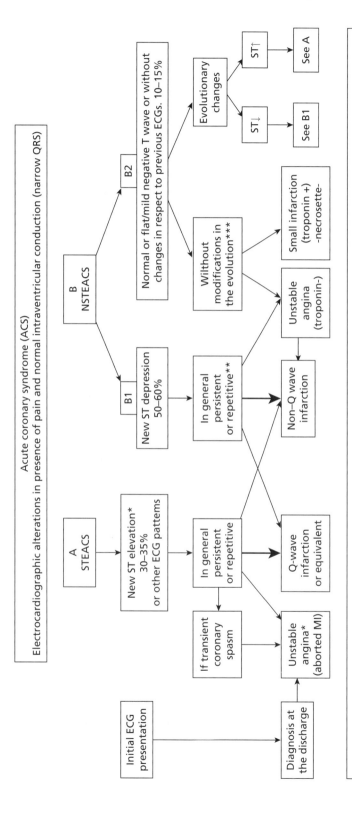

Figure 9.47 Acute coronary syndromes (ACS): ECG abnormalities at admission and diagnosis at discharge.

* Sometimes, thanks to quick treatment, in case of LAD occlusion, the STE changes to deep negative T wave and troponin levels remain normal despite important ST elevation in the initial ECG (aborted MI).
** InACS with ECG pattern of ST depression, troponin levels allow to distinguish between unstable angina (troponin-) and non-Q- wave infarction (troponin +).
*** According to ESC/ACC guidelines in patients presenting chest pain or its equivalent suggestive of ACS with accompanying nor mal ECG or flat/mild negative T wave, troponin level is a key to decide whether to diagnose small MI of unstable angina.

A

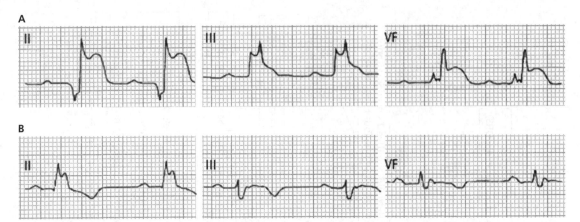

Figure 9.48 (A) Acute phase of infarction in a patient with advanced LBBB. Note the clear ST segment elevation. During the chronic phase (B), the symmetrical T wave in III (mixed repolarization disturbance pattern) suggests associated ischemia.

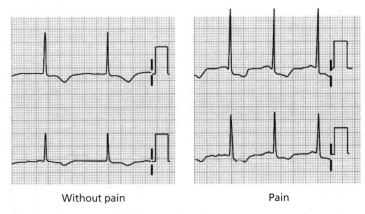

Without pain   Pain

Figure 9.49 A 62-year-old patient with arterial hypertension presenting NSTEACS. Left, Without pain, a LVH pattern with strain and a mixed negative T wave are observed. Right, During pain, a clear ST depression pattern appears.

B. Hemiblocks

Generally, myocardial infarction and ischemia may be diagnosed in the presence of hemiblocks, although some difficulties may occur. Perhaps the most challenging is to recognize, in a patient with left ÂQRS with Q waves in II, II, and VF, whether a superoanterior hemiblock associated with inferior infarction is present. Figure 9.51 shows how to perform the diagnosis of this association using the surface ECG thanks to the loop–hemifield correlation.

For more information on the association between necrosis and confusing factors see Bayés de Luna, 2012a.

9.7. Myocardial ischemia not due to atherothrombosis

We will comment on the three cases most frequently seen in clinical practice and which may

ZB

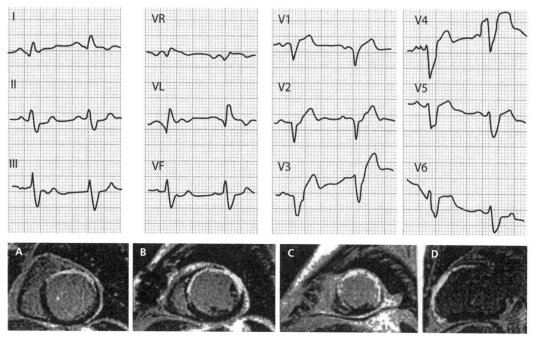

Figure 9.50 ECG of a patient with total LBBB and associated infarction. ECG criteria are suggestive of extensive anterior MI (qR in I, QR in VL, and low voltage in A in V3-V6 with slurrings indicating anteroseptal infarction). The CE-CMR patterns (A–D) show the presence of an extensive infarction in the anteroseptal zone (type A-3) (proximal LAD occlusion). The inferior wall is free of necrosis (D) because the LAD does not wrap the apex. In the transversal section of the CE-CMR (A–C) the infarction affects most of the anterior and septal walls with lateral involvement, although the high part of the lateral wall is preserved (A) because it is perfused by the CX. The inferior wall is preserved because LAD is not long (D).

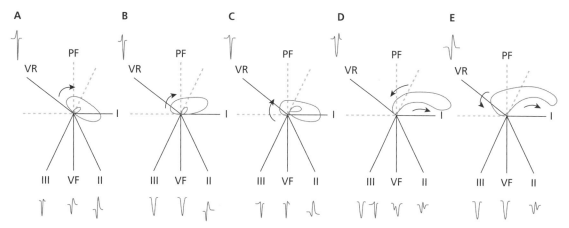

Figure 9.51 (A–E) ECG loops in different inferior infarctions associated in D and E with SAH. In these last two cases (D and E), the final part falls in the negative hemifield of II because of the special rotation of the QRS loop due to SAH and this explains the terminal 'r' in VR (D and E). Thus, the QS (qs) morphology without a terminal r in II, III, and VF (although qrs morphology may be seen) and with terminal 'r' in VR suggests associated SAH. In the absence of SAH, even if the entire VCG loop falls above 'X' axis (lead I) (B), there will always be a terminal r, at times small, at least in lead II, but never a terminal r in VR (A-C). (See Plate 9.51.)

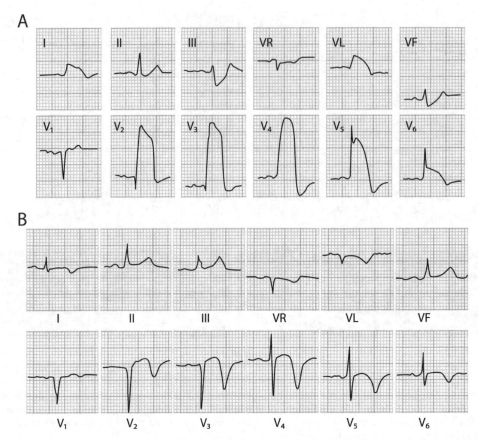

Figure 9.52 (A) Surface ECG of a 65-year-old patient with typical crisis of Prinzmetal angina that presents in the peak of pain an ST segment elevation like a transmembrane action potential (TAP). This case corresponds to a transitory complete proximal occlusion of the LAD above D1 (ST segment elevation from V2 to V6, I and VL with ST segment depression in inferior leads especially III and VF). The lack of ST segment elevation in VR, the small ST segment elevation in V1 and the clear ST segment elevation in V6 – if the placement of V6 is well done – is usually not seen when the occlusion is also above S1 (see Fig. 9.9). This is the first case of Prinzmetal angina seen by us in the early 1970s. Coronarography was not performed but enzymes were normal. (B) ECG some hours after the crisis with a typical pattern of very negative T wave in all precordial leads (reperfusion pattern).

correspond to true ACS. For more information, see Table 9.1 and Bayés de Luna, 2012.

9.7.1. Coronary spasm

(Figs 9.52 and 9.53)

The typical ECG abnormality seen in the very early phase is a high, peaked T wave followed by ST elevation lasting usually from 1 to 3 min (Bayés de Luna et al., 1985) (Fig. 9.53). If the spasm is very severe and reaches a large area of the myocardium, a brief, very negative T wave may appear at the end of the spasm (Fig. 9.51). When the spasm is severe and long in duration, potentially dangerous, ST disturbances (alternance of ST-T) and ventricular arrhythmias, may occur.

9.7.2. Takotsubo syndrome (Fig. 9.54)

Takotsubo syndrome is characterized by the presence of a transitory, apical achynesia related to brisk release of cathecolamine and/or increased coronary tone. Typical angiographic and ECG patterns are recorded as shown in Figure 9.54.

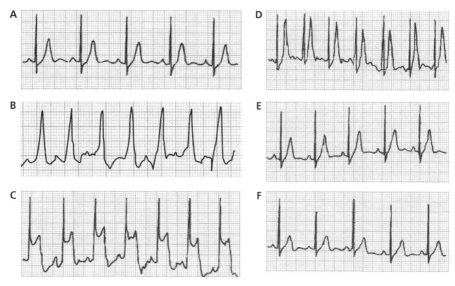

Figure 9.53 Crisis of coronary spasm (Prinzmetal angina) recorded by Holter ECG. (A) Control. (B) Initial pattern of a very tall T wave (subendocardial ischemia). (C) Huge pattern of ST segment elevation. (D–F) Resolution towards normal values. Total duration of the crisis was 2 minutes.

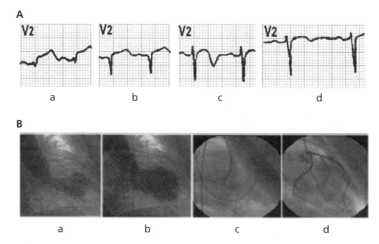

Figure 9.54 (A) ECG changes in V2 during the period of 3–4 days (a–d). Note the ECG pattern from ST elevation with Q wave to rS with deep negative T waves. (B) Typical angiographic image (a,b) and normal coronary tree (c,d).

9.7.3. X syndrome (Fig. 9.55)

Usually, X syndrome (angina-type pain related with disturbances in coronary microcirculation) appears during rest. The basal ECG is normal or with diffuse repolarization disturbances, especially T wave and/or small ST depression (Fig. 9.54A). During exercise (Fig. 9.55B) the ST depression may increase.

9.8. ECG in myocardial ischemia due to increased demand

ZC

Often, when precordial pain appears during a stress test, the ECG change is a certain degree of ST depression. This ST depression has special characteristics (Figs 9.12B and 9.56 A to C). If the

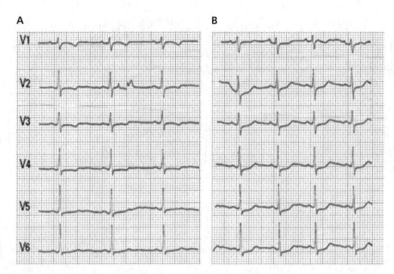

Figure 9.55 (A) A 60-year-old patient with typical X syndrome and normal coronary arteries. Observe the mild diffuse ST depression/flat flat T wave in the majority of the leads. (B) After exercise there is a clear ST depression, especially in horizontal leads.

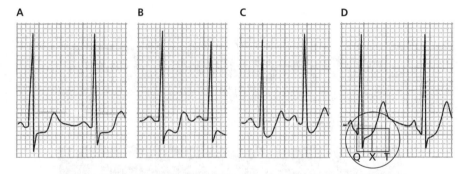

Figure 9.56 Various types of subendocardial severe ischemia patterns may appear in the course of an exercise test: (A) horizontal displacement of the ST segment; (B) descendant displacement of the ST segment; (C) concave displacement; and (D) ST segment depression from J point with ascendant morphology and rapid upslope: QX/QT<0.5 (Fig. 4.12). This usually is seen in normal cases. The coronary angiography was abnormal in A, B, and C, and normal in D. These changes are especially visible in leads with dominant R wave especially V3–V4 to V5–V6, I, and VL, and/or inferior leads with dominant R wave.

ST depression rapidly ascends (Figs 9.12A and 9.56D) it is considered normal. The same type of abnormal ST depression may be seen in spontaneous angina recorded during a Holter ECG (Fig. 9.57).

The ST depression occurs because the affected zone, the subendocardium, is already hypoperfused and this is reflected by increased blood demand.

Exceptionally, the ECG changes during a stress test can be ST elevation or high, peaked T wave (transmural involvement due to spasm). Arrhythmias may also be seen, usually ventricular extrasystoles, which indicate the immediate suspension of the test. Lastly, hyperventilation may alter repolarization, generally causing flat T wave, but without clinical relevance (Fig. 4.25).

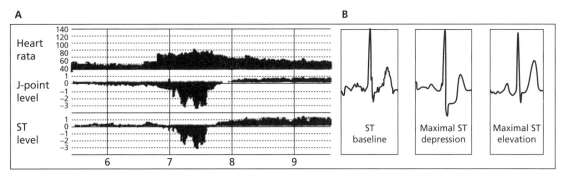

Figure 9.57 Changes of the ST segment in a patient with exercise angina. (A) The trend of ST segment changes and heart rate. (B) The different morphologies of ST.

In any case, false positive ST depression occurs both in stress tests and Holter recordings, and patients with angina may not present ECG changes (see Bayés de Luna, 2012).

ZD **9.9. Arrhythmias in ischemic heart disease (IHD)**

9.9.1. Acute phase

Acute ischemia may originate any type of active or passive arrhythmia. The most frequent types are:
(a) Supraventricular arrhythmias. Extrasystoles and atrial fibrillation occur in 10% of MI, especially in cases of atrial involvement.
(b) Ventricular arrhythmias. Ventricular extrasystoles are frequent and may trigger ventricular fibrillation (VF) and sudden death (SD), generally in patients with severe ischemia. The incidence of acute ischemia as the cause of SD is around 50% (Burke et al., 1997; Subirana, 2011; Bayés de Luna, 2012). Once the patient is in the Intensive Care Unit, if presents VF this may be usually resolved and this has no further prognostic relevance.
(c) AV block, especially due to RC occlusion before the artery of the AV node. This case may provoke complete AV block and occasionally SD.
(d) Ventricular block. In particular, RBBB which is very frequent in STEACS due to complete occlusion of the main trunk or LAD proximal to D_I and S_I.

9.9.2. Chronic phase

It is especially important to monitor the first months after infarction, when the risk of VT and VF is higher. In fact, 90% of cases of SD appear in patients with IHD, 50% in the acute phase. The rest in chronic phase, mainly due to sustained VT around one old scar of previous MI.

There is no relationship between the presence of VF in the acute phase and the risk of VT/VF later on. However, the ejection fraction (EF) is very relevant. VT and FV are more frequent in patients with low EF and the presence of a significant number of premature ventricular complexes in the Holter recording (Bayés de Luna, 2012a). In fact, in 80–90% of cases SD appears in the presence of IHD (50% in the hyperacute phase) (Subirana, 2010).

9.10. The significance of the flat or negative T wave in ischemic heart disease

The flat or negative T wave seen in the course   ZE
of acute ischemic heart disease (STEACS and NSTEACS) and chronic ischemic heart disease (post Q-wave MI) are not due to acute ischemia although it often appears just after that (reperfusion). We can no longer say that negative T wave means ischemia, and less subepicardial ischemia. Negative T wave due to subepicardial involvement only may occur in myopericarditis.

The negative T wave, whether very deep (atypical ECG in STEACS of after Q-wave MI) or shallow (NSTEACS) is a pattern that should be considered post-ischemic, often immediately after the ischemia (reperfusion), but not due to acute ischemia, because of the following:

(a) It appears in the evolutive phase of Q-wave MI once the pain has passed and necrosis has developed, even when some ST elevation remains. This represents left intraventricular pattern (Wilson's electric window effect) (Fig. 9.30A). If there is a subepicardial area free of infarction, which has been shown to occur frequently thanks to MRI (gadolinium), this area is usually hypokinetic or akinetic and presents a repolarization delay, and/or lack of TAP formation, that also explains in a practical sense the presence of a negative T wave and even a QS pattern. The normalization of negative T wave after MI, is a sign of functional recovery of viable myocardium in the infarct area. (Bayés de Luna, 2012a)

(b) It appears in cases of aborted STEACS (spontaneously, or after fibrinolysis or PCI especially in case of LAD) in which the pattern rs in V1-V2 is well recorded. In other words, without the development of a Q wave of necrosis (reperfusion pattern). It has been shown in a short series that it is due to transmural edema with TAP lengthening in the area, which disappears if the T wave is positive (Fig. 9.16). Occasionally, the artery may remain occluded, but in this case there is considerable collateral circulation.

(c) It appears at the end of severe coronary spasm, is short in duration, and is due to the reperfusion that lengthens the TAP in the affected zone (see b, Fig. 9.52).

(d) Cases of flat or negative T in the course of NSTEACS correspond to ACS with a better prognosis than when ST depression is present. In these cases the patient no longer feels pain, but this does not indicate that the artery will present important subocclusion, but still remains at least partially open, or with great collateral circulation (Fig. 9.25).

It is exceptional that a positive T changes to a clear negative T due to acute ischemia during a stress test. However, in some circumstances (i.e. hyperventilation) a flat/negative T wave may appear (false-positive) (Fig. 4.25). What is almost always observed during exercise testing, as a pathologic ECG criterion suggestive of ischemia, is that an ST depression appears that may pull down the positive T wave. In rare cases a peaked T wave may be recorded as an abnormal response.

Summary of ecg changes (QRS-ST-T) in patients with ischemic heart disease due to coron ary athe rot hrom bosis and narrow QRS

A. Acute phase
  1. **Changes in the T wave**
    1.1 High, peaked, and symmetrical T wave: hyperacute phase of STEACS (acute ischemia). Occasionally, it may last more time and then may be accompanied also of ST depression.
    1.2 Negative T wave
      – **Deep (≥3–4 mm) and symmetrical**
        ○ In case of Q-wave MI: left intraventricular pattern that appears in the evolutive phase of Q-wave infarction (electric window effect) (fig. 9.30)
        ○ Post-reperfusion: usually with rS pattern in case of LAD occlusion: a) Evolutive phase of STEACS with the artery at least partially open (fig. 9.17), spontaneously of after drug treatment; b) post PCI or fibrinolysis ; and c) post coronary spasm (fig. 9.52).
      – **Flat or slightly negative (< 2.5mm)** (fig. 9.25 to 9.27)
        ○ The evolutive phase of NSTEACS in general without pain: usually with R or RS pattern; may correspond to a reperfusion pattern and in the presence of angina may evolve to ST depression.
  2. **ST changes**
    2.1. ST elevation: Atypical sign of STEACS that without treatment tends to develop into Q-wave MI in a matter of hours.
      We must remember that there are mirror ECG patterns (LCX occlusion), that may mimick an SCASEST, and are atypical ECG patterns of STEML

If the ST elevation persists in subacute phase of STEACS, is a marker for possible rupture.

An ST elevation in VR and often in V1 is seen in NSTEACS.

2.2. ST depression with horizontal or descending slope: Typical sign of NSTEACS.

Often appears during anginal pain in a patient with normal basal ECG or with flat T wave or even with some ST depression. It may remain after the acute is chemia (pain) has passed. InVl-V3 may represent equivalent pattern of STEACS (LCX occlusion)

B. Chronic phase.

1. Q wave. STEACS evolves to Q-wave MI, starting in the subacute phase with often transmural invol vement.

2. Fragmented QRS. Appears in basal infarctions in particular.Often coexist with Q-**wave**

3. Repolarization abnormalities:

  – **Elevated ST** (rule out aneurysms) or **depressed ST** (residual pattern)

  – **Negative T:**

  a) **deep:** residual pattern in STEACS that is reperfused or is present in case of chronic Q-wave ML

  b) **flat or slightly negative:** Is seen in case of STEACS with Q-wave MI in certain leads, often co-existing with deep negative T waves in other leads.

In NSTEACS flat/mild negative T wave, may also be seen as a residual pattern in some leads.

  – **Symmetrical positive T:** In V1-V2, especially as a mirror image of chronic lateral infarction.

Self-assessment

A. What are the clinical settings due to decreased blood flow in patients with atherothrombosis-associated coronary occlusion?

B. What is the clinical setting of increased blood demand?

C. Describe the evolutive ECG changes in STEACS.

D. What is the electrophysiologic mechanism that explains the presence of high, peaked T wave of subendocardial ischemia appearing in the initial phase of STEACS?

E. How does ST segment elevation appearing after the high T wave in ACS-STE occur?

F. What are the characteristics of ST elevation in STEACS?

G. What is the significance of ST elevation characteristics in evaluating extension and intensity of the ischemia?

H. What are the mirror patterns of ST in STEACS and why are they relevant?

I. What are the atypical ECG patterns (without ST elevation) seen in the course of STEACS and

what is the electrophysiologic mechanism involved?

J. What is the differential diagnosis of high, peaked T wave of subendocardial ischemia?

K. What is the differential diagnosis of ischemic ST elevation?

L. Describe the ECG presented by patients with NSTEACS.

M. What is the electrophysiologic mechanism that explains the ST depression in NSTEACS?

N. What are the ECG criteria for ST depression due to ischemia?

O. What are the two ECG patterns with ST depression seen in NSTEACS?

P. Under what circumstances is a flat or negative T wave seen in STEACS?

Q. How is the differential diagnosis for ST depression made?

R. How is the differential diagnosis for a negative T wave in NSTEACS made?

S. What is the Q wave of necrosis and how does it originate?

T. How is the Q wave of necrosis diagnosed?

U. What is the correlation between the Q wave of necrosis and the infarction zone of LV?

V. Why is the prominent R in V1 explained by lateral infarction but not posterior infarction?

W. What is the differential diagnosis of Q wave of necrosis in infarction?

X. What is a fractionated QRS?

Y. How many types of infarction without Q wave exist?

ZA. How is myocardial ischemia in the presence of factors of confusion (branch block, LVH, etc.) manifested?

ZB. What are the most typical ECG disturbances presented in myocardial ischemia not due to atherothrombosis (coronary spasm, Takotsubo syndrome, X syndrome, etc.)?

ZC. What is the most frequent ECG presentation in myocardial ischemia due to increased blood demand?

ZD. List the most frequent arrhythmias observed in the IHD.

ZE. What is the relevance of a flat or negative T wave in IHD?

PART III
The ECG in Arrhythmias

In this third part, we review in Chapter 10 the basic concepts of arrhythmias, which aid in the understanding of how different arrhythmias originate.

Later, in Chapters 11, 12, and 13 we explain the most relevant surface ECG patterns that allow the active supraventricular and ventricular arrhythmias and passive arrhythmias to be diagnosed. We also briefly outline the ECG patterns of pacemakers.

Lastly, Chapter 14 contains a short summary of the above with the aim of outlining the best approach when interpreting a tracing showing arrhythmia.

We hope the reader is able to learn all of the above well enough to easily interpret arrhythmias in the ECG in the future. Please also consult the references.

ECGs for Beginners, First Edition. Antoni Bayés de Luna.
© 2014 John Wiley & Sons, Inc. Published 2014 by John Wiley & Sons, Inc.

CHAPTER 10

Concepts, Classification, and Mechanisms of Arrhythmias

A **10.1. Concepts**

Any cardiac rhythm that is not normal sinus rhythm is considered an arrhythmia (see Section 4.2.1 in Chapter 4).

The ECG is the gold standard pattern in the diagnosis of arrhythmias.

B **10.2. Classification and mechanisms: preliminary aspects**

Arrhythmias may be active or passive.

A. Active arrhythmias appear before the basal rhythm. These are due to:

  1. Anomalous origin of stimuli:

   (a) Increased automatism: ectopic focus extrasystoles and parasystoles;

   (b) Triggered electrical activity: after potentials.

  2. Reentry:

   (a) Classical: Anatomic reentry. This requires the following: (1) the presence of an anatomic circuit; (2) the presence of a unidirectional block; and (3) adequate conduction velocity. The circuit may be microscopic or macroscopic (see later).

   (b) Many arrhythmias may originate through a functional reentry (heterogene-

ous dispersion of repolarization, rotors, etc) (see later).

B. Passive arrhythmias appear in substitution of the basal rhythm. They are due to:

  1. Decrease in automatism;

  2. Decrease in conduction: blocks.

Each of these aspects will be discussed in this chapter.

10.3. Previous considerations

There are some previous considerations that must be taken in to account before examining an ECG tracing with an arrhythmia.

1. Both a magnifying glass and a compass are useful.

2. A long recording of 12-lead ECG is needed.

3. In paroxysmal tachycardia the ECG recording must be made during carotid sinus massage (Fig. 10.1). C

4. The clinical history of the patient is needed and the patient must be questioned about any characteristics relevant to the suspected arrhythmia.

5. Tests results performed to the patient (e.g. stress test, Holter, Tilt test) should also be reviewed.

6. The secret to an accurate diagnosis is determining the atrial and ventricular activity and finding the AV relationship. **Lewis diagrams** are very useful for this purpose (Fig. 10.2).

ECGs for Beginners, First Edition. Antoni Bayés de Luna.
© 2014 John Wiley & Sons, Inc. Published 2014 by John Wiley & Sons, Inc.

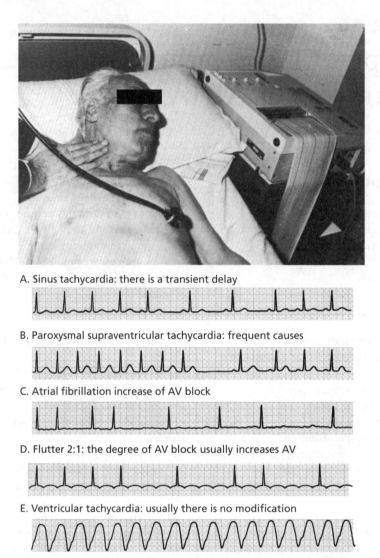

A. Sinus tachycardia: there is a transient delay

B. Paroxysmal supraventricular tachycardia: frequent causes

C. Atrial fibrillation increase of AV block

D. Flutter 2:1: the degree of AV block usually increases AV

E. Ventricular tachycardia: usually there is no modification

Figure 10.1 Note the correct procedure for carotid sinus massage (CSM). The force applied with the fingers should be similar to that required to squeeze a tennis ball, during a short time period (10–15 s) and the procedure should be repeated four to five times on either side, starting on the right side. Never perform this procedure on both sides at the same time. Caution should be taken in older people and in patients with a history of carotid sinus syndrome. The procedure must include continuous ECG recording and auscultation. (A–E) examples of how different arrhythmias react to CSM.

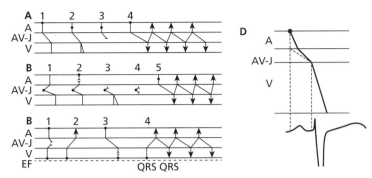

Figure 10.2 (A) 1: Normal atrioventriclar (AV) conduction; (2) premature atrial impulse (complex) with aberrant conduction; (3) premature atrial impulse blocked at the AV junction; (4) sinus impulse with slow AV conduction that initiates an AV junctional reentrant tachycardia. (B) (1) Premature junctional impulse with an anterograde conduction slower than the retrograde; (2) premature junctional impulse sharing atrial depolarization with a sinus impulse (atrial fusion complex); (3) premature junctional impulse with exclusive anterograde conduction and, in this case, with aberrancy (see the two lines in the ventricular space); (4) premature junctional impulse concealed anterogradely and retrogradely; (5) premature atrial impulse leading to AV junctional reentrant tachycardia. (C) (1) sinus impulse and premature ventricular impulse that cancel mutually at the AV junction; (2) premature ventricular impulse with retrograde conduction to the atria; (3) sinus impulse sharing ventricular depolarization with a premature ventricular impulse (ventricular fusion beat); (4) premature ventricular impulse triggering an AV junctional reentrant tachycardia. (D) Shows the path of the stimulus through the AV junction as per the diagram shown in the figure. The solid line shows the real path of the stimulus across the heart. In general the dashed line is used instead, because it is the place at which the atrial and ventricular activity starts. Thus, the time that the stimulus spends to cross the AV junction, the most important information, is more visible. EF: ectopic focus.

10.4. Response to carotid sinus massage (CSM) (Fig. 10.1)

This must be carried out on one side only using auscultation and an ECG. Figure 10.1 shows how to perform that and the responses in different tachycardias.

10.5 Lewis diagrams

These diagrams demonstrate the pathway of the electrical stimulus in sinus rhythm and specific active and passive arrhythmias. Figure 10.2 shows
C how to obtain Lewis diagrams in sinus rhythm (D) and in different active, atrial (A), junctional (B) and ventricular, arrhythmias (C). Throughout this book we will see the usefulness of Lewis diagrams in these active arrhythmias as well as passive arrhythmias (Chapters 11–13).

10.6. The mechanism of active arrhythmia (Bayés De Luna, 2011)

10.6.1. Increased automaticity

They are early impulses that appear before the basal rhythm and are originated in a supraventricular or ventricular extrasystolic or parasystolic focus. May be isolated (extrasystoles and parasystoles) or repetitive (automatic atrial and ventricular tachycardias, or triggers of reentrant supraventricular tachycardias and atrial or ventricular flutter and fibrillation).

Extrasystoles are related to the preceding impulse and thus have a fixed coupling interval. The focus in which the extrasystole originates remains depolarized after each impulse of the basal rhythm because this area is not protected by an entry block, as happens with parasystoles. As a result, a new stimulus may arise depolarizing the neighboring myocardium before

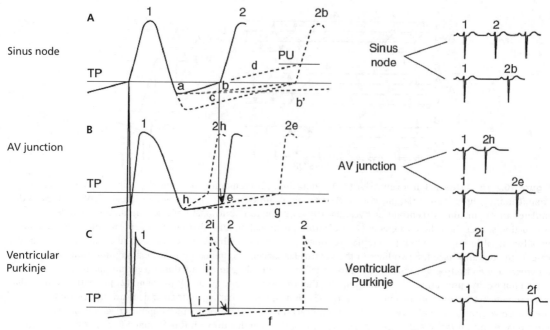

Figure 10.3 Left: see the lines joining the TAPs of the sinus node, the AV junction, and the ventricular Purkinje system. This figure shows the generation of active and passive arrhythmias due to disturbances of automaticity: (a) normal diastolic depolarization curve of the sinus node; (b) diminished diastolic depolarization curve; (c) diastolic depolarization curve of sinus node with normal rate of rise but starting at a lower level; (d) normal diastolic depolarization curve with a less negative TP; (e) normal diastolic depolarization curve of the AV junction; note that before this curve is complete (i.e. before it reaches the TP), the sinus stimulus (arrow) initiates a new AP (end of the continuous line in '3'); (f) normal diastolic depolarization curve of a ventricular Purkinje fiber (the same as in 'e' applies); (g) marked decrease of the automaticity of the AV junction; (h) increase of automaticity of the AV junction; (i) increased automaticity in ventricular Purkinje fibers. Therefore, under pathologic conditions, the increased automaticity of the AV junction (h) and the ventricular Purkinje system (i) may be greater than that of the sinus node (active rhythms). Alternatively, the normal automaticity of the AV junction (broken lines in 'e' and 'g') or the ventricle (broken line in 'f') may substitute the sinus depressed automaticity (b and b') (passive rhythms). **Right:** ECG examples of the different electrophysiologic situations commented on (normal sinus rhythm: 1-2; sinus bradycardia:1-2b; junctional extrasystole: 1-2h; junctional escape complex 1-2e; ventricular extrasystole: 1-2i and ventricular escape complex: 1-2f).

the next stimulus of the basal rhythm arrives. This explains the fixed coupling interval (Fig.10.3). **By contrast, parasystoles have a variable coupling interval**, because the focus automaticity is independent of the preceding impulse (see later) (Fig 10.4).

A. Extrasystolic impulses

D   The ectopic, atrial, AV junction, or ventricular foci present a sharper increase in phase 4 (TDP), which explains why the threshold potential is reached earlier originating an early impulse before the next basal stimulus can depolarize the ectopic foci. The fact that the coupling interval of successive extrasystoles is fixed is explained because the increase in the speed of phase 4 in all cases is related to the preceding impulse (Fig. 10.3h and 10.3i).

• Figure 10.3 explains the active arrhythmias (extrasystole) and passive (escapes) that are produced due to the different changes in the slope of the curve of phase 4 of the sinus node or the ectopic foci.

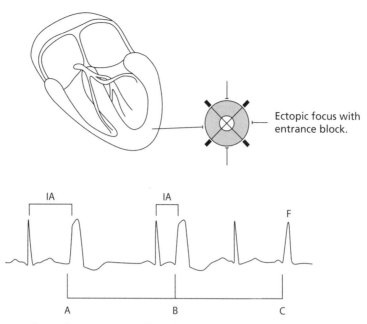

Figure 10.4 The parasystolic mechanism is generally explained by an entry block in the ectopic focus. The central point represents the parasystolic focus, surrounded by an area with an entry block (shaded area). Parasystolic stimuli may be conducted out of this zone but external stimuli cannot get into it. Usually, some degree of exit block also exists. Bottom: Scheme of parasystolic ventricular premature complexes with the characteristic three electrocardiographic features: variable coupling interval, multiple interectopic intervals and fusion complexes (see Chapter 12).

• Meanwhile, automatism of the ectopic focus, which is subthreshold, may originate an early impulse with a fixed coupling interval if it coincides with the supernormal excitability phase that occurs at the end of TAP.

• Approximately 10% of supraventricular tachycardias (Figs 11.4, 11.5, 11.9 and 11.10) are due to increased repetitive automatism of an ectopic focus. Lastly, it has been recently demonstrated that most paroxysmal atrial fibrillations are due to an atrial automatic focus (Fig. 11.15B).

B. Parasystolic impulses

E Parasystolic impulses are not related to the preceding complexes and thus have a variable coupling interval. Furthermore, they present an entry block that prevents it from being depolarized by the basal rhythm that is usually sinus rhythm (Fig. 10.4 above).

• When the parasystolic impulses find the surrounding tissue outside the refractory period, **an** ectopic complex with a variable coupling interval is recorded and **fusion complexes** often appear. Due to the independence of the basal rhythm the parasystolic impulses are multiple among themselves.

• Figure 10.4 shows the criteria of parasystoles previously described and Figure 12.3 shows a perfect example of ventricular parasystoles.

10.6.2. Triggered activity

In this case there is an abnormal capacity to originate stimuli in phase 3 of the TAP or at its end, producing the early or late (A, B, C) or (D and E) post potentials. These post potentials can initiate a propagated response with a fixed coupling interval (Fig. 10.5).

10.6.3. Reentry phenomena   F

Explain isolated impulses of extrasystolic origin and are the triggers of repetitive tachycardias.

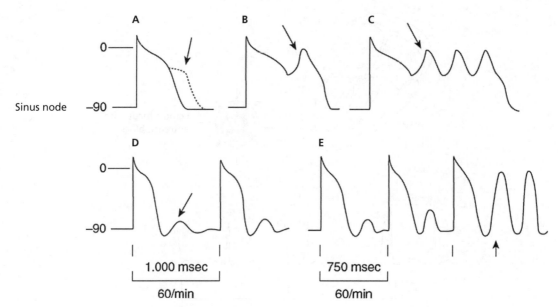

Figure 10.5 The presence of early (A-C) and late (D and E) post-potentials is the mechanism that explains the occurrence of early stimuli (complexes) caused by triggered activity.

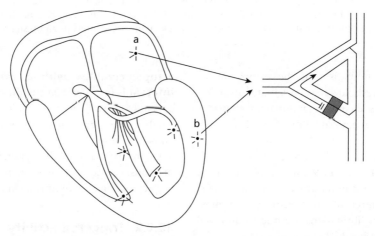

Figure 10.6 Circuits located in the Purkinje-atrial muscle junction (a) and Purkinje-ventricular muscle junction (b) (micro-reentry). These circuits show the formation of atrial or ventricular extrasystoles with a fixed coupling interval (see Section 10.6.3.1).

10.6.3.1. Classical reentry

This mechanism consists of a determinate circuit; in the case of extrasystoles, an atrial or ventricular microcircuit is formed, for example, by the junction of three or more cardiac cells, and the preceding stimulus can, at the moment of depolarization of this circuit, originate a new impulse. Because this new impulse is related to the preceding one, it has a fixed coupling interval.

The conditions necessary for a classical reentry are listed below (Moe & Méndez, 1966) (Figs 10.6 and 10.7).

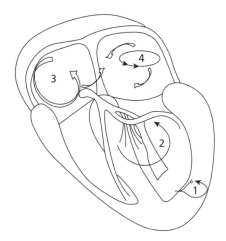

1: see Fig. 12.8 and 12.9
2: see Fig. 12.10A
3: see Fig. 11.17 – 11.19
4: see Fig. 11.21

Figure 10.7 Example of a circuit located in a necrotic area of the ventricle (1), or of a circuit involving the left specific intraventricular system (2), or the atria (3) flutter, or (4) macro-reentrant tachycardia (see Chapter 11).

1. There must be a circuit in which the reentrant stimulus can circulate. Generally, in isolated impulses, this is a microcircuit, as previously mentioned.
2. There must be a unidirectional block zone in some part of this circuit.
3. The conduction speed in the circuit must be appropriate, neither too fast, because in this case the stimulus would block in some part of the circuit that would still be in the refractory period, or too slow, because here the next sinus stimulus would have already depolarized the circuit.

Microreentrant circuit
Figure 10.6 shows how an atrial or ventricular extrasystole is originated in a microreentrant mechanism.

The sinus stimulus (SS) (1) reaches the focus where the microcircuit is located. It passes easily to pathway 3, but is blocked in pathway 2 where a unidirectional block exists. Sinus stimulus from pathway 3 passes to two sides of the circuit (4) to stimulate the rest of the myocardium. However, upon reaching the opposite part of the unidirectional block in pathway 2, the sinus stimulus crosses it and reenters through pathway 3 to originate a new impulse, which is an atrial extrasystole if the circuit is atrial, and ventricular extrasystolic if the circuit is ventricular.

If this phenomenon is repeated, an atrial, junctional or ventricular tachycardia, depending on the location of the microcircuit, occurs instead of an isolated extrasystole.

From a clinical point of view, most extrasystoles are of microreentrant origin (see above). Microreentrant extrasystole is also a mechanism that may trigger some types of atrial and ventricular fibrillation (Chapters 11 and 12).

Macroreentrant circuits
These circuits originate different types of arrhythmia that are described below.
1. Ventricular circuits: Originate ventricular tachycardia (VT) in macrocircuits located in the ventricles surrounding scar tissue (postinfarction VT) (Fig. 10.7-1) or between two branches of the specific conduction system (branch–branch reentry) (VT branch–branch) (Fig. 10.7-2). The latter are difficult to diagnose using surface ECG because they resemble LBBB.
2. Atrial circuits (Figs 10.7-3 and 4, and 10.8): Macroreentry at the atrial level explains atrial flutter, and macroreentrant atrial tachycardia, which may be considered atypical flutter, (see later).
• **Atrial flutter:** Figure 10.8 shows the reentry circuits explaining the appearance of **common atrial flutter:** right atrial circuit with anticlockwise conduction (A), and **uncommon or**

reverse flutter, which is an atrial circuit with clockwise conduction in the right atria (B). The same figure shows the most common ECG patterns in leads II and V1 in both types of flutter. **In common flutter**, in leads II, III, and VF there is clearly no isoelectric line between the waves (Fig. 11.17) (see lesson 11).

• Like all arrhythmias caused by reentry, flutter is triggered by an atrial extrasystole that finds an area of the circuit in the refractory period and triggers, in the two most common types of atrial flutter, the macroreentrant mechanism, shown in Figure 10.8A and B. Other types of atypical flutter may exist (Garcia Cosio et al., 1990). Figs 10.8C and 11.21 show an example of atypical flutter arising in left atria.

• **Atrial tachycardias caused by atrial macroreentry** present isoelectric lines between the waves in leads II, III, and VF. **They differ from atypical flutter** mainly in the rate of the atrial waves (>200–220 bpm is considered atypical flutter). The mechanism is a macroreentry located around an atrial circuit that is often related to post-surgery or ablation scarring (Fig. 10.7-4).

3. Reentrant circuits of the AV junction: these originate the reentrant tachycardia of the AV junction (JRT):

• **The most frequent are the paroxysmal.** Rarely, they are **permanent or repetitive**. These infrequent cases, start with a critical shortening of the sinus RR interval and originate a reciprocating tachycardia using an accessory pathway with slow retrograde conduction. For this reason they are referred to as **fast–slow** (the stimulus goes fast from the atria to the ventricles through the AV junction and goes from the ventricles to the atria through a slow accessory pathway) ($RP' > P'R$) (Farré et al., 1979) (Fig. 11.8).

• **Paroxysmal tachycardia caused by reentry.** In paroxysmal tachycardia, the AV junction is involved in the circuit (80% of supraventricular paroxysmal tachycardia with narrow QRS) and a slow–fast type conduction occurs ($RP' < P'R$) (Figs 10.9, 11.6, and 11.7).

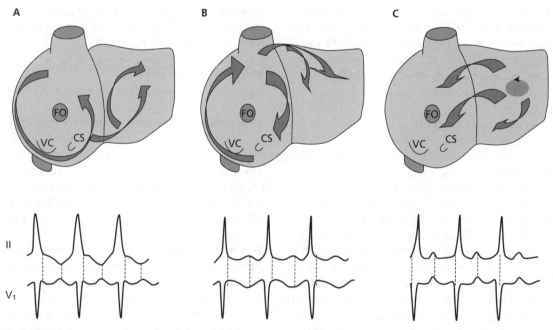

Figure 10.8 Circuits explaining the presence of common flutter with counterclockwise rotation (A); non-common (reverse) flutter with clockwise rotation (B); and one case of atypical flutter arising in the left atrium (C). (See Plate 10.8.)

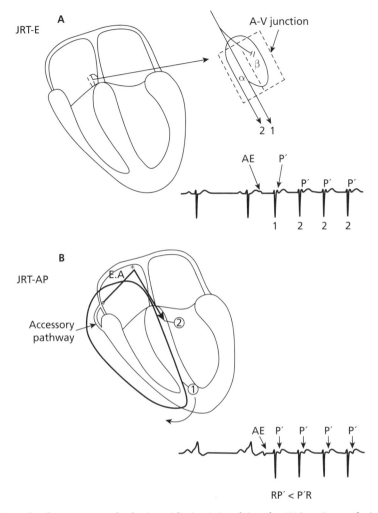

Figure 10.9 (A) Example of re-entrant arrhythmias with circuit involving the AV junction exclusively (JRT-E) (A) or also involving an accessory pathway (JRT-AP) (B). In the first case (A), the premature atrial extrasystole (AE), which does not undergo anterograde conduction on the β pathway is conducted with longer P′R, only through the α pathway (slow conduction),but with fast atrial retrograde activation (P′), which may be concealed within or at the end of the QRS complex (it may mimic an r′ or S wave). In the second case (B) the circuit has the following composition: His-Purkinje system–ventricular muscle–accessory pathway–atrial muscle–His–Purkinje system. An atrial extrasystole (AE) is blocked in the accessory pathway that shows a unidirectional block, thus being conducted through the normal pathway. Consequently, the resulting complex (1) does not show a delta wave. This impulse reenters retrogradely over the accessory pathway, activates the atria, and initiates a re-entrant tachycardia with narrow QRS complexes (2) (without delta wave). In this case, the premature atrial beat is conducted with shorter P′R than in the case of JRT-E (see A), and due to longer retrograde conduction over the accessory pathway, the P′ is recorded close but at a short distance from the QRS (RP′ < P′R).

The circuit may be exclusively in the AV junction (Fig. 10.9A) **or it may participate in the same an accessory pathway** (Fig. 10.9B). Therefore, the paroxysmal tachycardias may present a circuit **exclusively in the AV junction (junction reentrant paroxysmal tachycardia-exclusive) (JRT-E) or in the AV junction with an accessory pathway (JRT-AP)**. In English literature the reentrant tachycardias of AV junction exclusively are usually named AVNRT, and the ones with participation of an accessory pathway, AVRT. We prefer JRT-E and JRT-AP as they are named in this book; however both terms may be used. Figure 10.9 shows the mechanism involved in establishing both cases of tachycardia triggered by an atrial extrasystole (AE) that find the beta pathway of the AV node (Fig. 1.3C) or the accessory pathway in the refractory period, which allow the reentrant tachycardia to start, as seen in the figure diagrams (Fig. 10.9).

Note how in JPT-AP the P′ is somewhat separated from QRS but with RP′ < P′R (slow–fast), while in JPT-E, P′ is hidden or attached to QRS, and is not visible. This is due to the fact that the retrograde conduction through the accessory pathway is longer than in case of JPT-E (Figs 10.9, 11.6, and 11.7).

10.6.3.2. Other forms of reentry

They are many other types (Bayés de Luna, 2011). We only describe the following:
• **Rotors theory.** The rotor is a spiral wave that when it has a high-frequency, may be one of the mechanisms that may explain atrial and ventricular fibrillation (Fig. 10.10).
• **Heterogeneous dispersion of repolarization (HDR).** There are also reentrant tachycardias pro-duced by heterogeneous distribution of repolarization (HDR) that originates a voltage gradient between two ventricular zones. One of these has a longer TAP, and the other has a shorter TAP and/or different morphology, producing a reentry at the beginning of phase 2 of the TAP that triggers VF (Fig. 10.11). HDR explains ventricular arrhythmias (VF) that induce sudden death in cases of inherited heart disease (long and short QT syndrome and Brugada syndrome) (Fig. 10.11) (see Chapter 16).

10.6.4. The mechanism of atrial fibrillation (Fig. 10.12)

Atrial fibrillation (AF) may be explained by three mechanisms: **(a) multiple reentries in the atria; (b) ectopic focus located in the pulmonary veins with fibrillatory conduction** (the most common mechanism in paroxysmal AF); and **(c) a high frequency rotor (energy source)** initiated by an atrial extrasystole.

10.6.5. The mechanism of ventricular fibrillation (Figs 10.10 and 10.11)

Ventricular fibrillation (VF) usually begins due to a ventricular impulse (generally extrasystole) that originates **multiple reentries** as in AF. Recently, it has been suggested that **VF is caused by a spiral wave (rotor)** (Fig. 10.10) that conducts in a meandering pattern (B) and results in chaotic conduction and finally fibrillatory conduction (C and D). It may also trigger VT or VF; a heterogeneous dispersion of repolarization (Fig. 10.11 and Section 10.6.3.2).

VF is often preceded by VT or ventricular flutter. Ventricular flutter may also be considered very fast VT (250–300 bpm) showing only repetitive QRS complexes without visible repolarization waves.

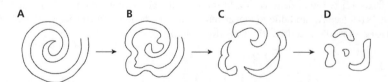

Figure 10.10 Here we see how a spiral wave (rotor) (A) is disrupted and turned into a meandering (B), and later increasingly chaotic conduction until it completely breaks up, resulting in a fibrillatory conduction (C and D).

Reentry due to hetereogeneous dispersion of repolarization (phase 2)*

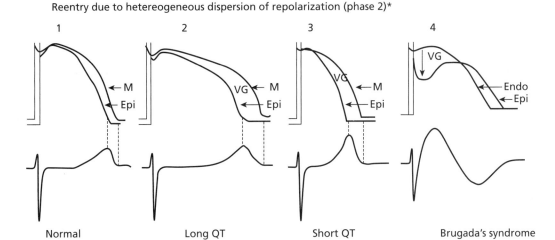

*According to Antzelevitch at transmural level

Figure 10.11 Example of phase 2 reentry due to heterogeneous dispersion of repolarization (HDR). According to Antzelevitch, dispersion takes place at a transmural level and the AP of M cells is the longest compared with the AP of the rest of the wall areas. This HDR produces a ventricular gradient (VG) between the areas with longer AP and the area with shortest AP and accounts for the possible occurrence of VT/VF in patients with long QT syndrome (2) and short QT syndrome (3). In the Brugada syndrome (4) the HDR takes places between the endocardium and the epicardium of the RV at the beginning of phase 2 (VG), because of the transient predominance of outward I_{to} current. Epi: Epicardium; M: M cells.

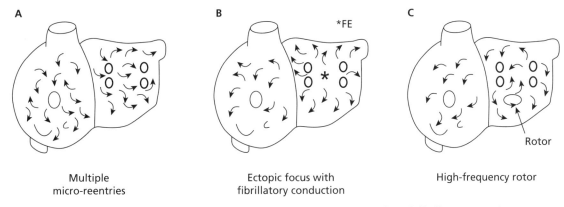

Figure 10.12 The three mechanisms dealing with the onset and perpetuation of atrial fibrillation. (A) Micro-reentry located in an ectopic focus induces multiple reentries (classical concepts). (B) Ectopic focus (EF) with increased automaticity (pulmonary veins) (asterisk) and fibrillatory conduction. (C) Atrial extrasystole located in an ectopic focus initiates a high-frequency rotor that perpetuates the arrhythmia with fibrillatory conduction.

10.7. Mechanisms of passive arrhythmias

These include decreased automaticity, classical block at the sinoatrial and atrioventricular level, and the concepts of conduction aberrancy and concealed conduction. Block at the atrial and ventricular level is described in Chapters 5 and 7.

10.7.1. Decreased automaticity

These are cases of bradycardia due to reduced sinus node discharge (sinus bradycardia) (Fig. 10.3 and Chapter 13). Rarely, sinus bradycardia is produced by active associated arrhythmia, as does the presence of concealed ventricular extrasystoles that depolarize the sinus node and change its cadence (Section 13.2 in Chapter 13).

10.7.2. Heart block

L   As explained in Chapter 5, this refers to any difficulty in carrying the stimulus to any area of the heart. Classical heart block may take place in the sinoatrial junction, the atria (Chapter 5), the AV junction, and in the ventricles (Chapter 7). They may be first-degree (the stimulus passes slowly), third-degree (completely blocked stimulus), and second-degree (the stimulus, whether in presence of normal conduction or first-degree block) sometimes passes and sometimes not. We will now explain **heart block at the sinoatrial and atrioventricular level** (AV block).

We will also discuss the concepts of aberrancy at the ventricular, and less often atrial level, as well as the concealed conduction concept in patients with some conduction disturbances in the heart. We must remember that reentry (active arrhythmia) always involves a unidirectional block in some area of the heart (Fig. 10.6).

10.7.2.1. Sinoatrial block (Fig. 10.13)

In this case the stimulus block occurs between the
M   sinus node and the atria. Like atrial and ventricular block, first- (A), second- (B), or third-degree (C) sinoatrial block may exist. Second-grade sinoatrial and also atrioventricular block may be classified into two types: (1) the block is progressive, Wenckebach- or Mobitz 1-type block; or (2) abrupt, Mobitz 2-type

block. Figure 10.13 shows the different types of sinoatrial block (Chapter 13 and Fig. 13.3).

10.7.2.2. AV block (Fig. 10.14)

This type of block takes place in the AV junction. Figure 10.4 shows the different types of AV   N block that may also be first-, second-, or third-degree. To define the exact location of the block (supra, infra, or intrahisian) the HISIAN deflection must be recorded using intracavitary methods (Chapter 13) and Figure 13.4.

10.7.3. Conduction aberrancy

This is the abnormal and transitory distribution of a supraventricular impulse through the ventricles   O (Singer and Ten Eick, 1971; Rosenbaum, 1973) or atria. We will focus on ventricular conduction aberrancy. Chapter 5 mentions atrial aberrancy (abrupt and transitory changes in the P morphology that meet the criteria for intermittent atrial block, although it requires a differential diagnosis with other processes such as escape and fusion complexes, artifacts, etc).

Ventricular aberrancy: usually presents as aberrancy of the early complexes (EC) (phase 3 aberrancy) when there is a short coupling interval (CI) and the EC falls in the refractory period of one branch (the longest under normal conditions is the right branch). Therefore, the E′ complex in Figure 10.15 (B) will be blocked, and the E complex in (A) not. Aberrancy is also related to the preceding diastole, because the longest diastoles are followed by longest TAPs. As a result, there are more chances of aberrancy when an early complex has a short coupling interval and a long preceding diastole (**Gouaux–Ashman criteria**). Figure 10.15C shows how both E and E′ complexes presents aberrancy in this situation.

In the presence of atrial fibrillation (AF), the Gouaux-Ashman criteria are not useful because many f waves penetrate the AV junction to some degree and change the refractory period. However, the QRS morphology helps to distinguish between aberrancy and ectopy in cases of early complexes in AF (as well as sinus rhythm). If the morphology in V1 is ⩗ it indicates aberrancy, and if it is ⩘ it favors ectopy. The morphology in V6 is also useful. If is ⩗ it favors ectopy and if is ⩘ aberrancy (Fig. 10.16).

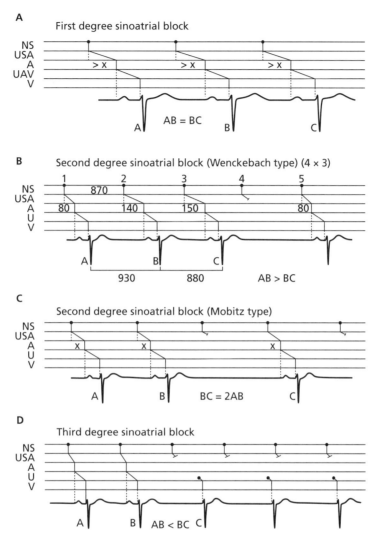

Figure 10.13 (A) First-degree sinoatrial block. The sinoatrial conduction is consistently slowed down (>x), but this does not translate onto the surface ECG (x = normal sinoatrial conduction time). (B) Second-degree sinoatrial block (Wenckebach type, 4 × 3). The sinoatrial conduction time progressively increases from normal (80 ms) to absolute block (80 = x, x + 60, x + 70) and block. The distance between the first two RR (930 ms) is greater than that between the second and the third RR (880 ms). The sinoatrial conduction cannot be determined. However, considering that distances 1-2, 2-3, 3-4, and 4-5 are the same and assuming that the sinus rhythm cadence is 870 ms, 1, 2, 3, 4, and 5 theoretically represent the origin of the sinus impulses. Therefore, as we have assumed that the first sinoatrial conduction time of the sequence is 80 ms, the successive increases in the sinoatrial conduction which explain the shortening of RR duration and the subsequent pause should be 80 + 60 (140) and 140 + 10 (150). Thus, it is explained that in Wenckebach sinoatrial block the greatest increase occurs in the first cycle of each sequence, after reach pause (AB > BC). The PR intervals are constant. The second RR interval is 50 ms shorter, since this is the difference between the increases of sinoatrial conduction between the first and the second RR cycles. Actually, the first RR cycle equals 870 + 60 = 930 ms, while in the second cycle it equals 930–50 (50 is the difference between the first increment 60 and the second one 10) = 880 ms. (C) Second-degree sinoatrial block (Mobitz type). Sinoatrial conduction (normal or slowed down) is constant (x) before the stimulus is completely blocked (BC = 2AB). (D) Third-degree sinoatrial block. An escape rhythm appears (in this case, in the AV junction) with no visible P waves in the ECG (AB < BC). The escape rhythm may retrogradely activate the atria (not seen in the scheme).

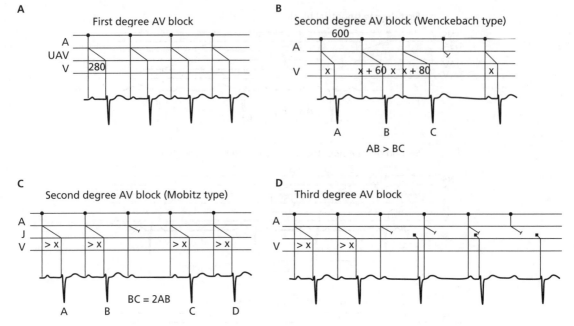

Figure 10.14 (A) First-degree AV block. The PR interval is always prolonged (>200 ms); (B) second degree AV block 4 × 3 (Wenckebach type). The criterion AB > BC also applies in this case (see text and Fig. 13.4); (C) second-degree AV block (Mobitz type) (BC = 2AB); (D) third-degree AV block. A clear AV dissociation may be seen. After two conducted QRS complexes there is a pause, followed by escape QRS rhythm (at slow rate) dissociated from P waves. In this case the QRS complexes are junctional (narrow).

Delayed complexes (**phase 4 aberrancy**) may also present aberrancy (see Bayés de Luna, 2011 and 2012a).

The ventricular aberrancy may also be repetitive and occurring in sinus rhythm related to tachycardization, or the bradycardization of sinus rhythm or even without changes in heart rate. These cases constitute the second degree BBB (Figs 7.9 and 7.19), and have been already commented on in Chapter 7. There are also supraventricular tachycardias or escape rhythms with aberrancy (Figs 12.10B and 13.1).

10.7.4. Concealed conduction

Occasionally, a structure (e.g. the AV junction) remains partially depolarized by a stimulus that does not finish crossing it. This partial depolarization is unseen in surface ECGs, but modifies the next stimulus. For example, a ventricular extrasystole partially conducted in the AV junction lengthens the conduction (PR interval) of the next sinus stimulus (Fig. 10.14). The presence of unexpected wide or narrow QRS in AF may be explained by different degrees of concealed conduction in previous 'f' waves (Bayés de Luna, 2011 and 2012a).

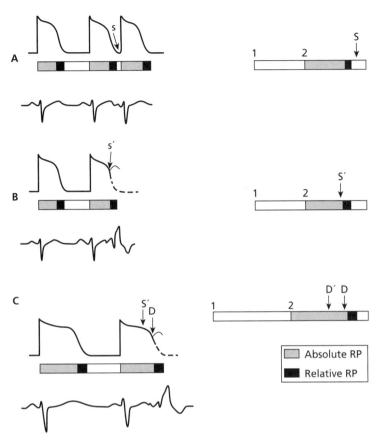

Figure 10.15 (A), (B) and (C). In each case the TAP of right bundle branch (RBB), length of absolute and relative refractory period (RP) of RBB, and the surface ECG in three different situations of one premature atrial stimulus (S). The premature stimulus E does not present aberrant conduction because it falls outside the refractory period of the right bundle branch (RBB). (B) However, the stimulus E′ that is earlier is conducted with RBBB aberrancy because it falls within the ARP of the RBB. (C) In C as the previous RR the interval is longer, the following TAP of RBB is also longer, and consequently both stimuli D and D′ are conducted with aberrancy because they fall in the ARP of the right branch.

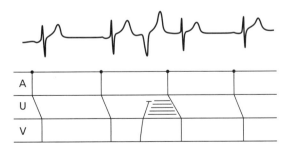

Figure 10.16 Interpolated ventricular extrasystole. The following P wave is conducted with a longer PR due to the concealed conduction of the ventricular extrasystole at the AV junction.

Self-assessment

A. Describe the concept of arrhythmia.

B. Remember the classification of arrhythmias.

C. Remember the Lewis diagrams.

D. What are the mechanisms of extrasystole with fixed coupling intervals and regular tachycardias?

E. What is a parasystole?

F. Explain the classical reentry phenomenon.

G. How many types of macroreentrant circuits exist?

H. What is the mechanism of atrial flutter?

I. What is the mechanism of re-entrant tachycardia of the AV junction?

J. What is the mechanism of atrial fibrillation?

K. What is the mechanism of ventricular fibrillation?

L. Explain the concept of heart block.

M. How many types of atrioventricular block exist?

N. How many types of sinoatrial block exist?

O. What is ventricular aberrancy?

CHAPTER 11

ECG Patterns of Supraventricular Arrhythmias

In this chapter we describe the ECG characteristics of supraventricular arrhythmias. Their mechanisms have been explained in Chapter 10.

A

11.1. Premature complexes (Fig. 11.1)

These are early complexes, usually extrasystoles (atrial paraxystole are very rare – see Bayés de Luna, 2011) due to atrial microreentry (Fig. 10.5). They may be conducted to the ventricles normally or with aberrancy, or be concealed in the AV junction. They may present normal or aberrant morphology (Fig. 11.1 A-C).

It is important to make a differential diag-
B **nosis between aberrancy and ectopy in cases of wide premature QRS.** Table 11.1 lists the ECG criteria for each condition (see Chapter 10).

11.2. Sinus tachycardia
(Figs 11.2 and 11.3)

Sinus tachycardia (ST) occurs when the sinus rate automaticity exceeds 90 to 100 x′. Very rarely the mechanism is sinoatrial reentry. ST may be seen in patients with spontaneous or induced sympathetic overdrive and associated with many processes (e.g. fever, hyperthyroidism, heart failure) (Figs 11.2 and 11.3). It is often related to exercise and emotions, in which cases the sinus acceleration is quick and progressive and with more or less deceleration depending on the degree of exercise or emotion.

Figure 11.2 shows an example of acceleration and deceleration during an intense emotional experience (a parachute jump). On rare occasions, they appear without evident cause (inappropriate sinus tachycardia).

11.3. Monomorphic atrial tachycardia (E-AT) (Fig. 10.4)

In this case the P wave is not sinus but ectopic (often peaked and narrow) and is due usually to **C** an increase in automatism of an ectopic focus or to atrial micro or macro reentry. Its rate tends to accelerate and decelerate at the start and end of the episode (Fig. 11.4). The site of origin of the tachycardia can be located using the morphology of the ectopic P wave; if the P′ wave is − or ± in V1, the origin is in the right atrium, and if P′ is + or −+ in V1, it is located in the left atrium. If P′ is negative in II, III, and VF, the origin is in the lower part of the atria in the AV junction or surrounding area. In general, the P′ wave is located before QRS with the following relationship: P′-QRS < QRS-P′ (Fig. 11.4). Often, the P′ wave presents a certain degree of AV block (Fig. 11.5).

11.4. Reentrant tachycardia of the AV junction (see Fig. 11.6)

The mechanism is explained in Chapter 10 (Fig. 10.9).

ECGs for Beginners, First Edition. Antoni Bayés de Luna.
© 2014 John Wiley & Sons, Inc. Published 2014 by John Wiley & Sons, Inc.

A

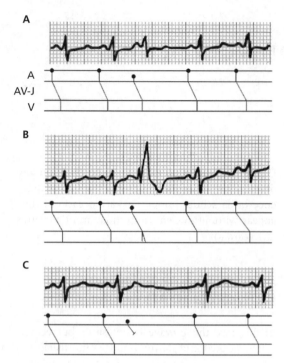

A
AV-J
V

B

C

Figure 11.1 A patient in sinus rhythm with paroxysmal atrial fibrillation (AF) episodes and frequent premature supraventricular complexes (PSVC). (A) A PSVC is conducted normally. (B) A PSVC is conducted with aberrancy because it occurs earlier. (C) A PSVC is blocked (arrow), because it occurs even earlier and the preceding diastole is a little longer. The pause is due to an active, not to a passive, arrhythmia.

Table 11.1 ECG evidence indicative of the presence of ectopy or aberrancy when early wide isolated QRS complexes are observed in the presence of sinus rhythm

---

Indicative of ectopy: ventricular extrasystoles
• Wide QRS complex not preceded by a P′ wave (premature ectopic P) (it should be confirmed that the P′ it is not concealed within the previous T wave)
• QRS morphology in V1 ⋀ ⋀ ⋀: and QRS morphology in V6:

• Presence of complete compensatory pause.
Indicative of aberrancy: supraventricular extrasystoles
• P′ wave preceding a wide QRS complex (slight changes in the previous T wave should be identified)
• QRS morphology in V1: ⋀ , particularly if QRS morphology in V6 is

• In the presence of wide and narrow premature QRS complexes, it should be checked that only wide QRS complexes meet Gouaux–Ashman criteria (see text).

Specificity ≥90%.

A   B   C   D

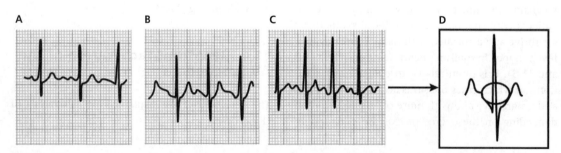

Figure 11.2 Holter recording of a 32-year-old man at different moments during a parachute jump A before, B and C during jump a typical ECG sympathetic overdrive pattern is observed (140 bpm), where PR and ST are part of an arch circumference (drawing, D).

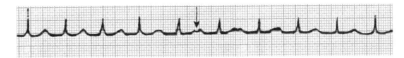

Figure 11.3 Sinus tachycardia (100 bpm) in a patient with fever. The P wave is hidden in the previous T wave and may be seen during breathing (arrow).

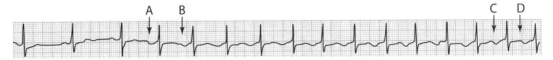

Figure 11.4 A 20-year-old patient with dilated cardiomyopathy and incessant atrial tachycardia due to an ectopic focus with warming up of the ectopic focus (AB = 0.64 s and CD = 0.52 s).

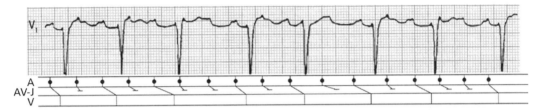

Figure 11.5 A digitalis-intoxicated patient with atrial tachycardia due to an ectopic focus at 175 bpm, with P waves that are different from the preceding sinus waves but not narrow. The atrial waves have some variable cadence and different degrees of AV block.

11.4.1. Junctional reentrant paroxysmal tachycardia with circuit exclusively in the AV junction (JRT-E)

(Fig. 11.6 A-1 and B)

In Chapter 10 (Fig. 10.9A) we have discussed the mechanism for this type of slow–fast tachycardia and the start and end of a crisis.

In this case, as the atrial activity is usually not seen separated from QRS, the P'-R relationship cannot be studied (Fig. 11.7).

11.4.2. Junctional reentrant paroxysmal tachycardia with a circuit involving an accessory pathway (JRT-AP) (Figs 11.6 A.2 and C)

The mechanism has been already discussed in Fig. 10.9B and there is a RP' < P'R relationship.

Figure 11.6 C-1 shows QRS alternans during tachycardia that indicates the involvement of an accessory pathway (20% incidence). We also see

how after the QRS complex, retrograde P' is closely seen, with P'QRS > QRS-P'.

At the end of the tachycardia (Fig. 11.6 C-2) in the second complex, there is a clear delta wave (pre-excitation).

11.4.3. Significance of P' location in the diagnosis of supraventricular paroxysmal tachycardia (Fig. 11.7)

To make the differential diagnosis between different types of paroxysmal tachycardia with regular RR, the location of the P' wave is very important. Figure 11.8 contains a summary of all these possibilities (see figure legend).

11.4.4. Antidromic tachycardia. Antegrade conduction through accessory pathway

This type of tachycardia has to be differentiated from VT (see Section 8.2.4 in Chapter 8 and Section 12.2.3.2 in Chapter 12).

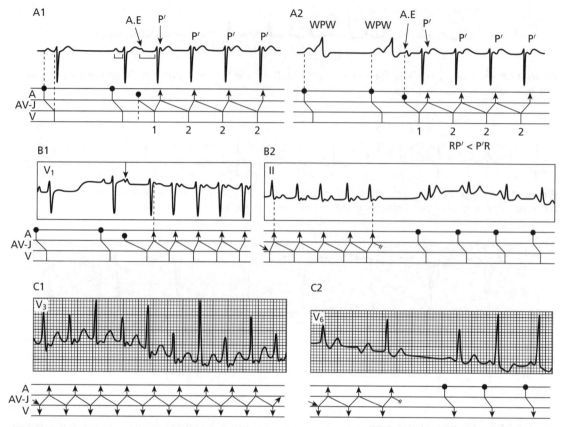

Figure 11.6 (A1) Onset of junctorial reciprocating exclusive tachycardia (JRT-E). See the atrial extrasystole leading to a long PR interval, the P' stuck at the end of QRS and Lewis diagram. (A2) Onset of JRT-AP. See the atrial extrasystole leading to a long PR interval, although not as long as in the previous case. See also the Lewis diagram, with RP' < P'R (where P' is separated from R and not attached to it, as in JRT-E). (B) Onset and termination (B₁ and B₂) of a JRT-E episode. We can observe the initial P'R lengthening and often the small QRS changes during the episode due to the P' overlapping (R' in V1 and in II and VF. (C) JRT-AP.C1:V3, where alternance of QRS complexes are observed. (C2) V6, where the termination of the episode of JRT-AP with anterograde block in AV junction is observed, after the tachycardia, the onset of preexcitation in the second sinus complex.

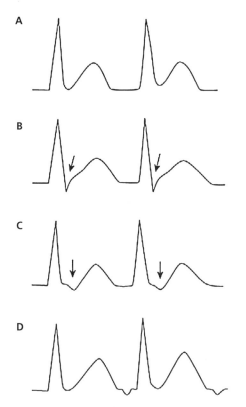

Figure 11.7 Location of P′ waves in paroxysmal supraventricular tachycardias. (A) Non-visible P′ wave, hidden by the QRS (circuit exclusively involving the AV junction). (B) P′ wave that distorts the end of the QRS (simulating that it ends with an S wave) (circuit exclusively involving the junction as well). (C) P′ wave separated from the QRS, but with RP′ < P′R (reentrant) (circuit involving an accessory pathway). (D) P′ wave preceding the QRS with P′R < RP′ (atrial circuit or atrial ectopic focus).

11.4.5. Repetitive reentrant tachycardia of the AV junction (Fig. 11.8)

This type of tachycardia, described by Coumel in 1974, is very rare and is more common in children. It begins with a critical shortening of the sinus RR. It is a fast–slow-type tachycardia with the anterograde arm in the SCS and the retrograde arm in a slow accessory pathway (Farré et al., 1979).

11.5. Ectopic tachycardia of the AV junction (JT-EF)

This tachycardia may be paroxysmal (Figs 11.9 and 11.10) or non-paroxysmal (progressive start and end). This tachycardia is often seen in the past due to digitalis intoxication. Today, it is very rare. **G**

AV dissociation is often present. The basal atrial rhythm may be **sinus** (A) (Fig. 11.9), **atrial flutter** (A) or **atrial fibrillation** (B) (Fig. 11.10). When the ectopic tachycardia in the AV junction is dissociated from atrial flutter, it presents regular RR and irregular FR intervals (Fig. 11.19B). In cases of atrial fibrillation, the presence of regular RR with a fast rate may be explained by dissociated ectopic tachycardia in the AV junction (Fig. 11.10A).

11.6. The differential diagnosis of supraventricular paroxysmal tachyarrhythmias with narrow QRS and regular RR intervals
H
(Fig. 11.11 and Table 11.2)

The algorithm in Figure 11.11 shows the differential diagnosis of all these types of tachyarrhythmias with regular RR interval and narrow QRS based on whether or not an atrial wave is seen and where it is located and the Table 11.2 shows the different ECG characteristics of different regular supraventricular tachycardias with narrow QRS.

11.7. Chaotic atrial tachycardia
(Fig. 11.12)

The diagnostic criteria of this infrequent tachycardia seen particularly in patients with decompensated cor pulmonale (hypoxia) are as follows (Fig. 11.12): **I**

1. Variable PP and PR intervals that produce irregular rhythm. The differential diagnosis of atrial fibrillation through palpation is very difficult to perform;

2. The presence of three or more P wave morphologies;

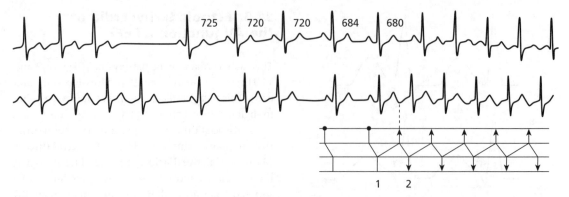

Figure 11.8 Holter continuous recording. Incessant junctional reentrant tachycardia with the fast–slow circuit type AVRT. The accessory bundle with slow conduction constitutes the retrograde arm of the circuit. Bottom: Lewis diagram corresponding to the onset of one episode.

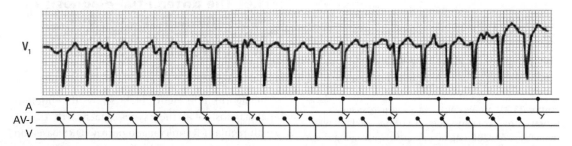

Figure 11.9 Example of a fast junctional ectopic focus tachycardia (180/min) with complete atrioventricular dissociation. Atrial rhythm is sinus rhythm.

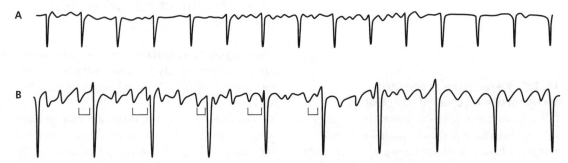

Figure 11.10 (A) Atrial fibrillation with regular RR. The ECG is from a patient with a junctional tachycardia and digitalis intoxication who showed atrial fibrillation as an atrial rhythm. (B) F flutter waves of variable morphology and changing FR intervals coinciding with fixed QRS intervals. This supports the existence of a junctional ectopic focus that is dissociated from the atrial rhythm (atrial flutter).

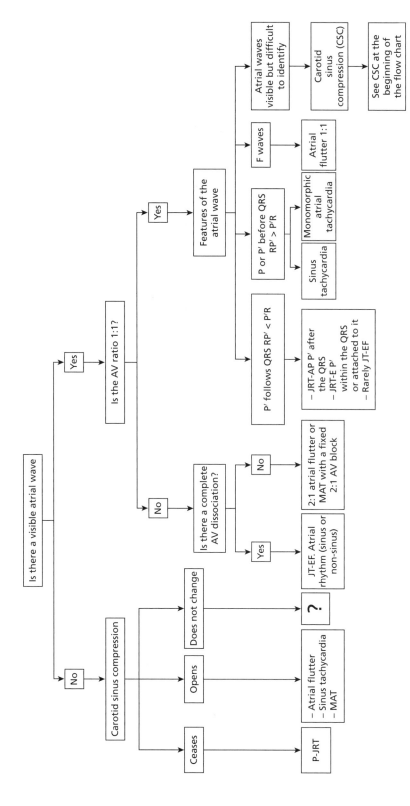

Figure 11.11 Algorithm for the diagnosis of active supraventricular arrhythmias with regular RR intervals and narrow QRS (see Table 11.2).

Table 11.2 Electrocardiographic characteristics of the different types of paroxysmal supraventricular tachyarrhythmias with regular RR and narrow QRS complexes[1]

ONSET DURING TACHYCARDIA	Atrial flutter	Junctional reeentrant tachycardia (JRT)[1] JRT-E[2]	JRT-AP[3]	Sinus tachycardia	Monomorphic atrial tachycardia (MAT)[4]	Junctional tachycardia due to an ectopic focus (JT-EF)
Beginning of tachycardia	Usually initiated with a premature supraventricular impulse	P' wave Initiating the tachycardia shows a different morphology compared with the subsequent P' waves	P' initiating the tachycardia is also different to subsequent P' waves	Progressive P wave does not feature significant changes	Initial P' wave is identical to the subsequent P' waves	Initiation and termination usually abrupt may be gradual. Initial P' wave is Identical to the following P' waves
Status of the atrial activity wave (P, P' or F) during tachyarrhythmia	Flutter waves. generally two waves for QRS complex. Almost never 1 × 1	P' with-in the QRS complex = 65%. P' after but very close QRS = 30%	P' following the QRS complex in 100% of the cases, but with RP' < P'R	P preceding the QRS complex shows a sinus polarity. Almost always P-QRS < QRS-P	P' wave usually precedes the QRS complex, with P'-QRS < QRS-P'	It is generally concealed in the QRS complex or. more frequently, an AV dissociation is observed
Presence of ventricular block	Depends on the underlying disease and the heart rate	Rarely seen. Almost always features a RBBB morphology	Sometimes observed	Depends on the underlying disease and the heart rate	Depends on the underlying disease and the heart rate	Depends on the underlying disease and the heart rate
QRS alternans (voltage difference >1 mm)	No	No	20% of the cases	No	No	No
AV dissociation	Usually a 2 × 1 AV block Is present	Never, unlike that observed in JT-EF	Never	Generally not present	2 × 1 AV block may be present	Frequently, in many cases it is observed in heart disease patients. Incessant types may be observed
Mechanism and clinical presentation	Atrial macro-reentry usually in heart disease patients.	Reentry exclusively in the AV Junction. Almost always paroxysmal	Reentry through an accessory pathway. Almost always paroxysmal	Generally, it is due to a physiologic increase of automatism.	It may be due to EF (paroxysmal or incessant) or to macro-reentry (MR).	

[1] Basal ECG with or without WPW-type pre-excitation.

[2] JRT with circuit exclusively involving the AV Junction, (JRT-E) also named AVNRT.

[3] JRT with a circuit also involving an accessory pachway, (JRT-AP) also named AVRT.

[4] MAT may be due to an ectopic focus (MAT-EF) or an atrial macro-reentry (MAT-MR).

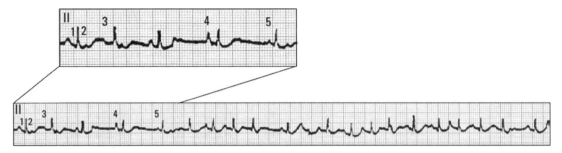

Figure 11.12 A patient with decompensated chronic obstructive pulmonary disease showing all the features of multimorphic or chaotic atrial tachycardia. Note the five different types of P waves in the first five QRS complexes.

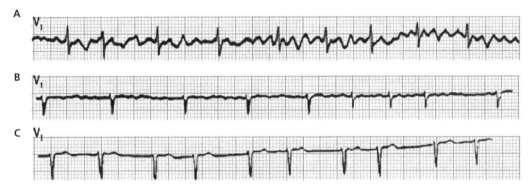

Figure 11.13 (A) Atrial fibrillation (AF) with 'f' waves with prominent voltage. (B and C) 'f' waves with lower voltage.

3. **An iso-electric line between P waves;**
4. **The absence of a dominant rhythm.**

11.8. Atrial fibrillation

This mechanism has been explained in the previous chapter (Fig. 10.12).

The ECG characteristics of this common atrial tachycardia are as follows:

J 1. **The presence of fibrillation waves (f wave)** that have low voltage and a rate of between 350 and 700 bpm (Fig. 11.13).

2. **An irregular ventricular rhythm** due to the variable penetration of the f waves in the AV junction. The ventricular rate also depends on the degree of AV block that exists (Fig. 11.13).

3. **The QRS can be narrow or wide** (aberrancy or fixed bundle branch block).

4. **It cannot coexist with atrial extrasystoles** but often there are early wide QRS complexes (ventricular extrasystoles or aberrancy) (Fig. 11.16) or late wide QRS complexes (ventricular escapes).

5. **Occasionally, the f waves are so small that they are not clearly visible.** They are better seen in V1 (Figs 11.13 and 11.14).

6. **At the end** of an episode of AF there is sometimes a **long pause** that may or may not be followed by a sinus P (**sick sinus syndrome**).

7. **The bradytachycardia syndrome** (Fig. 17.9)   K presents long pauses in sinus rhythm with episodes of atrial flutter or fibrillation.

8. **The AF may be paroxysmal or permanent** (Fig. 11.15).

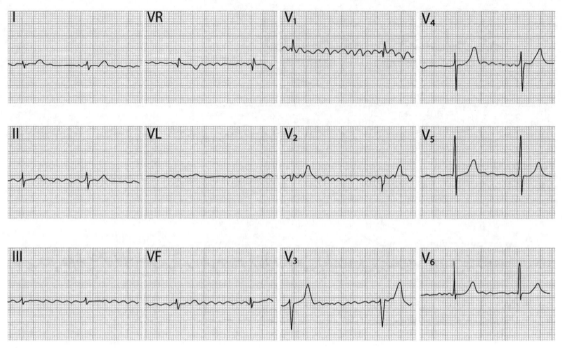

Figure 11.14 A 45-year-old patient with a tight mitral stenosis and mild aortic regurgitation. Note the typical atrial fibrillation (AF) medium-sized waves, which are especially visible in V1.

L **9. Episodes of paroxysmal AF usually start with a very early atrial extrasystole** (Fig. 11.15). At present, if this condition is not resolved by change of habits (no alcohol intake) and/or adequate medication, ablation of the pulmonary veins may be carried out.

11.9. Atrial flutter

M This mechanism has been explained in the previous chapter (Fig. 10.8). **The ECG characteristics of this common arrhythmia, which is often transitory, include:**

1. This is a well-organized and regular **fast arrhythmia** (250–300 bpm) that presents identical atrial waves (flutter waves) with no isoelectric lines between them.

2. The flutter waves are slowed (≈200 bpm) by certain drugs.

3. The AV conduction is usually 2 × 1 and fixed, but the conduction may also be 1 × 1, 3 × 1, or greater, and often the conduction is variable from one moment to the next (Figs 11.17 and 11.20).

4. In common flutter, the F waves originate from an anticlockwise reentry in the right atrium and in **no common flutter (reverse flutter)** are originated from a clockwise reentry in this atrium (Fig. 11.8 A and B).

5. The F waves are seen in the ECG as follows: N
• **Common flutter:** (a) II, III, and VF. Flutter (Fl) waves without an isoelectric line, presents a sawtooth morphology with clear negativity; (b) V1 Fl waves are positive (Fig. 11.18).
• **No common flutter (reverse):** (a) II, III, O and VF. Fl waves are generally wide and positive without isoelectric line; (b) V1. Fl waves are predominantly negative F waves (Fig. 11.19).
• There other types of flutter with different P morphologies included in the group of **atypical**

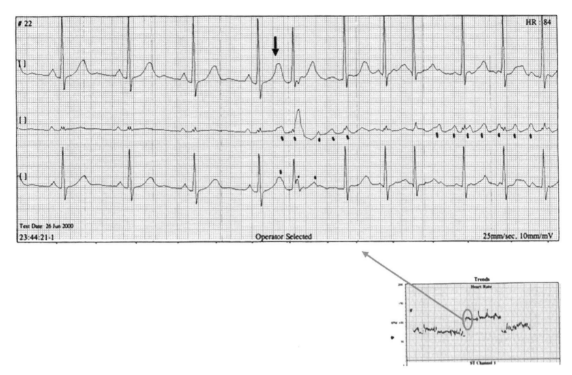

Figure 11.15 A 37-year-old patient who showed frequent paroxysmal atrial fibrillation (AF) episodes despite drug therapy and who was a good candidate for ablation. We see the onset of an episode of paroxysmal AF after a very premature atrial systole that distorts the preceding T wave and is conducted with an aberrant QRS (arrow). Bottom: Onset and end of the episode in the heart rate trend of a Holter recording.

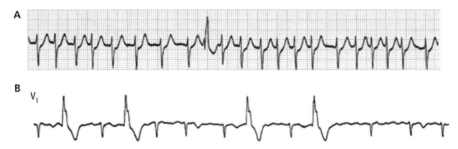

Figure 11.16 Two cases of AF with wide QRS. In (A) atrial fibrillation (AF) patient with one wide premature QRS complex with a distinct morphology in V1. in general, the Gouaux–Ashman criteria in the presence of wide QRS complexes during AF are not as useful to distinguish between aberrancy and ectopy as in sinus rhythm. Nevertheless, the rsR′ morphology in V1, as seen in this case, suggests that the aberrancy is more probable. (B) A patient with atrial fibrillation (AF) showing wide QRS complexes with a single R in V1. The notch in the descending arm of the QRS and the fixed coupling interval definitely point to an ectopic origin, ruling out aberrant conduction.

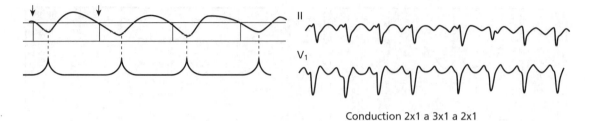

Conduction 2x1 a 3x1 a 2x1

Figure 11.17 Morphology correlation between II and V1 in a common 2 × 1 flutter, with an eventual 3 × 1 conduction.

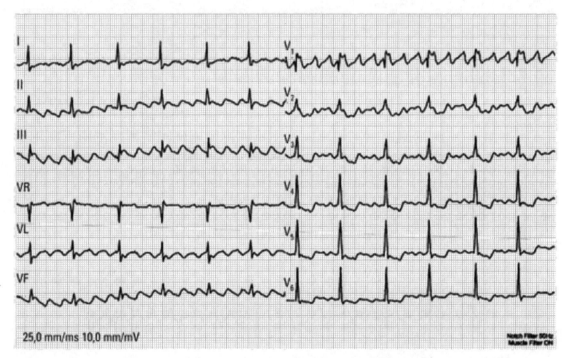

25,0 mm/ms 10,0 mm/mV

Figure 11.18 A 15-year-old patient with Ebstein's disease. Note the sawtooth morphology of the common 3 × 1 flutter waves, which show a voltage greater than usual because of the large size of the atria.

flutter (see before). The characteristics of left arium atypical flutter have been explained in Chapter 10. The ECG presents positive T waves in V1 and II, III, VF and negative in lead I at >200–220 bpm. At least in some leads there is an isoelectric line (Figs 10.8C and 11.21). In fact, macroreentrant tachycardias originated in the left atrial may present similar morphology, but with a slow atrial rate (<200 bpm) (see above).

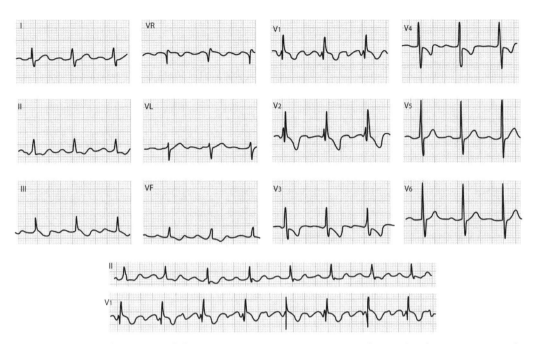

Figure 11.19 Example of reverse atrial flutter (positive 'F' waves in I, II, III, and VF, and wide negative in V1) that appeared after surgery for anomalous drainage of pulmonary veins.

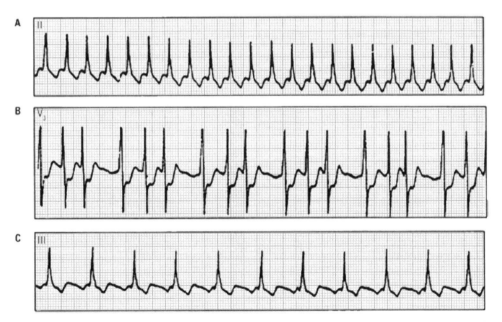

Figure 11.20 A patient with tight mitral stenosis taking antiarrhythmic agents who presented with a 1 × 1 flutter that turned into a Wenckebach-type 4×3 conduction (B) and finally a 2 × 1 flutter (C).

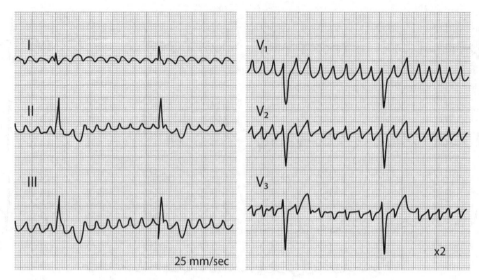

Figure 11.21 Example of atypical flutter with fast atrial waves (≈280x′) and predominantly negative waves in I and positive waves in I, II, III, VF and V1. This type of flutter is very often recorded in patients with advanced interatrial block with retrograde activation of the left atrium.

Self-assessment

A. Describe the concept of the premature supraventricular complex (PSVC).

B. In cases of wide premature supraventricular complexes, how is the differential diagnosis between aberrancy and ectopia made?

C. How is the diagnosis of ectopic atrial tachycardia made?

D. How is the diagnosis of junctional of reentrant paroxysmal tachycardia with circuit exclusively in the AV junction (JRT-E) made?

E. How is the diagnosis of junctional reentrant paroxysmal tachycardia with an accessory pathway (JRT-AP) in the circuit made?

F. Why is the location of P′ important in the diagnosis of paroxysmal tachycardia?

G. How is the diagnosis of ectopic tachycardia in the AV junction made?

H. List the key points in the differential diagnosis of regular supraventricular tachycardia with narrow QRS.

I. List the key points of chaotic atrial rhythm.

J. List the key points of atrial fibrillation.

K. What is bradytachycardia syndrome?

L. How does an episode of paroxysmal AF begin?

M. What are the ECG characteristics of atrial flutter?

N. How do the flutter F waves appear in common flutter?

O. How do the F waves appear in reverse flutter?

P. How do the F waves appear in atypical flutter?

CHAPTER 12

ECG Patterns of Ventricular Arrhythmias

In this chapter, we describe the ECG characteristics of ventricular arrhythmias. Their mechanisms have been explained in Chapter 10.

12.1. Premature ventricular complexes

12.1.1. Ventricular extrasystoles (VE): fixed coupling interval

This mechanism is explained in Chapter 10. We will now look at how it appears in the ECG.

• **The morphology depends on the site of origin.** If VEs start in the right ventricle (RV), the morphology resembles that of LBBB, and if they start in the left ventricle (LV), R wave may be present in V1 as in the case of RBBB. Often, the morphology does not resemble branch block (e.g. all positive or negative in the HP).

• **In healthy individuals, QRS does not present notches and repolarization is opposite to QRS and asymmetrical.** When there is associated pathology, notches are frequent, especially in the plateau of QRS. Figure 12.1 shows the three types of conduction of ventricular extrasystoles (VE) in the atria: (A) VE remains cancelled in the AV junction, with the next sinus impulse also blocked, and a complete compensatory pause originates (BC = 2AB); (B) the VE is conducted to the atria and depolarizes the sinus node, changing its cadence (incomplete compen-

satory pause [BC < 2AB]; and (C) VE remains blocked in the AV union, but the next P may be conducted, generally with a longer PR due to the concealed conduction phenomenon (interpolated VE) (Chapter 10).

12.1.2. Lown classification of VE from low to high degrees of severity

Lown and Wolf (1971) classified five types of VE: (1) isolated; (2) frequent (>30 per hour); (3) polymorphic; (4) repeating forms: (a) pairs and (b) runs; and (5) with R/T phenomenon (Fig. 12.2).

In practical terms, the risk for the patient is mostly related to the clinical context in which it appears. The most serious cases occur during the course of acute ischemia and in patients with a low ejection fraction (<30%). In these patients a VT/VF may be produced, especially when Lown classification is high. The R/T phenomenon is especially dangerous in acute ischemia.

12.1.3. Ventricular parasystole: variable coupling interval

They are very infrequent, and only in rare cases are presented in the form of runs, usually slow, of VT.

Figure 12.3 provides an example of ventricular parasystole: **variable coupling intervals** (from 560 to 1000 ms), **multiples ectopic spaces, and the presence** (third row) **of fusion complexes (F)** when the cadence of sinus and ectopic focus coincide.

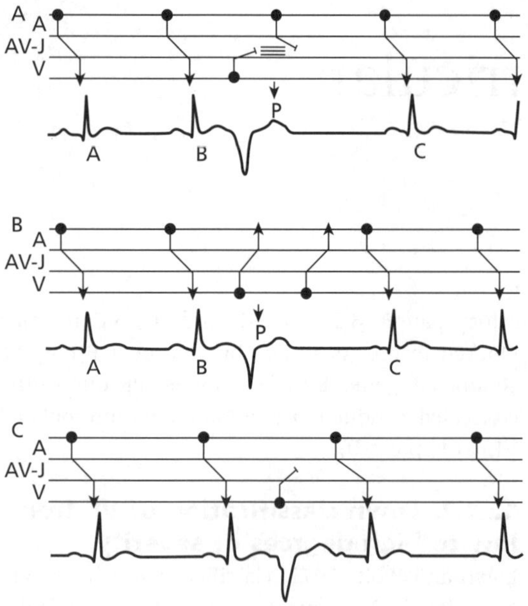

Figure 12.1 (A) Premature ventricular complexes (PVCs) with concealed junctional conduction, which hinders the conduction of the following P wave to the ventricles. (B) PVC with retrograde activation to the atria with depolarization of the sinus node. A change starts in the sinus cadence. (C) PVC with partial atrioventricular (AV) junctional conduction that permits the conduction of the following sinus P wave to the ventricles, albeit with longer PR.

12.2. Ventricular tachycardia

The mechanisms are explained in Chapter 10. They may be sustained or appear in runs.

12.2.1. Classification

D **Monomorphic**
We refer mainly to **classical VT** (QRS $\geq$ 120 ms). It may be idiopathic, usually of a focal origin ($\uparrow$ automaticity or microreentry), or appear in patients with heart disease (may be focal or due to a macroreentry (scar or branch-to branch) (Fig. 10.6).

Rarely, VT originates in the upper part of one fascicle with narrow QRS (<120 ms) and morphologies resembling intraventricular conduction disturbances and, exceptionally, VT may be of parasystolic

origin. These forms of VT are not discussed in this book (see Bayés de Luna, 2011 and 2012a).

Polymorphic
The most frequent types are *torsades de pointes* VT. There are also other types such as bidirectional VT, catecholaminergic VT, etc (see Bayés de Luna, 2011–2012).

12.2.2. Idiopathic monomorphic ventricular tachycardia

Idiopathic monomorphic ventricular VT may originate in both ventricles (Table 12.1), explaining the morphology resembling LBBB (generally starting in VD) or RBBB (always starting in VI).　　　　E

If it originates in the inferoposterior fascicle of the LV, it is sensitive to verapamil and due to microreentry; if it is sensitive to adenosine it is due to triggered activity; and if it is sensitive to propranolol it is due to increased automaticity.

It may present in the form of sustained VT or in runs. Table 12.1 shows the most important ECG characteristics of different types of idiopathic VT, according to the place of origin, and Figures 12.4 and 12.5 are two examples of idiopatic VF with right and left BBB morphology.

12.2.3. Classical monomorphic VT in patients with heart disease

Sustained monomorphic VT is a relatively common arrhythmia that occurs especially in ischemic heart disease (acute and chronic phase), inherited heart diseases and when heart failure is present. In some cases VT may trigger VF and sudden death.

The VT in these cases may be triggered by different factors alone or in combination (increased automaticity, HDR, rotors, macroreentrant circuits) (see Chapter 10).

12.2.3.1. ECG diagnosis (Figs 12.6 to 12.12)
(See also Bayés de Luna, 2012a.)

By definition, QRS in classical VT is wide ($\geq$120 ms), its morphology varies, and it is usually different from typical bundle branch block. The type most similar to BBB is the branch-to-branch VT. In fact, this type of VT is very difficult to distinguish from a supraventricular tachycardia with

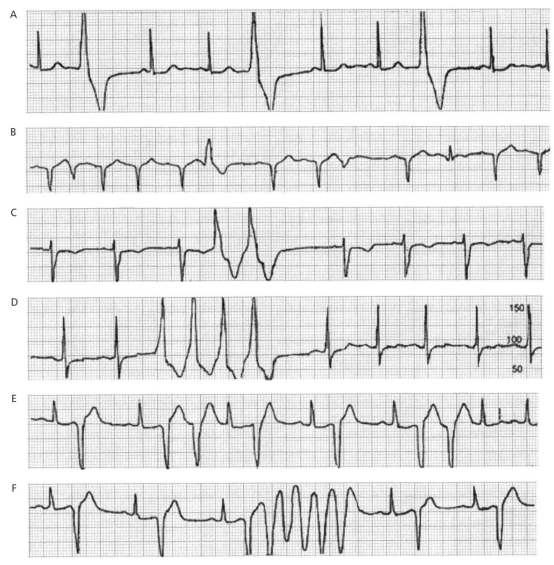

Figure 12.2 Different types of premature ventricular complexes (PVC) according to Lown's classification: (A) frequent PVCs; (B) polymorphic PVCs; (C) a pair of PVCs; (D) run of ventricular tachycardias (VT); (E and F) examples of R/T phenomenon with a pair and one run.

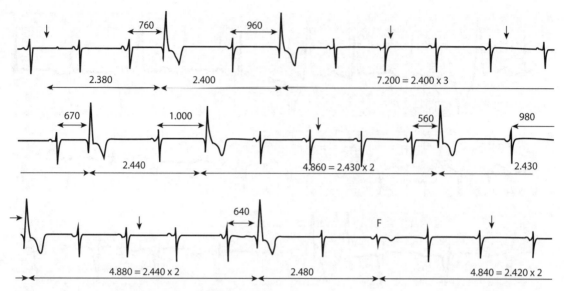

Figure 12.3 An example of parasystole. Note the variable coupling intervals, 760 ms, etc., the interectopic intervals that are multiples 2380, 2400, 2400 × 3, etc., and the presence of a fusion complex (F). The diagnosis of parasystole may be already performed before the appearance of the fusion complex.

Table 12.1 ECG characteristics, place of origin and incidence of different types of idiopathic monomorphic VT

Place of origin and incidence	ECG Pattern	ÂQRS	Left. If right-handed, the origin is in the superoanterior fascicle. ORS in the frontal plane	QRS morphology in V1	RS transition in precordial leads
• Tricuspid ring 5–10%	LBBB	Never right-handed. Between ≈+60° + 30°	R in I and VL	QS o rS	Beyond V_3
• RV outflow tract, pulmonary valve and high septum 60–65%	LBBB	Right	R in II, III and VF	QS or rS	Generally beyond V_3
• Below the aortic valve ≈5%	LBBB	Right	R in II, III and VF	– qrS – RS – rS	In V_2–V_3
• Mitral ring	Atypical LBBB	Right	R in II, III and VF	∿, ⋀	Generally in V1,V3
• Fascicular. Generally inferoposterior 10–20%	RBBB	Left. If right-handed, the origin is in the superoanterior fascicle.	It depends on the ÂQRS	R	R in V_1

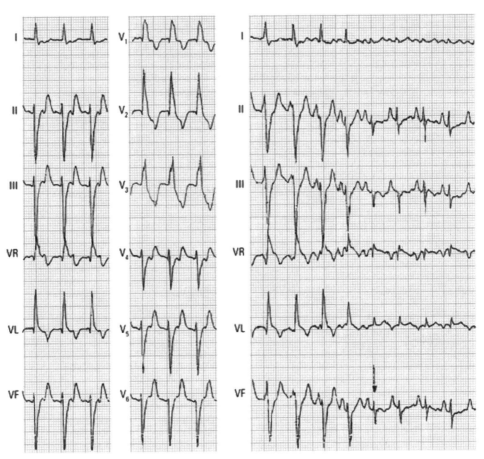

Figure 12.4 An example of verapamil-sensitive ventricular tachycardia (VT). Note the morphology of right bundle branch block + superoanterior hemiblock (RBBB + SAH), but with qR morphology in V1. In the right panel it can be appreciated how the sinus tachycardia exceeds the VT rate during exercise testing. (See Plate 12.4.)

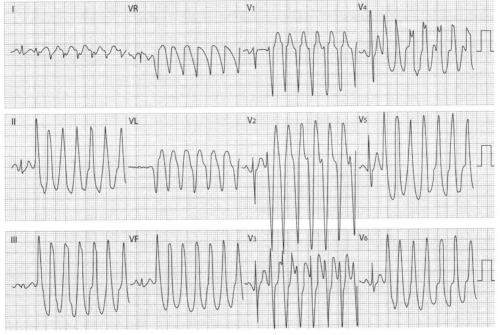

Figure 12.5 An example of left bundle branch block (LBBB)-type ventricular tachycardia (VT) with rightwards QRS occurring as repetitive runs during exercise testing in an individual without heart disease. (See Plate 12.5.)

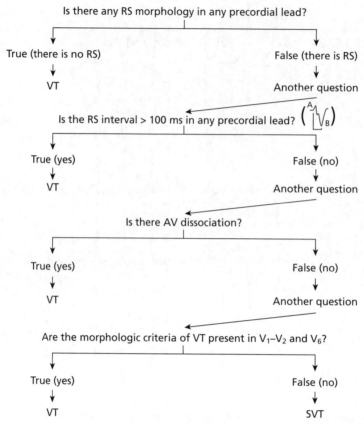

Is there any RS morphology in any precordial lead?

True (there is no RS)   False (there is RS)

VT   Another question

Is the RS interval > 100 ms in any precordial lead?

True (yes)   False (no)

VT   Another question

Is there AV dissociation?

True (yes)   False (no)

VT   Another question

Are the morphologic criteria of VT present in V_1–V_2 and V_6?

True (yes)   False (no)

VT   SVT

Figure 12.6 Algorithm for the diagnosis of wide QRS tachycardia. **Step 1:** When an RS complex is not visible in any precordial lead, we can make a diagnosis of ventricular tachycardia (VT).**Step 2:** When an RS complex is present in one or more precordial leads, the longest RS interval should be measured (from start of the R wave to S wave nadir—see inside the figure). If the RS interval is greater than 100 ms, we can make a diagnosis of VT. **Step 3:** If the RS interval is shorter than 100 ms, the next step is to check the presence of atrioventricular (AV) dissociation. If it is present, we can make a diagnosis of VT. **Step 4:** If AV dissociation not present, the morphologic criteria for the differential diagnosis of VT should be checked in V1 and V6 leads. According to these, we will diagnose VT or supraventricular tachycardia. (Source: Brugada et al., 1991. Reproduced with permission of American Heart Association, Inc.)

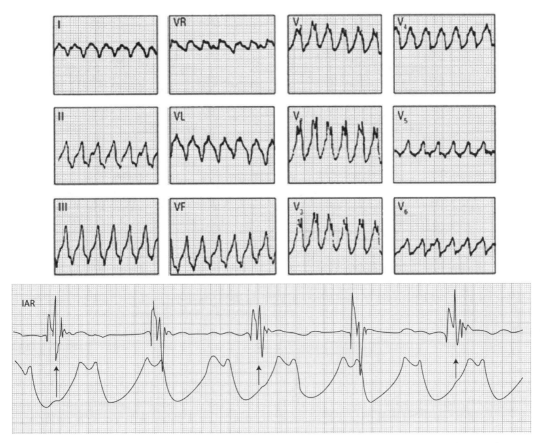

Figure 12.7 Example of monomorphic sustained ventricular tachycardia (VT). An atrioventricular (AV) dissociation is shown with the use of a right intra-atrial lead (IAR) and the higher speed of ECG recording, allowing us to see better the presence of small changes in QRS that correspond to atrial activity (arrow). The morphologies of V1 (R) and V6 (rS) also support the ventricular origin.

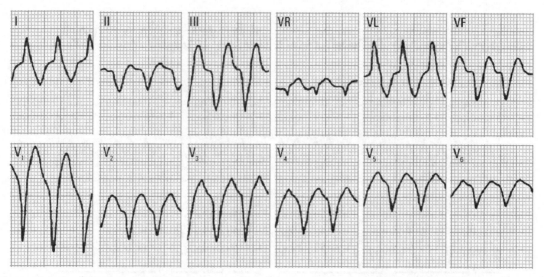

Figure 12.8 The ÂQRS is deviated to the left in the frontal plane, similar to that observed in some cases of left bundle branch block (LBBB). However, all the QRS are negative in the horizontal plane (morphologic concordance in precordial leads), which is not observed in any type of bundle branch block, and this supports diagnosis of ventricular tachycardia (VT).

LBBB aberrancy (Fig. 12.9). In other cases when VT resembles LBBB, there is usually an rS morphology in V1 with wide r >1 mm (Fig. 12.9).

The diagnosis must be made after ruling out aberrant supraventricular tachycardia. This may be carried out following the sequential algorithm of Brugada et al. (1991), based on some morphological criteria (steps 1, 2 and 4 of the algorithm) and in the presence of AV dissociation. The other criteria explained below are also helpful.

F **A. Morphological criteria:** Table 12.2 shows the classical morphologies that indicate aberrancy or ectopy in tachycardia with wide QRS including the criteria used in the Brugada algorithm (step 4) and those of Pava et al. (2010) (favors ectopy a peak time of R in lead II > 50 ms), and Vereckei et al. (2008) (favors ectopy the presence in VR of slow recording of first 40 ms of R or Q with slurrings).

B. Presence of AV dissociation (Fig. 12.7). This is a crucial diagnostic criterion. Step 3 of Brugada algorithm.

C. The sequential algorithm by Brugada, based partially on some of the mentioned criteria,

is useful to make the differential diagnosis between VT with wide QRS and high Se and SP, as explained   G in Figure 12.6. The first step is to look for the presence of RS morphology in precordial leads. If none are found, VT is indicated (Fig. 12.10). Second, if RS is present in the precordial leads, the duration of the R/S interval is measured (Fig. 12.6). If greater than 100 ms, VT is indicated. If less than 100 ms, the third step is taken: looking for AV dissociation (Fig. 12.9). If not found, we move to the fourth step, which involves morphological criteria as shown in Table 12.2 and below.

Figures 12.7 to 12.9 show three clear examples of VT based on morphologic criteria and Brugada's algorithm (Figs 12.7 and 12.9, first criteria and 12.8, second and third criteria).

D. Other important criteria
  • **Capture and fusion complexes.** The presence of these complexes confirms the presence of VT (Fig. 12.11).
  • **Atrial activity occurring before the first complex of wide QRS tachycardia** confirms that this type of VT is supraventricular (Fig. 12.12).

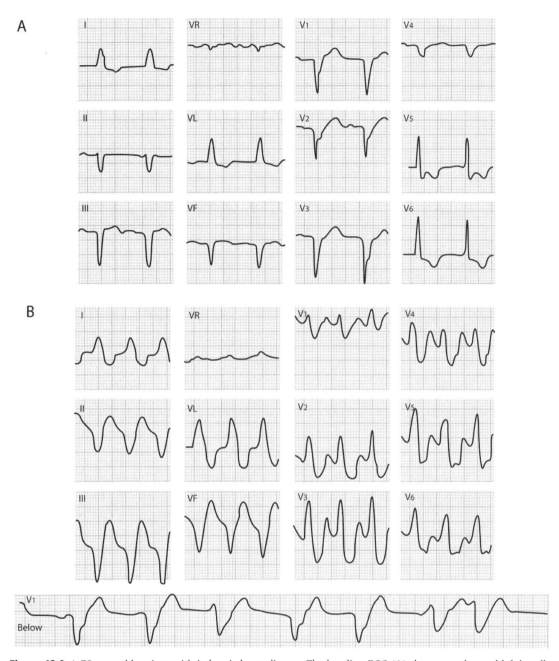

Figure 12.9 A 75-year-old patient with ischemic heart disease. The baseline ECG (A) shows an advanced left bundle branch block (LBBB), with an extremely leftwards ÂQRS and poor progression of R wave from V1 to V4, with a notch in the ascending limb of the S wave, suggestive of an associated myocardial infarction. The patient suffered an episode of paroxysmal tachycardia at 135 bpm, with advanced LBBB morphology (B). Despite the fact that the ECG pattern is of LBBB type and the patient presented with baseline LBBB, we diagnose ventricular tachycardia (VT) because of the following: (1) the R wave in V1 was, during the tachycardia, clearly higher than the R wave in V1 during sinus rhythm. Additionally, the bottom panel shows that, in the presence of sinus rhythm, the patient showed premature ventricular complexes (PVC) with the same morphology as those present during the tachycardia. The first and second PVC are late (in the PR), and after the second one, a repetitive form is observed; and (2) according to the Brugada algorithm (Fig. 12.6), in some precordial leads featuring an RS morphology, this interval, measured from the initiation of the R wave to S wave nadir, is >100 ms.

A

B

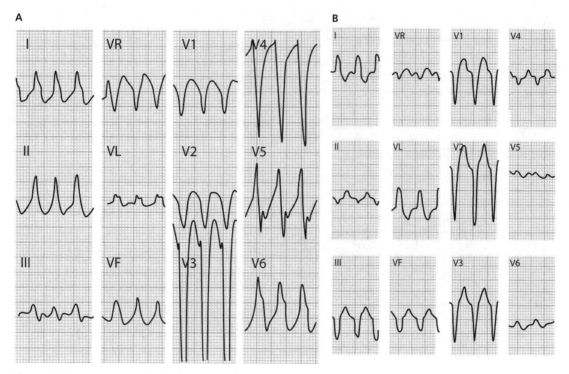

Figure 12.10 (A) An example of a bundle branch ventricular tachycardia (VT) with a typical advanced left bundle branch block (LBBB) morphology (see V1 with a QS pattern) (see Fig. 10.7-2). (B) An example of patient with a paroxysmal supraventricular tachycardia with LBBB morphology that already presented in sinus rhythm, and also QS morphology in V1. The ECG is very similar to the baseline one.

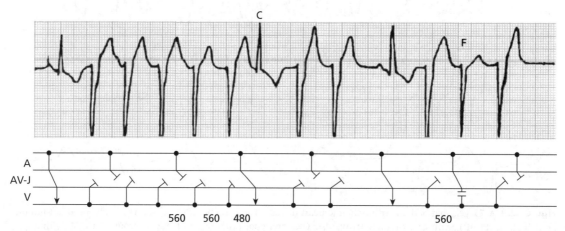

Figure 12.11 After a sinus complex, a ventricular tachycardia (VT) run lasting seven beats occurs. The Lewis diagram represents the complete atrioventricular (AV) dissociation. Between the fifth and sixth complexes of the VT, there is a typical ventricular capture (C) (early QRS with the same morphology as the baseline rhythm). Afterwards, after a normal sinus stimulus (not early), there is a short VT run (three QRS complexes). The complex in the middle is a fusion complex (D), as it has a different morphology from the other two (narrower QRS and a less sharp T wave), and the RR interval is not modified.

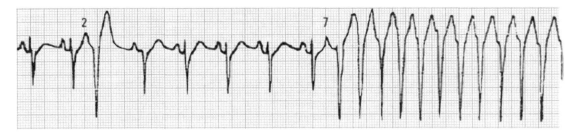

Figure 12.12 Taken from a 51-year-old woman who showed frequent paroxysmal tachycardia episodes. Note how the second and seventh T waves prior to arrhythmia onset are much sharper than the remaining waves, because an atrial extrasystole causes, respectively, an isolated or repetitive aberrant conduction.

Table 12.2 Aberrancy versus ectopy in tachycardia with wide QRS

In favor of ectopy:

1. V_1

2. V_1 ⁓ ⁓ especially if in V_6

3. II Delay in recording R wave (Pava et al., 2010)

4. VR (Vereckei et al., 2008)

5. VF:

    (1) In presence of wide QRS and RBBB pattern

    (2) In presence of wide QRS and LBBB pattern

6. All the complexes are positive or negative in precordial leads

In favor of aberrancy:

1. V_1 if in V_6

2. VR

3. VF:

    (1) presence of wide QRS and RBBB pattern

    (2) In presence of wide QRS and LBBB pattern

4. Typical morphologies of right or left BBB (excluding branch-to-branch VT)

12.2.3.2. Summary of differential diagnosis of wide QRS tachycardia

The criteria explained before (Brugada sequential algorithm and others) are useful for performing the correct diagnosis between aberrancy and ectopy in cases of wide QRS tachycardia with high SP and Se.

The most difficult cases are the branch-to-branch TV, because usually the QRS morphology is very similar to LBBB (see Fig. 12.10).

On the other hand, both **the antidromic tachycardia due to the Kent bundle and to atriofascicular fibers** may be difficult to differentiate from sustained VT. However, the antidromic tachycardia due to the Kent bundle compared with the one due to atriofascicular fibers, present in the precordial leads transition to R wave before V4 (see Section 8.2.4 in Chapter 8). The Brugada algorithm is not useful for performing differential diagnosis between junctional reentrant antidromic tachycardia and VT. We may use the criteria of Steurer (1994). According to these, the following criteria favor VT: (1) Negative QRS from V4 to V6; (2) QR pattern in one lead from V2 to VL; and (3) ÂQRS located between −60 to +150°.

12.3. Polymorphic ventricular tachycardia (Fig. 12.13)   H

The most important type of polymorphic VT is '*torsades de pointes* VT'. This tachycardia is characterized by **a change in polarity of the QRS (Dessertene, 1966), which is more visible in**

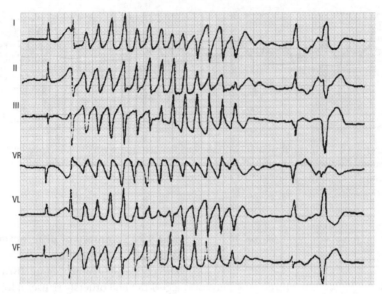

Figure 12.13 A run from a typical torsades de pointes ventricular tachycardia (VT). Taken from a patient with long QT syndrome. Note the typical pattern that is particularly evident in some leads (III, VF, and VL).

"Torsades de pointes" VT   Monomorphic VT

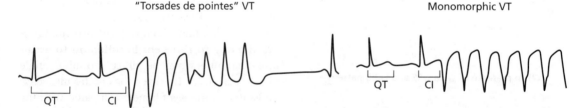

Figure 12.14 Characteristic morphologies of a run of a *torsades de pointes* ventricular tachycardia (VT) and of a classic monomorphic VT. CI: coupling interval.

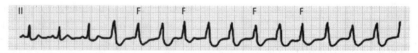

Figure 12.15 Example of different fusion degrees (F) in the presence of an accelerated idioventricular rhythm (about 100 bpm).

certain leads, and a long QT interval. Figure 12.13 shows a run of *torsades de pointes* VT in a patient with long QT syndrome.

The differentiating characteristics between classical VT, monomorphic VT, and *torsades de pointes* VT are shown in Figure 12.14.

For more information on other types of polymorphic VT see Bayés de Luna, 2011 and 2012a).

12.4. Accelerated idioventricular rhythm (Fig. 12.15)

Ventricular rhythm with wide QRS that does not surpass 100 bpm indicates accelerated idioventricular rhythm (AIR), because true ventricular tachycardia only exist when the rate is above this threshold.

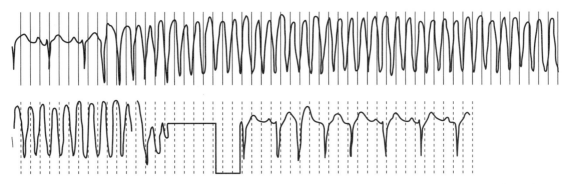

Figure 12.16 Ventricular flutter in a patient with an implantable cardioverter defibrillator (ICD). The discharge from the defibrillator terminates the arrhythmia.

In the presence of AIR, fusion complexes occur, presenting a morphology between ventricular rhythm and sinus rhythm that can have a similar rate. Based on the quantity of ventricular mass activated by ventricular or sinus rhythm, different degrees of complexes of intermediary morphologies (Fig. 12.15) (fusion complexes) exist. The morphology goes from capture complexes (the entire complex is sinus, see Fig. 12.7), to different intermediate patterns between the sinus complex and the ventricular extrasystole (VE) that depolarize the entire ventricular mass. The fusion complexes depolarize more or less the quantity of the ventricular myocardium, and according to that will be more or less within a degree of similarity with the basal rhythm (Fig. 12.13).

12.5. Ventricular flutter (Fig. 12.16)

J   Ventricular flutter **is a fast (≈300 bpm) and regular ventricular arrhythmia. The QRS complexes do not have an isoelectric line between them and repolarization is not observed**.

The differential diagnosis with fast VT is difficult to perform, although the repolarization signs are not seen in ventricular flutter. In addition, it may be confused with 1 × 1 atrial flutter with aberrancy (Bayés de Luna, 2012a).

Ventricular flutter usually triggers VF/SD unless it appears in the intensive care setting (Fig. 12.16).

12.6. Ventricular fibrillation
(Figs 12.17 and 12.18)

Ventricular fibrillation **is a fast, irregular arrhyth-   K mia with a rate greater than 300–400 per minute that may be originated by (a) multiple reentries; (b) spiral wave (rotor), or c) HDR (see Chapter 10)**. It does not generate mechanical activity and leads to cardiac arrest and death, with the exception of rare self-limiting cases or situations where the patient is resuscitated with cardioversion or previously with an implantable cardioverter–defibrillator (ICD).

The ECG shows (Fig. 12.17) **a fast and irregular rhythm, with QRS varying in morphology and height and without visible repolarization**. When voltage is low, recuperating the basal rhythm is proportionally more difficult.

Ventricular fibrillation may be preceded by sustained VT, generally in patients with chronic ischemic heart disease (Holter recorder) (Fig. 12.18A). On other occasions (Fig. 12.18B) ventricular fibrillation is primary and occurs during the course of myocardial infarction and, less frequently, in ambulatory patients (Bayés de Luna et al., 1985). Ventricular fibrillation is triggered by VE (*) (Fig. 12.18C) and on very rare occasions is self-limiting. If may be resolved with cardioversion (Fig. 12.16C) if it appears in the intensive care unit or in ambulatory patients with an implanted ICD (see Bayés de Luna, 2011 and 2012a).

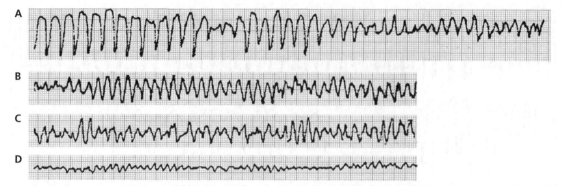

Figure 12.17 (A) Very fast ventricular rhythm of intermediate characteristics between ventricular tachycardia (VT) (it is too fast) and ventricular flutter (typical QRS do not appear in this lead), which quickly turns into ventricular fibrillation (VF). (B, C, and D) Different types of VF waves.

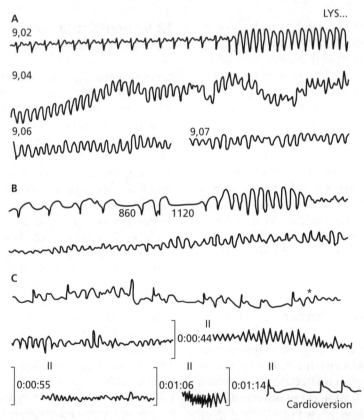

Figure 12.18 (A) Ambulatory sudden death due to a ventricular fibrillation (VF) in an ischemic heart disease patient treated with amiodarone for frequent premature ventricular complexes (PVCs). At 9:02 a.m. he presented with a monomorphic sustained ventricular tachycardia (VT), followed by a VF at 9:04 a.m. after an increase in VT rate and width of QRS complex. (B) Ambulatory sudden death due to a primary VF triggered by a PVC with a short coupling interval, after a post-PVC pause (1120 ms) longer than the previous one (860 ms). Note that the sequence of events started with an atrial premature complex, which caused the first shorter pause. (C) Ventricular fibrillation in a patient with acute MI in CCU that was finished with cardioversion.

Self-assessment

A. Describe the ECG of ventricular extrasystole.

B. What is the Lown classification?

C. What are the ECG criteria that distinguish an extrasystole from a ventricular parasystole?

D. Describe how VT is classified.

E. What are the most typical morphologies in idiopathic VT?

F. What are the most important morphologic criteria to keep in mind to diagnose VT in patients with heart disease?

G. Describe the Brugada algorithm used to differentiate ventricular tachycardia from wide QRS tachycardia with aberrancy.

H. What are the characteristics of *torsades de pointes* VT?

I. What is accelerated idioventricular rhythm?

J. Define ventricular flutter and list its ECG characteristics.

K. Define ventricular fibrillation and list its ECG characteristics.

CHAPTER 13

The ECG Patterns of Passive Arrhythmias

13.1. Complex and escape rhythm (Fig. 13.1)

A Escape complexes and escape rhythms **originate in a structure below the sinus node when the sinus node is depressed** or sinoatrial or AV block exist. Generally, escape rhythm is from the AV junction at its normal discharge rate (40–50 bpm), but if the AV junction is also depressed, a ventricular complex or escape rhythm may appear at a discharge rate that is very slow (20–30 bpm).

B Occasionally, complexes of capture appear alone or as escape rhythm. **Capture** refers to the early sinus complexes that occur earlier than the VT (Fig. 12.9) or escape rhythm (Fig. 13.1).

13.2. Sinus bradycardia

Sinus bradycardia during sleep or in athletes or in the presence of vagal overdrive is physiological, but may be very important. Figure 13.2A shows sinus bradycardia in an athlete, also presenting a marked arrhythmia in relation to breathing coinciding with a visible reduction of the heart rate.

Quite frequently, the sick sinus node (or sinoatrial block) produces **pathologic sinus bradycardia**. If accompanied by recurrent supraventricular tachyarrhythmias, they constitute the brady-tachycardia syndrome (Fig. 17.9).

Rarely, sinus bradycardia may be due not to depressed sinus automatism, which may also exist,

but to concealed atrial bigemy. Figure 13.2B shows severe sinus bradycardia at about 30 bpm that is **C** reduced abruptly in the last RR to about 50 bpm. This is due to the disappearance of concealed atrial bigeminy, which was present in the first three complexes. The arrow indicates the hidden P' wave.

13.3. Sinoatrial block

The different types of sinoatrial block have been discussed in Chapter 10 (Fig. 10.13).

Figure 13.3 shows a case of 4 × 3 sinoatrial block **D** in which the sinoatrial conduction delay cannot be measured, contrary to what happens in AV block, in which the PR interval allows this measurement to be made. However, we know that it is around 80 ms (see Fig. 13.3). In sinoatrial block, the PR is normal but RR is progressively shorter until a pause is reached (Fig. 13.3).

The 3 × 2 sinoatrial block is a bigeminal rhythm that it is difficult to differentiate from the parasinusal bigeminal rhythm. In the case of the 3 × 2 sinoatrial block, the RR intervals previous to the bigeminal rhythm are similar to the short RR intervals of the bigeminal rhythm, and in the case of the parasinusal bigeminal rhythm, they are similar to the long RR interval of the bigeminal rhythm (Bayés de Luna et al., 1991).

Lastly in the case of severe bradycardia, exercise may help to differentiate whether it is due to depressed automaticity or to sinoatrial block. In the

ECGs for Beginners, First Edition. Antoni Bayés de Luna.
© 2014 John Wiley & Sons, Inc. Published 2014 by John Wiley & Sons, Inc.

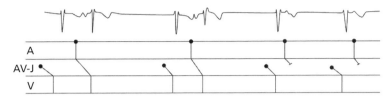

Figure 13.1 An example of incomplete AV dissociation with slow escape rhythm (first, third, fifth, and sixth complexes) and sinus captures (second and fourth complexes). After the two last QRS complexes, we observe how the P waves are not conducted because they are closer to the QRS complex than the two first P waves, therefore falling in the junctional refractory period.

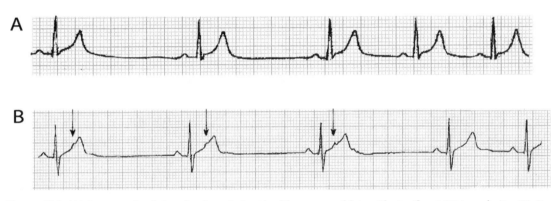

Figure 13.2 (A) An example of sinus bradycardia in a healthy young athlete with significant RR irregularity. (B) One continuous strip in sinus rhythm with frequent concealed atrial extrasystoles (notch in T wave ascending limb, see arrow), which give the impression that the basal rhythm, which is already slow, is much more bradycardic.

first case the increase in heart rate is progressive and in the second, if the block disappears, it is brusque.

13.4. Atrioventricular block

E • The mechanisms of the various types of AV block are explained in Chapter 10 (Figure 10.4). **Figure 13.4** shows examples of first-degree AV block (A), second-degree Wenkebach-type block (A) and Mobitz 2 block (C), type 2 × 1 block (D), and third-degree block (E). The P wave-QRS relationship best explains the various degrees of block (Fig. 13.4).

• **Sinus tachycardia during the day associated with the appearance of second-degree**
F **Wenkebach-type AV block at night is frequent in athletes,** but it is not particularly dangerous, although reducing athletic activity is recommended

if the degree of AV block is high. During the day, the patient presents tachycardia during exercise and the AV block disappears (normal PR and no blocked P wave) (Fig. 13.5).

• **The congenital AV block** usually appears in relation to systemic disease of the mother during pregnancy, which results in fetal myocarditis involving the AV node. It is not easy to decide the best moment to implant a pacemaker (Fig. 13.6) (consult Bayés de Luna, 2012).

13.5. ECG in patients with pacemakers

The implantation of a pacemaker has undoubtedly become a very useful treatment for syncope and sudden death, due to depression of automatism and sinoatrial and AV block.

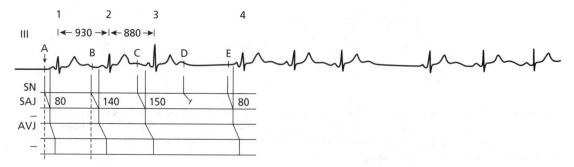

Figure 13.3 Second degree Wenckebach-type sinoatrial block (4 × 3). The sinoatrial conduction time progressively increases from normality (80 ms) (from A to onset of first P wave) until a complete block occurs (D not followed by a P wave). The distance between the first two RRs (930 ms) is greater than the distance between the second and third RRs (880 ms). Sinoatrial conduction cannot be determined. Theoretically, A, B, C, D, and E represent the origin of the sinus impulses. A–B, B–C, C–D, and D–E distances are the sinus cadence (870 ms). In addition, assuming that the first sinoatrial conduction time in the sequence is 80 ms (distance from the arrow to A), the successive increases observed in the sinoatrial conduction (80 + 60 = 140 and 140 + 10 = 150) account for the shortening of RR and explain the following pause. Therefore, it is confirmed that the more significant increase in the Wenckebach-type block (a sinoatrial block in this case) occurs in the first cycle of each sequence, following a pause (1–2 > 2–3). PR intervals do not change. The second RR interval is 50 ms shorter than the first (930 vs. 880 ms), as this is the difference between the sinoatrial conduction increases of the first and second cycles. In fact, the first RR is 870 + 60 = 930 ms, while the second cycle is 930 − 60 + 10 = 880 ms (see Fig. 10.13).

G **The spike of stimulation, an abrupt and short recording and the ventricular depolarization and repolarization waves must be examined in the ECG of patients with an implanted pacemaker.** These spikes may be monopolar or bipolar. Monopolar spikes have a higher voltage.

When the stimulation electrode is placed on the right ventricle, which is more common, the QRS morphology resembles LBBB (Fig. 13.7).

The stimulated cavity may be the ventricles (V), the atria (A) or both (A + V) (D); the detected cavity (sensed) may be in the ventricles (V), the atria (A), or both (A + V) (D), and the type of response can be triggered or on demand (inhibited) (I). **In this way, according to the stimulated cavity, the detected (sensed) cavity, and the type of response, pacemakers may be classified by a 3-letter code** (I = cavity stimulated; II = cavity detected (sensed) and III = type of response). Table 13.1 shows the characteristics of the three types of pacemaker currently most in use: VVI, AAI and DDD (Fig. 13.8).

At present, **pacemakers adapt to the needs of daily life,** increasing discharge rate on demand. For this purpose, biosensors, such as the P wave or muscular activity, are used. This type of response is called rate responsiveness (R), and occurs in both DDD pacemakers (DDD-R) and VVI pacemakers (VVI-R) (Fig. 13.9).

Furthermore, the pacemaker can be shown in an algorithm which explains the minimizing of ventricular pacing (MVP). This makes it possible to reduce the disynchronization due to pacing (Fig. 13.10).

Figure 13.10 illustrates the algorithm that may be used to choose the best type of pacemaker in different cases of bradycardia. In recent years, pacemaker implantation in the LV, located in a coronary vein accessed through the coronary sinus, is very common. The aim is to stimulate the LV from the lateral wall and resynchronize ventricular contraction (**resynchronizing pacemaker**), which is very useful in heart failure with LBBB and QRS >130–140′ms. Figure 13.11 shows an example of this situation. There is a spike and initial negative complex in VL and a positive complex in V1 that indicates stimulation of the left lateral wall. The width of QRS is reduced, in this case from 160 ms, when the patient was in sinus rhythm with LBBB,

H

I

J

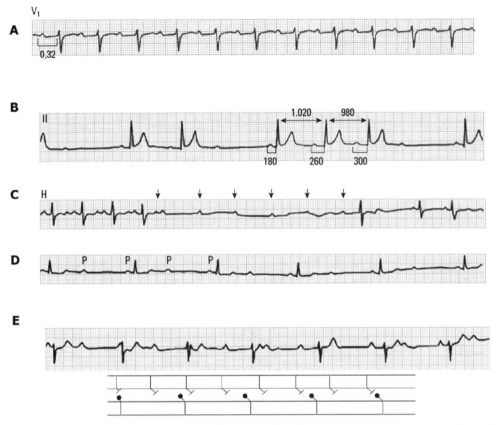

Figure 13.4 (A) First-degree atrioventricular (AV) block (PR 0.32 s) (B) Second-degree type I atrioventricular (AV) block (see Wenckebach phenomenon). (C) Paroxysmal second-degree AV block (Mobitz II type). Note the six blocked P waves without a prior increase of the PR interval. The first QRS complex following the pause is an escape QRS complex as it feature a very long PR interval. The last two P waves are conducted. (D) Second-degree 2 × 1 AV block. (E) Third-degree or advanced atrioventricular (AV) block. A complete AV dissociation is observed.

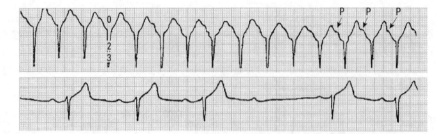

Figure 13.5 A 25-year-old athlete without significant bradycardia with clear ECG signs of sympathetic overdrive during the day (top) and frequent atrioventricular (AV) Wenckebach episodes at night due to the preferential involvement of the left vagus nerve (below).

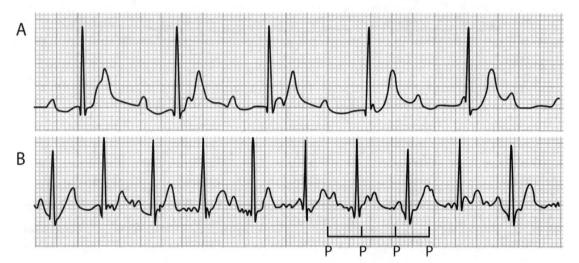

Figure 13.6 (A) Congenital atrioventricular (AV) block with clear AV dissociation in a 20-year-old patient. P waves are independent from QRS complexes, with an escape rate >60 bpm. Note the high and sharp T waves. (B) During exercise there is still AV dissociation, although the sinus heart rate is >130 x' (see P–P) and the accelerated escape rhythm is over 100 x'. This is a clear example of congenital AV block not yet requiring pacemaker implantation.

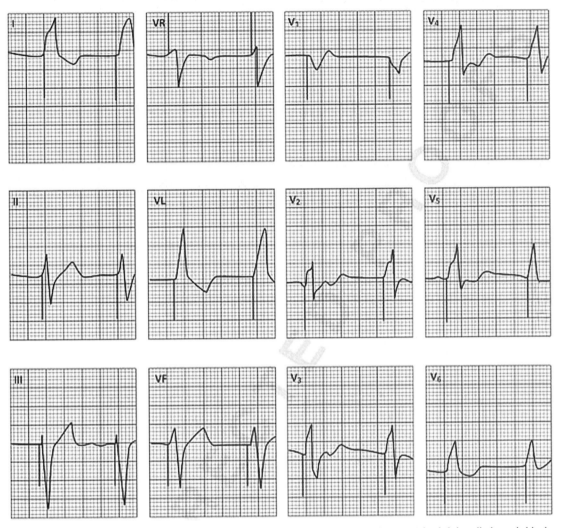

Figure 13.7 Pacemaker rhythm with electrode implanted in the apex of the right ventricle (left bundle branch block (LBBB) morphology).

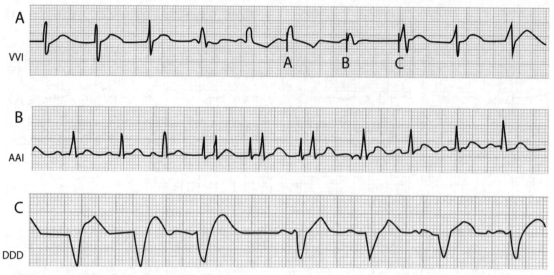

Figure 13.8 (A) VVI pacemaker. Ventricular on-demand pacemaker. The pacemaker is activated when the spontaneous rhythm is slower than its discharge rate. There are fusion impulses (4 and 7). After two sinus impulses (5 and 6), the pacemaker rhythm starts again. The first pacemaker impulse is delayed with regard to the programmed stimulation rate (hysteresis) (AB > BC). (B) AAI pacemaker. The three first complexes and the three final complexes are sinus complexes, start with an atrial spike, followed by an atrial depolarization wave (P wave). From the eighth complex, the sinus activity is again predominant and the pacemaker is inhibited. (C) DDD pacemaker. Example of physiologic (sequential) pacemaker. First, we observe three complexes caused by the pacemaker ventricular stimulation ('atrial sensing'). Next, the sinus rate decreases and starts the pacing by complexes initiated by the physiologic atrioventricular sequential stimulation (two spikes).

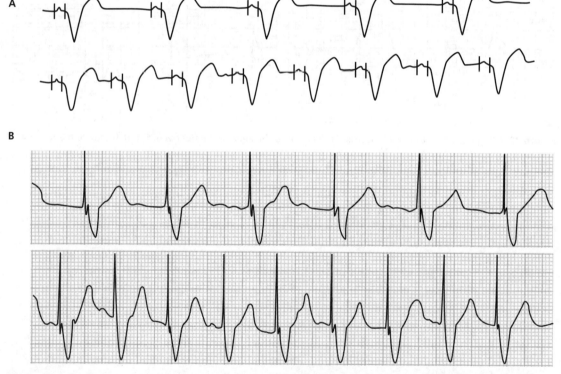

Figure 13.9 (A) A: DDDR pacemaker in a patient with sick sinus and atrioventricular (AV) block. Note how the pacemaker pacing increases with exercise: B. (B) VVIR-type pacemaker in a patient with atrial fibrillation (AF) and atrioventricular (AV) block. Note how the pacemaker pacing increases with exercise.

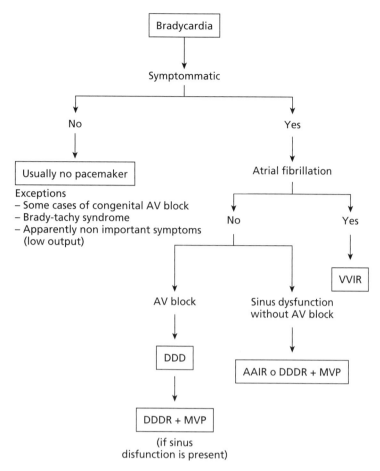

Figure 13.10 Decision tree. Selection of stimulation for all cases of bradycardia, regardless of their origin (see Nielsen, 2010) (see Table 13.1). MVP = minimizing ventricular pacing.

Table 13.1 Characteristics of the three types of pacemaker currently most used

Letter position (I II III)	Mode description	Use
VVI	Ventricular on demand pacemaker (inhibited by R wave) (Fig. 13.8A). The spontaneous QRS complex is detected by the device. If this does not occur, a pacemaker impulse at predetermined heart rate arises. On-demand tachycardization. Capability type VVI-R biosensors) (Fig. 13.9B).	It is especially indicated for patients with atrial arrhythmias, particularly atrial fibrillation, slow ventricular rate, advanced age, sedentary lifestyle, infrequent bradycardia episodes and recurrent tachycardia mediated by the pacemaker.
AAI	Atrial on demand pacemaker (inhibited P wave) (Fig. 13.8B). Capability type AAI-R biosensors.	Especially indicated for sinus node disease with intact AV conduction, and presumably with no atrial fibrillation in the short-term follow-up.
DDD	Universal. Atria and ventricles sensed and paced (Fig. 13.8c). Different types of programmable parameters may be included. Capability of on-demand tachycardization (DDD-R type) (Fig. 13.9A).	Sinus node disease and all types of AV block. It does not provide additional benefits over the VVI in case of persistent atrial fibrillation. Pacemaker-mediated tachycardias may occur in the presence of retrograde conduction, which could be prevented by programming the pacemaker without atrial detection.

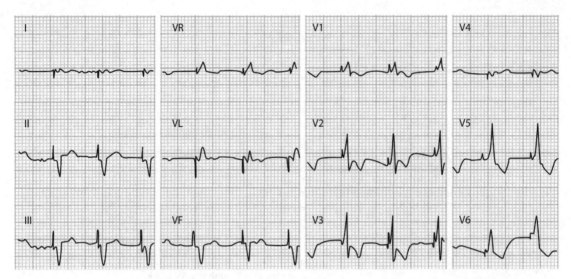

Figure 13.11 Patient with biventricular stimulation (resynchronization pacemaker). The QRS is definitively shorter than the previous QRS in sinus rhythm. The left ventricular stimulation explains the ÂQRS and the QRS complex morphologies (R in V1 and QR in VL) in the different leads. Patient with biventricular stimulation (resynchronization pacemaker). The QRS is definitively shorter than the previous QRS in sinus rhythm. The left ventricular stimulation explains the ÂQRS and the QRS complex morphologies (R in V1 and QR in VL) in the different leads.

to 115 ms after fitting with the pacemaker, indicating that resynchronization is taking place successfully. For more information, see Bayés de Luna, 2011 and 2012a.

Self-assessment

A. Define complex or escape rhythm.

B. Define ventricular capture.

C. Define pathologic sinus bradycardia.

D. List the basic concepts used to diagnose sinoatrial block.

E. List the basic concepts of AV block.

F. What type of second-degree AV block is found in athletes?

G. What are the components of a pacemaker ECG?

H. What are the 3-letter codes used to classify different types of pacemaker?

I. How do pacemakers adapt to the needs of daily life?

J. What is a resynchronization pacemaker?

CHAPTER 14

How to Interpret ECG Tracings with Arrhythmia

This very brief chapter may in fact require a lot of time if the student reads the chapter slowly trying to remember all the concepts previously commented upon.

When a recording with arrhythmia appears in clinical practice, the recommendations described below should be used to reach the correct diagnosis. The information in Chapters 10 to 13 is to be used in this process.

1. Confirm the presence of atrial activity and determine the type of rhythm (sinus or ectopic), rate, morphology, and location of atrial activity in the RR cycle.

2. Analyze the QRS complexes: rate and morphology.

3. Analyze the AV relationship and identify normal or retrograde conduction (Fig. 10.2).

4. Analyze the premature complexes (extrasystoles, parasystoles, sinus capture) and determine the presence of repeating complexes (automatic or reentrant).

5. Analyze pauses. Identify decreased automaticity, blocks, or concealed atrial bigeminy.

6. Analyze the delayed sinus complexes and the complexes and escape rhythms.

7. Analyze bigeminal rhythm. Figure 14.1 shows the most frequent causes.

8. Analyze the QRS with variable morphology in the presence of regular RR. It may indicate true alternans when changes in QRS-ST-T are due to intrinsic disturbances in the myocardium (Fig. 14.2). Alternatively, a pseudo-alternance may be present when it is the result of a change in cardiac activation (e.g. 2×1 branch block or 2×1 pre-excitation). It may also be confused with very delayed ventricular bigeminy with PVC in the PR interval.

If this sequence is followed, the information in Chapters 10 to 13, along with references when in doubt, may be used to make the correct diagnosis in nearly all cases of arrhythmia. Furthermore, it may be used to determine the most adequate treatment and better estimate the prognosis. If necessary, additional testing (e.g. Holter recording, stress test, tilt test, electrophysiologic study) can be used.

ECGs for Beginners, First Edition. Antoni Bayés de Luna.
© 2014 John Wiley & Sons, Inc. Published 2014 by John Wiley & Sons, Inc.

Bigeminy rhythm

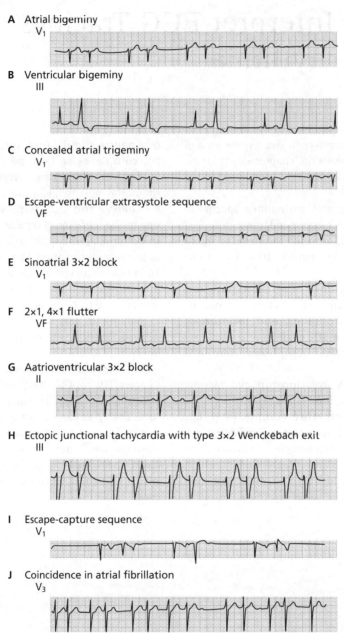

Figure 14.1 Different types of bigeminal QRS complexes. The different mechanisms are shown within the figure, except for the case K.

Complexes with variable morphology

Note: There is no self assessment in this chapter because the contents are a form of self-evaluation.

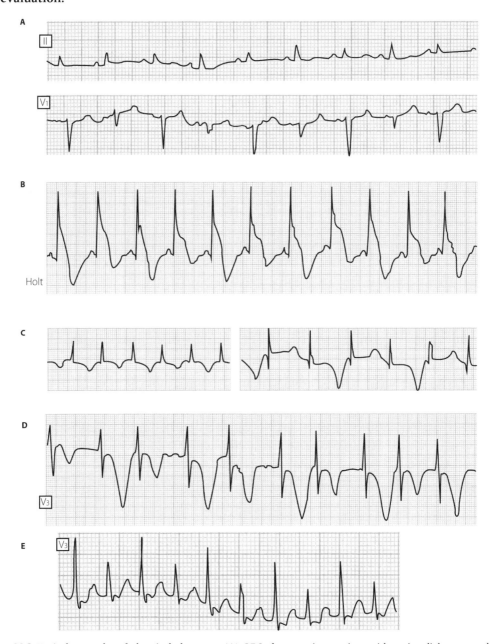

Figure 14.2 Typical examples of electrical alternans. (A) QRS alternans in a patient with pericardial tamponade. (B) ST/T alternans in Prinzmetal angina. (C) Repolarization alternans in a congenital long QT syndrome. (D) Repolarization alternans in significant electrolytic imbalance in a patient with atrial fibrillation. (E) QRS alternans during a reentrant atrioventricular junctional tachycardia involving an accessory pathway (JRT-AP).

PART IV
ECG in Clinical Practice

The ECG is very useful in clinical practice. We have already seen how the ECG is the gold standard for the management of arrhythmia (Part III) as well as atrial and ventricular block and pre-excitation in Chapters 5, 7, and 8.

In Chapter 9 we have also seen its importance in the description of not only the electrophysiologic mechanisms, but also the importance of the ECG in the clinical diagnosis of different syndromes related to ischemia and necrosis.

ECG is also very valuable in the diagnosis of atrial and ventricular hypertrophy, although imaging techniques are superior in these cases. However, the information provided by the ECG often has more prognostic value.

As part of this final section of the book, **Chapter 15** analyzes the importance of the ECG in relation to the symptoms presented by the patient. In this case we emphasize the importance of 'precordial pain' and the usefulness of the ECG in the global evaluation of this symptom, as already widely discussed in Chapter 9. The correlation among clinical presentation, ECG pattern, and biomarkers in patients with precordial pain is very important. Also the ECG is very useful in the follow-up of patients after an ischemic attack. Furthermore, we will discuss the ECG in the context of dyspnea, palpitation, and syncope.

In Chapter 16 we analyze the importance of the ECG in other heart diseases and diverse situations.

Chapter 17 outlines the main ECG patterns that by themselves indicate a poor prognosis in the absence of symptoms. It includes the patterns of genetically induced heart diseases and other groups of ECG patterns that even in the absence of symptoms during the ECG recording indicate a poor prognosis. In all these cases, it is important to take a detailed medical history and carry out a physical examination in order to complete the importance of the ECG findings.

Finally, in **Chapter 18** we comment on the importance of abnormal ECG in patients with normal history and physical examination, and how frequently the ECG is normal in patients with even advanced or serious heart disease.

CHAPTER 15

From Symptoms to the ECG

ECGs in the presence of precordial pain or other symptoms

15.1. Chest pain

15.1.1. Ischemic heart disease versus pericarditis or other causes of chest pain

Patients with chest pain in the emergency room may have of three types of origin:

A **1. Clearly ischemic pain, in which case medical history and ECG changes (Chapter 9) together with biomarkers** are the key to confirming the diagnosis.

2. Non-ischemic pain that may or may not be cardiovascular. The former includes pathologies which are usually benign, such as pericarditis, or very dangerous, such as aortic dissection. A detailed medical history together with the evaluation of a clinical examination, together with the ECG and the imaging techniques are all very important in

B reaching a definitive diagnosis. Table 15.1 shows the keys to the **differential diagnosis between acute coronary syndromes (ACS), pericarditis, miocarditis, pulmonary embolism and aortic dissection, the five most important cardiovascular pathologies involving chest pain.** Along with a description of the ECG, the relevance of the medical history and biomarkers are also outlined.

Non-cardiovascular pathologies include: (i) pain due to chest wall and skeletal muscle problems (very frequent); (ii) respiratory pain (pneumothorax, pleuritis, etc.); (iii) pain in the digestive tract,

and colecistitis; and (iv) psychogenic pain (anxiety, hyperventilation, etc.). It should be remembered that hyperventilation may change the ECG, especially inducing a flat/negative T wave (Fig. 4.25).

3. Chest pain in 25–30% of patients who arrive at hospital is difficult to diagnose. The course of the episode of pain must be followed and the ECG findings and, if necessary, additional tests are needed before clarifying these cases.

15.2. Acute dyspnea

The presence of acute dyspnea may be explained by the following processes as outlined below. The ECG findings are very important in the diagnostic deduction of the causal process.

1. Left ventricular failure. Edema or subedema of the lungs during the course of **ACS or fast tachyarrhythmia** most likely indicates atrial fibrillation or, less frequently, ventricular tachycardia. It is accompanied by anginal pain in ACS **C** and sometimes also in tachyarrhythmias without ischemic heart disease. The medical history and the ECG findings are very important in the diagnosis.

2. Pulmonary embolism. There is more dyspnea than pain. Risk factors must be identified, if they exist.

The ECG is very important because it may show typical ECG abnormalities such as: $S_I Q_{III} T_{III}$

ECGs for Beginners, First Edition. Antoni Bayés de Luna.
© 2014 John Wiley & Sons, Inc. Published 2014 by John Wiley & Sons, Inc.

Table 15.1 Differential diagnosis with ACS, pericarditis, aortic dissection and pulmonary embolism: role of ECG

	ACS	Pericarditis	Myocarditis	Aortic dissection	Pulmonary embolism
History of respiratory infection	NO	YES	NO	NO	NO
Pain characteristics	Precordial angina with spreading to the upper limbs, jaw, back, stomach, etc.	Precordial that increases with breathing	More dyspnea than pain. Increase with inspiration.	Mainly located in the back	More dyspnea than pain
ECG	1. Presents the typical or atypical characteristics described in ACS-STE and ACS-NSTE (see Chapter 9). 2. It is possible that the acute ischemia is not due to athero-thrombosis (see Table 9.1).	1. It may present ST elevation in the initial phase and be confused with STE ACS. The ECG evolves to negative T wave that persists over time (Fig. 15.1). 2. PR segment elevation in VR and depression in II*: without Q wave, which is sometimes the only anomaly 3. No changes during the stress test. In early repolarization ST elevation is reduced with exercise. See Figure 15.2.	• Low voltage • Sinus tachycardia • Repolarization abnormalities • Sometimes Q wave of necrosis	1. No typical ECG pattern. 2. ECG in relation to the associated disease (hypertension, etc). 3. Sometimes ST elevation in V1-V2 as a mirror image of LVE with strain in V5-V6 (see Fig. 15.3).	1. Sinus tachycardia 2. $S_1 Q_3 T_3$ negative (Fig. 5.4) 3. RBBB with ST changes (Fig. 15.5). 4. Negative T wave in V1-V3.
Biomarkers (troponins)	Generally high but they may be normal (unstable angina)	Generally normal but they may be elevated by associated myocarditis.	Usually positive	Generally, negative troponins. Increase in Dimer-D (high SE, low SP)	Troponin usually negative Dimer-D positive
Clinical course	Dependent on treatment It may lead to Q infarction or non-Q infarction.	Good. Often, negative T due to decrease of the subepicardial involvement. No Q wave.	Often good. Occasionally evolution to CM and even SD.	Often poor. Urgent surgery.	Variable May be very poor. Sometimes sudden death.

*ST elevation followed by a negative T may be explained by the direct involvement of the subepicardium, which first originates an ST elevation (pattern of an important subepicardial injury). Later, the residual pattern shows negative T, similar to that which appears after acute ischemia (Bayés de Luna 2012)

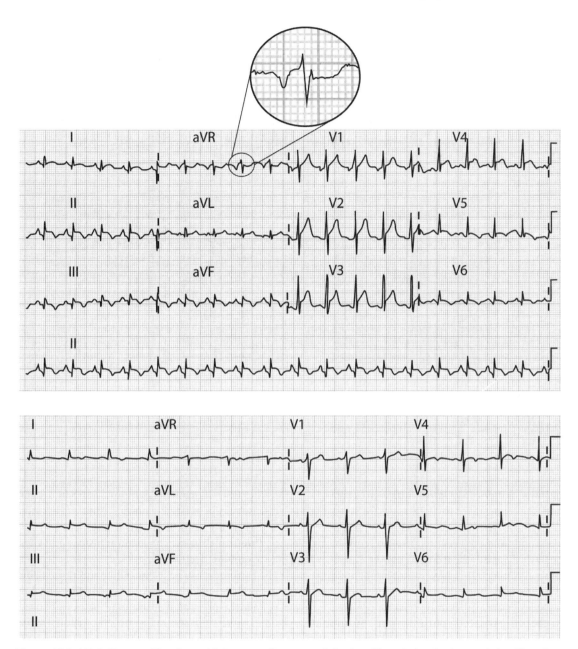

Figure 15.1 (A) A 39-year-old patient with long-standing precordial pain without ischemic characteristics. There is an ST segment elevation in many leads in someone with a final negative T wave but without Q waves and with PR elevation in VR with depression in II (myopericarditis). The clinical history and the follow-up (B) with the ECG show an evolution compatible with pericarditis (flat negative T wave without Q wave) and suggests this diagnosis.

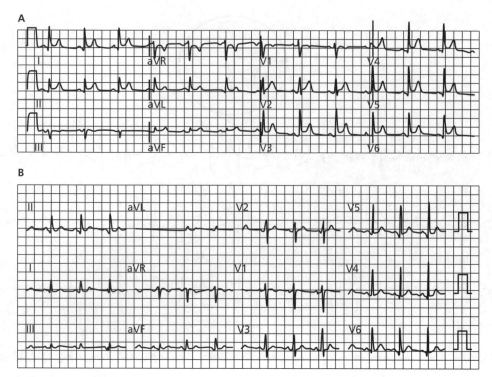

Figure 15.2 (A) A patient with thoracic pain and mild ST segment elevation in many leads. ECG was considered by automatic interpretation as pericarditis. (B) The ST segment elevation disappears with exercise, which favors the diagnosis of early repolarization pattern. This is an example of misdiagnosis of automatic interpretation.

negative pattern (McGinn-White sign) (Fig. 15.4) and the appearance of advanced RBBB pattern (Fig. 15.5). Where there is an abrupt appearance of symptoms and the very frequent presence of sinus tachycardia (with the exception of the elderly with sinus dysfunction) it is very important to suspect the diagnosis. The additional testing and imaging techniques are particularly important.

3. Decompensated chronic cor pulmonale. This is generally due to a presentation of an additional respiratory infection in patients with chronic obstructive pulmonary disease.

The physical examination, medical history, oxygen saturation, ECG and biomarkers are important in the diagnosis (Fig. 6.5).

4. Episode of bronchial asthma. This may be seen in young people. The medical history and physical examination are key.

The ECG in patients without associated heart disease may be relatively normal (sinus tachycardia and peaked P with the P axis to the right).

5. Pneumothorax. The medical history and chest XR exam are decisive.

The ECG may also be useful. Often it is normal, but in the left pneumothorax a right ÂQRS and low voltage in precordial leads may be seen. Sometimes, reversible and rarely striking, repolarization disturbances may occur.

6. Dyspnea as an equivalent to angina. In the presentation of acute ischemic attack cardiopathy, dyspnea may be the protagonist as the equivalent to anginal pain.

The medical history and ECG together with biomarkers can usually clarify the situation.

7. Chronic heart failure may present an exacerbation of the symptoms of dyspnea due to either

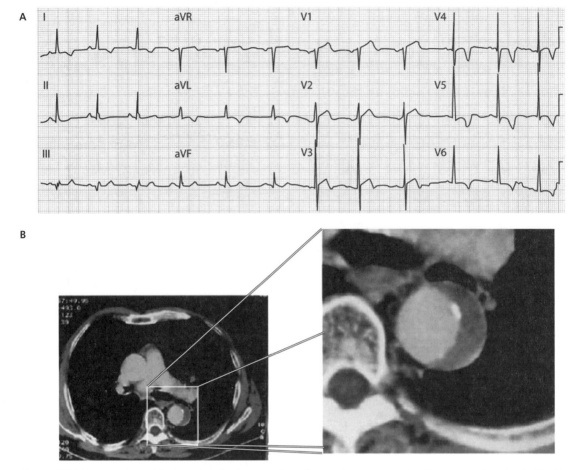

Figure 15.3 (A) A patient with thoracic pain due to a dissecting aortic aneurysm. An ST segment elevation in V1–V3 can be explained by the mirror pattern of an evident left ventricular enlargement (V6) due to hypertension. This ST segment elevation has been erroneously interpreted as due to an acute coronary syndrome. As a consequence, fibrinolytic treatment was administered, which was not only unnecessary but even harmful. (B) The CAT scan imaging shows the dissecting aneurysm of the aorta. This case demonstrates that before accepting a diagnosis of STE-ACS, other diseases that may cause ST segment elevation should be ruled out.

the clinical course of the disease or the association of some added factor previously mentioned, especially tachyarrhythmia, respiratory infection, or pulmonary embolism.

The ECG, the clinical course, and the biomarkers (NT-pro-BNP) are very important in reaching the correct diagnosis and most accurate prognosis.

15.3. Palpitations

If the patient presents with palpitations it may be possible to identify a specific arrhythmia based on the medical history and physical examination, but **the ECG is the definitive tool** confirming the diagnosis if the patient presents with arrhythmia, or

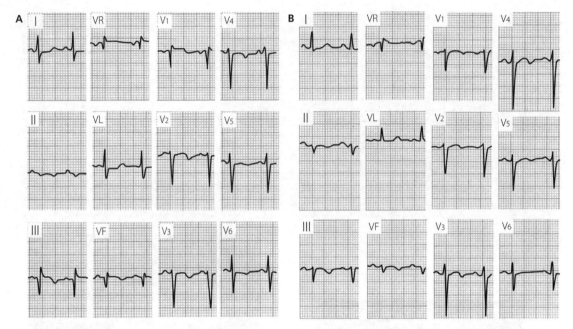

Figure 15.4 (A) A 59-year-old patient with pulmonary embolism and typical McGinn–White morphology: SI, QIII, negative TIII. (B) The ECG after the patient recovered.

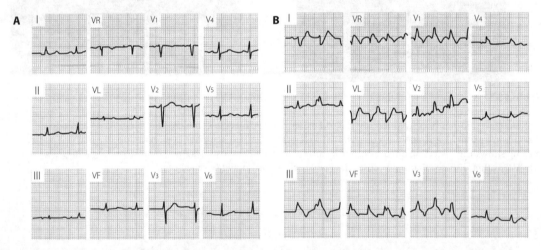

Figure 15.5 (A) Preoperative ECG of a 58-year-old female with no heart disease. (B) During the postoperative period, the patient presented with a massive pulmonary embolism with an ECG that showed a sharply right-deviated ÂQRS, advanced RBBB, and sinus tachycardia. The patient died a few minutes later.

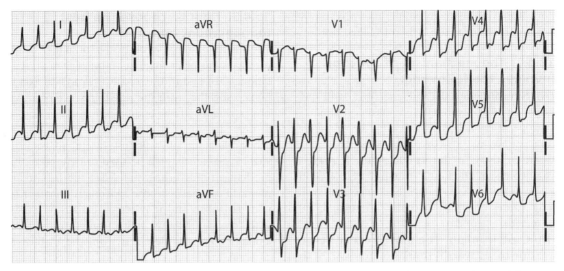

Figure 15.6 This is a case of young man with a very rapid re-entrant tachycardia with a circuit exclusive of the atrioventricular junction (AVNRT). The patient presents with chest discomfort, and shows evident ST depression as may be seen in the absence of ischemic heart disease in the case of fast heart rate.

suggesting it if is not present (e.g. WPW morphology, Brugada pattern, P± wave in II, III, VF). It is important to know that in the presence of rapid tachyarrhythmias the ST may present depression usually with ST upsloping. However, sometimes even in young people without heart disease, the ST may present, at least in some leads, an horizontalized ST depression (Fig. 15.6). In the absence of arrhythmia during examination, medical history plays a crucial role. A correctly taken medical history can lead to the following conclusions:

1. The patient presents a sensation of early isolated contractions that leave a void or give a sensation of the heart missing a beat. This is very likely due to extrasystoles.

2. The problem is the abrupt appearance in the elderly of the fast and irregular arrhythmia (atrial fibrillation) or regular arrhythmia (probably atrial flutter). In these cases, sometimes the patient complains of chest discomfort more than palpitations, and if the crisis lasts a long time may be considered as a possible ACS.

In the case of regular paroxysmal tachycardia that appears in a young person, it is probably a reentrant tachycardia with the circuit exclusively in the AV junction, if the patient feels the palpitation in the neck. If episodes began during childhood, it is probably paroxysmal tachycardia due to reentry of the AV junction with involvement of an accessory pathway. At the same time, the ventricular rate in the case of atrial flutter can vary when some F waves are blocked, while in paroxysmal tachycardia it is fixed and generally above 150–160 bpm (Figs 11.7 to 11.10). Figure 11.11 shows an algorithm used for differential diagnosis with regular tachycardias with narrow QRS, based on careful study of the ECG findings.

If in the physical examination and ECG no arrhythmia is detected despite suggestive data in the medical history, additional tests must be carried out starting with a Holter recording and stress test. Other tests may also be necessary (Bayés de Luna 2011, 2012).

15.4. Syncope

15.4.1. Concept

This is the abrupt and transitory loss of consciousness caused by a sudden reduction in cerebral blood **G** flow. It may be a benign symptom or a marker of serious arrhythmia with a risk of sudden death.

15.4.2. The mechanism of syncope involves the following:

(A) Neuromediated (>50% of cases) with participation of a vagal reflex. It includes coughing syncope, miccional syncope, syncope by vein puncture, orthostatic syncope, and syncope due to hypersensitivity in the carotid sinus. It may be vasodepressive (the most common type), cardioinhibitory (that occurs rarely but sometimes with long pauses requiring pacemaker implantation), or mixed.

(B) Cardiac origin. The most frequent types are due to tachyarrhythmias of bradyarrhythmias. The most serious syncopes are those provoked by VT/VF because they can produce sudden death in the first syncope (ischemic heart disease, heart failure, genetically induced heart disease) (see Chapter 17).

• Generally, **syncope due to bradyarrhythmias** (severe sinus bradycardia or sinoatrial or AV block) are preceded by a sensation of dizziness or instability, and the **first episode does not usually result in sudden death**. The more serious cases appear during the course of acute infarction (RC occlusion before exiting of the AV node artery). It is important to consider the possibility of syncope due to bradyarrhythmia in patients who present advanced branch block, especially LBB or bifascicular block and if PR is long (see Bayés de Luna, 2012). Naturally, the presence of trifascicular block (RBB alternating with two hemiblocks) requires, like many types of syncope associated with bradyarrhythmia, pacemaker implantation.

Syncope due to blood flow obstruction (e.g. aortic stenosis, hypertrophic cardiomyopathy, myxoma) can also occur.

(C) Neurological syncope. This type of syncope or feeling of instability may appear in situations related to transitory cerebral ischemic disturbances.

15.4.3. How to choose the best management approach

The medical history (family history of sudden death or vagal syncope in childhood), the type of presentation at rest or during exercise, the physical examination together with the ECG (presence of active or passive arrhythmia and branch block, especially if they are of high risk) (see Chapter 17), an echocardiogram, and tilt test (useful to confirm vagal syncope) may all be used to determine the mechanism of syncope and select the best treatment. In athletes, exercise syncope is a marker of poor prognosis and requires an exhaustive study with coronarography and imaging techniques, among others, to rule out ischemic heart disease, coronary and aortic anomalies, and genetically induced heart disease (see Bayés de Luna, 2011).

Self-assessment

A. How many types of chest pain may be encountered in the emergency room? How is ischemic pain diagnosed?

B. List the CV pathologies that are most often confused with ischemic pain.

C. Is the stress test useful in distinguishing between ST elevation in early repolarization and that of pericarditis?

D. List the most frequent causes of acute dyspnea and describe the utility of the ECG in its differential diagnosis.

E. What are the atrial repolarization disturbances observed in the acute phase of pericarditis?

F. Why is the ECG important in patients who present with palpitations?

G. Why is the ECG important in patients who present with syncope?

CHAPTER 16

The ECG in Genetically Induced Heart Diseases and Other ECG Patterns with Poor Prognosis

16.1. Concept

There are **ECG patterns in sinus rhythm** that by themselves, in the absence of current symptoms, indicate heart disease with a poor prognosis generally due to a risk of potentially serious arrhythmia.

Naturally, **the presence of active or passive arrhythmia, especially third-degree AV block or VT, already constitute a risk factor.** They will not be discussed in this chapter.

These ECG patterns may be classified in two groups: (A) ECG patterns with poor prognosis that are genetically induced; and (B) ECG patterns with poor prognosis that are not genetically induced (Table 16.1).

16.2. Genetically induced ECG patterns

These patterns are all markers of processes that can give rise to VT/VF and that require ICD implantation (Bayés de Luna, 2011).

16.2.1. Long QT syndrome

This is a channelopathy (disease of the ionic channels with no structural involvement) due to a slow activation of the K channels and incomplete inactivation of the Na channels. This explains the long QT interval and the tendency for malignant ventricular arrhythmia and sudden death to occur (Moss and Robinson, 1992; Schwartz et al., 1993).

Table 4.2 shows the limits of normal QT according to age and sex. It is important to measure QT in a recording with various leads in order to determine when they start and when they finish (an average of five cycles). QT must be corrected according to the heart rate. Generally, QTc >460 ms is always pathologic (Chapter 4).

A

16.2.1.1. ECG patterns

Figure 16.1 shows the most typical ECG morphologies (genotype–phenotype correlation) of the three types of congenital long QT syndrome best studied (I, II, and III) (Zareba et al., 1998; Zareba and Cygankiewicz, 2008).

As seen in Figure 16.2, the presence of ST-T alternance is a very characteristic ECG pattern.

A malignant ventricular arrhythmia is usually *torsades de pointes* VT, which is often preceded by long and negative T/U waves.

16.2.2. Short QT syndrome

B

This is a rare channelopathy characterized by the presence of **short QT (<300 ms) and some high and symmetrical T waves** (Fig. 16.3). It is sometimes associated with atrial fibrillation in young people and with early repolarization.

ECGs for Beginners, First Edition. Antoni Bayés de Luna.
© 2014 John Wiley & Sons, Inc. Published 2014 by John Wiley & Sons, Inc.

Table 16.1 ECG patterns with poor prognosis

(A) Genetically induced
- **Disturbance in the ionic channels with no structural involvement (channelopathies)**
  1. Long QT syndrome
  2. Short QT syndrome
  3. Brugada syndrome
  4. Other types: cathecolaminergic VT; inherited *torsades de pointes* VT, etc.
- **Specific types of myocardiopathy**
  1. Hypertrophic cardiomyopathy
  2. Arrhythmogenic right ventricular dysplasia (ARVD)
  3. Non-compacted cadiomyopathy

(B) Not genetically induced
  1. Severe sinus dysfunction
  2. Advanced interatrial block
  3. AV block with second-degree risk
  4. Pattern of ventricular enlargement with poor prognosis
  5. High risk ventricular block
  6. WPW syndrome
  7. High risk ECG in patients with chronic and acute ischemic heart disease
  8. Hypothermia
  9. Ionic disturbances
  10. Acquired long QT
  11. Pacemaker

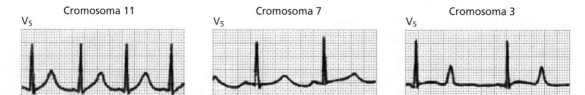

Cromosoma 11   Cromosoma 7   Cromosoma 3

V₅   V₅   V₅

Figure 16.1 Three examples of ECG patterns in long QT syndrome clearly associated with different chromosomal alterations: LQT1, LQT2, and LQT3.

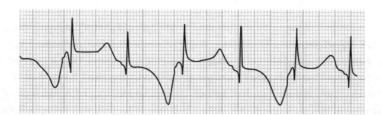

Figure 16.2 Repolarization alternans in a congenital long QT syndrome. (See Plate 16.2.)

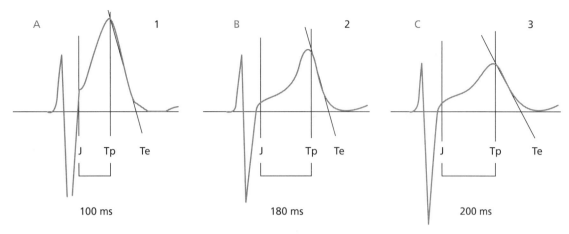

Figure 16.3 Symptomatic short QT pattern (A), asymptomatic (B), and normal QT (control) (C) (see text) (Adapted with permission from Anttonen et al., 2009). (See Plate 16.3.)

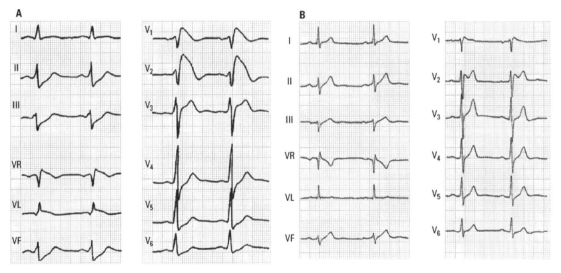

Figure 16.4 Typical ECG patterns of Brugada type I (coved) and type II (saddle-back) (see text).

16.2.3. Brugada syndrome

This is a genetically induced syndrome (Brugada and Brugada, 1992) due to inactivation in the outflow tract of the RV, of Na channels, with the K current having transitory predominance (Ito). It originates a voltage gradient between the epicardium and the endocardium of this zone in the RV, giving rise to malignant arrhythmia and sudden death (multiform VT/VF).

16.2.3.1. ECG patterns

Although the presentation of three ECG patterns has been described, it is currently accepted that there are only two well-defined ECG patterns with characteristic patterns in V1-V3 (Fig. 16.4) (Bayés de Luna, 2012a,b).

A. Type I pattern (coved): A rounded ascent appears at the end of QRS with a height that is generally ≥2 mm (dubious cases between 1 and

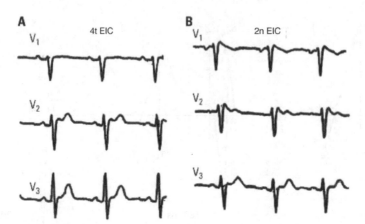

Figure 16.5 A patient with syncope episodes and an atypical ECG that present a clearly more typical pattern of Brugada type 2 in the second ICS (B) than in the 4th ICS (A).

2 mm) followed by a concave or rectilinear descending curve. May mimic an ACS-STE like pattern in asymptomatic patients. This pattern is the most dangerous which presents as VT/VF (Fig. 16.4A).

B. Type II pattern (saddle-back pattern): This presents r' (sometimes called the J wave) that is rounded and ≥2 mm, followed by a downsloping descending branch that gives way to ST elevation measuring at least 0.5 mm. ST is followed by a T wave that is positive in V2 and varies in morphology in V1 (Fig. 16.4B).

• **In both types QRS is longer in V1 than in V6** (Fig. 16.6), as occurs in ARVD. This is not observed in cases with r' in V1, due to variants of normality, such as pectus excavatum, athletes, or patients with partial RBB.

• Characteristically, **the QRS morphology can vary from one intercostal space to another**. It is always necessary to record V1-V2 in the second and fourth intercostal spaces (Fig. 16.5).

• The ECG pattern is dynamic and there are various factors behind it (e.g. fever, some drugs) (see www.brugadasyndrome.net/). Drugs that act on the sodium channels (ajmaline or some equivalent) are useful in determining whether the Brugada pattern is revealed or whether a change from type 1 to type II pattern occurs.

• **Phenocopies of the Brugada pattern: this term, proposed by Perez Riera and Baran-** **chuk, represents** ECG patterns identical to Brugada patterns (Baranchuk, 2013) that are not due to a genetic origin. These patterns appear transiently, usually in relation with environmental factors that preferentially affect RV such as ischemia of RV, tumors, pulmonary embolism, etc. The prognosis of this pattern is not well known; it is most probably different from the true Brugada pattern.

16.2.3.2. Differential diagnosis of the Brugada pattern in the ECG

Figure 16.6 shows the differences between different morphologies that present rSr' in V1. The bottom four patterns are pathologic (Brugada type I and II), and arrhythmogenic RV dysplasia (ARVD); hyperkalemia and the last four are variants on normality (V1 lead located in high position, pectus excavatum, athletes and partial RBBB).

• The differential diagnosis between type II Brugada pattern and other patterns with r' in V1 (Fig. 16.6) is sometimes very difficult. To evaluate the characteristics of r' is very important (Bayés de Luna, 2012a). The angle of the ascendant and descendent branch of r' is wider in the Brugada pattern (Chevalier, 2011). We have proposed the measurement of the base of r' at 5 mm from the vertex of r' (AB of Fig. 16.7) that is usually ≥4 mm in the Brugada II pattern and <4 mm in pectus excavatum, partial RBBB and athletes (Bayés de

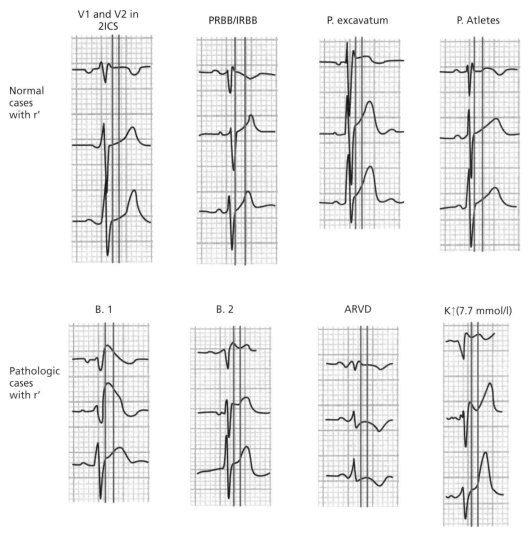

Figure 16.6 This figure shows clearly (first vertical line) the difference in the duration of QRS in V1 compared to V3 in Brugada patterns 1 and 2 ARVD and hyperkalemia (lower row). However, in four variants of normality (upper row) the duration of QRS in V1-V3 is the same. The second vertical line measured 80 ms later, clearly shows that in the two Brugada patterns the ST segment is downsloping (ratio ST↑ at J point / ST↑ 80 ms later >1) (Corrado index), but it is upsloping in at least V2 in normal variants (upper row) (ratio <1) (see text and Fig. 17.10). (See Plate 16.6.)

Luna et al., 2012b; Serra et al., 2014). This criterion is easier to measure than the β angle.

• ARVD may present a positive wave in V1 (ε wave) that is somewhat separate from QRS and generally without ST elevation.

• In pectus excavatum the P wave is usually negative in V1 and r′ is narrow. This is also seen in athletes and partial RBB.

• Figure 16.6 also shows, in the first vertical line, the differences in duration of QRS between V1 and

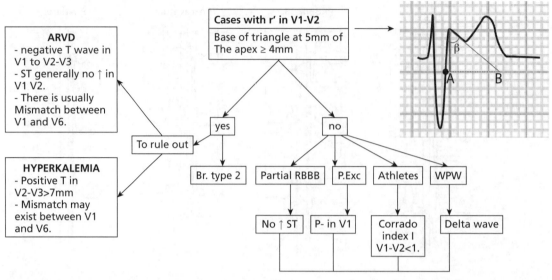

Figure 16.7 Flow chart for performing differential diagnosis of patients with r' in V1-V2 based on the measurement of the base of triangle of r'. If AB ≥ 4 mm, this is very suggestive of Brugada type 2 (see text and Baranchuk et al., 2014). (See Plate 16.7.)

middle/left leads in the ECG of the two types of Brugada pattern, hyperkalemia and ARVD. This does not occur in the four remaining examples of rSr' in V1, which are variants on normality. The second vertical line located 80 ms from the first shows how in the two Brugada patterns the curve of S-T in V_1–V_2 descends, while in athletes, pectus excavatum, and partial RBB it is ascending, at least in V_2 (Corrado index) (Corrado et al., 2010; Bayés de Luna et al., 2012b).

• Figure 16.7 shows the algorithm that we consider most useful for this differential diagnosis (Baranchuck et al., 2014).

16.2.4. Hypertrophic cardiomyopathy

• This is a genetic disease characterized by abnormalities in the proteins of the sarcomere, resulting in a disarray of the fibers, LV hypertrophy, and a risk of VT/VF (McKenna, 2002; Maron, 2010).

• **The ECG is abnormal in 95% of patients** and is sometimes found to be already abnormal before

detecting LVH by echocardiography. Unlike long QT syndrome, there is no clear genotype/phenotype correlation. **E**

• Often, a high-voltage LVH pattern with strain exists, that is difficult to differentiate from LVH due to other etiologies.<\bl>

However, two typical patterns may be found: (A) high voltage R followed by a very negative and peaked T wave (apical hypertrophy) and (B) a fine and sometimes deep Q wave (QS) due to septal hypertrophy, sometimes with low voltage (Fig. 16.8).

16.2.5. Arrhythmogenic right ventricular dysplasia (ARVD)

This is a genetic disease characterized by a fatty infiltration and fibrosis in the RV that can originate VT/VF. **The ECG is abnormal in 80% of patients.** **F** **The most characteristic ECG abnormalities (Marcus, 2009) include:**

• Atypical RBB pattern with a QRS duration in V1 > V6 (Fig. 16.9).

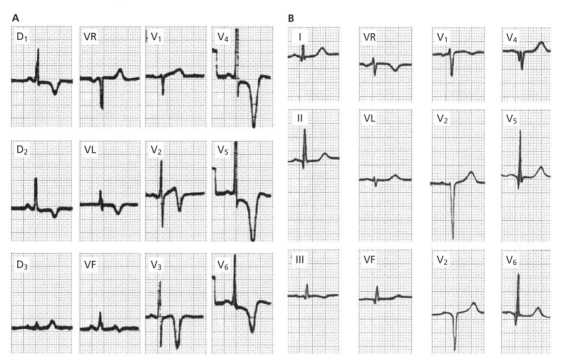

Figure 16.8 (A) Apical hypertrophic cardiomyopathy (HCM). The large negative T waves lead us to make a differential diagnosis with ischemic heart disease (IHD). (B) Hypertrophic cardiomyopathy (HCM). Deep 'q' waves are seen in the anterolateral leads, which may be mistaken for those observed in ischemic heart disease. However, they are usually are narrow and fine.

• In some cases (≈ 10% of cases), there is delayed activation in the RV that is recorded as a wave somewhat separate from QRS (ε wave) and which may mimic partial RBBB (Fig. 16.6). The late potentials that expressed this activation, are positive (see below). Sometimes the ε wave is very small, but its presence is very important for the diagnosis.

• Frequent right ventricle PVCs that may trigger VT with LBBB morphology are frequently with left ÂQRS.

• ST segment in V1-V2 is not usually elevated, or the elevation is very small.

• The T wave is negative and symmetric in V1 to V2-V4.

16.2.6. Non-compacted cardiomyopathy

• This is a genetic disease that is diagnosed today thanks to CV-MRI. It is characterized by an increase in the trabeculated mass in the right ventricle.

• The ECG is abnormal in 95% of cases and **the most characteristic abnormality (70%) is a symmetrical negative T wave in precordial leads beyond V2** (V1 to V3–V5) (Fig. 16.10).

G

• This pattern must not be confused with the normal pattern of a negative T wave seen in young people, which is usually asymmetrical and not present beyond V2.

• Intraventricular conduction disturbances, LVH, and long QT are also frequent.

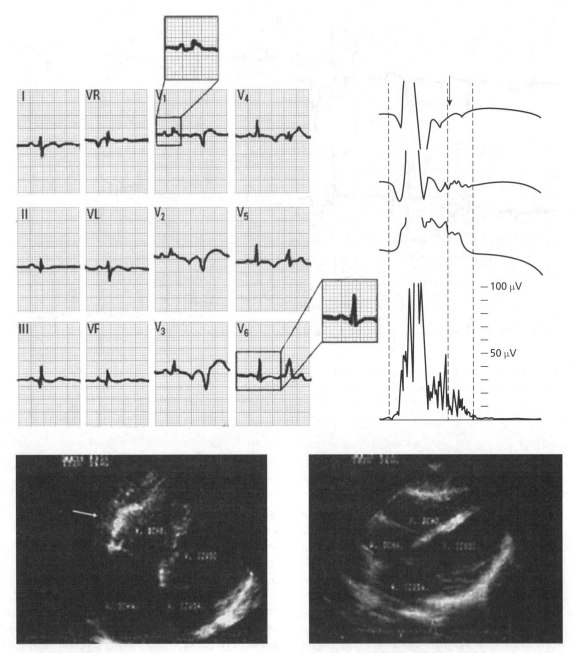

Figure 16.9 Typical ECG pattern of a patient with arrhythmogenic right ventricular cardiomyopathy (ARVC). Note the atypical right bundle branch block (RBBB), premature ventricular complexes (PVCs) from the right ventricle and negative T wave in V1–V4. We also see how QRS duration is clearly longer in V1–V2 than in V6. The patient showed very positive late potentials (right). Below: typical echocardiographic pattern showing the distortion of the right ventricular contraction (arrow).

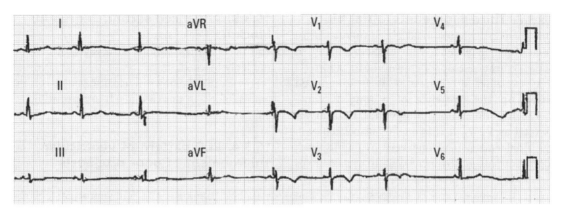

Figure 16.10 ECG of an 18-year-old patient with repetitive sustained ventricular tachycardia (VT). In sinus rhythm a clear QT prolongation is observed (>500 ms), as well as a negative T wave up to lead V3 with a flat T wave in V4–V6. This ECG may be mistaken for a normal ECG variant in a healthy subject. However, the long QT interval, the negative T wave up to V3 and the flat T wave in V4–V6 raise the suspicion of abnormal pattern. The echocardiogram indicates a diagnosis of spongiform cardiomyopathy.

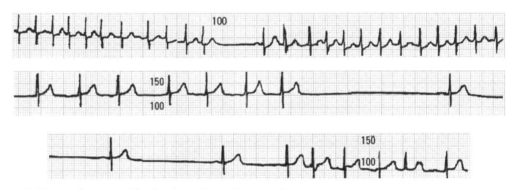

Figure 16.11 Typical pattern of brad-tachycardia syndrome (Holter ECG) (see text).

• Other types of genetically induced VT (Table 16.1) are very rare and are not described here (see Bayés de Luna, 2011 and 2012a).

16.3. High risk ECG patterns that are not genetically induced

H ### 16.3.1. Severe sinus dysfunction
Although it may be of genetic origin, it is generally found in the elderly due to degeneration of the sinus node and is sometimes associated with the use of some drugs.

The ECG shows the presence of marked bradycardia. This constitutes **sick sinus syndrome**, which is frequently associated with depressed automatism in the AV junction and frequent crisis of supraventricular tachyarrhythmia. This gives rise to symptoms ranging from those due to tachyarrhythmia to syncope due to severe bradyarrhythmia (**brady-tachycardia syndrome**). Pacemaker implantation is needed in order to avoid very slow rate and to properly treat the rapid tachyarrhythmias.

Figure 16.11 shows a Holter recording in which runs of tachyarrhythmias with very pronounced sinus pauses may be seen.

16.3.2. Third-degree interatrial block

This is especially found in advanced valvular heart disease and in patients with cardiomyopathy or ischemic heart disease, often with heart failure.

I   As explained in Chapter 5, **it is diagnosed based on the presence of a long P wave (>120 ms) and ± morphology in II, III, and VF, as well as V₁–V₂.** It is frequently associated with left atrial enlargement and very frequently with supraventricular tachyarrhythmia (especially atypical flutter). This represent a true cardiological syndrome (Bayés de Luna et al., 1985; Conde and Baranchuck, 2014) (Fig. 16.12).

16.3.3. Advanced second-degree AV block (Chapter 13)

This occurs when various successive P waves are suddenly blocked.

Figure 13.4C shows a clear example of this type of block, in this case needs urgent pacemaker implantation.

16.3.4. ECG pattern of ventricular enlargement of poor prognosis
(Chapter 6)   J

• In both the right and left ventricular enlargement the presence of high R and strain-type

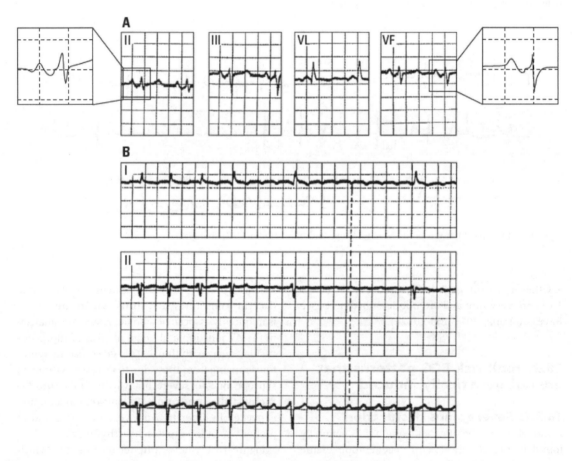

Figure 16.12 (A) Example of advanced interatrial block with retrograde conduction (P ± in II, III, and VF). (B) Associated atypical flutter.

repolarization morphology indicates severe and advanced ventricular enlargement.

• In RVE a pattern of rsR' with QRS <120 ms may be an expression of poor prognosis as in the isolated pattern of advanced RBB (in V_1 rSR' with QRS >120 ms).

• The presence of atrial fibrillation adds another risk factor, as does the presence of frequent ventricular extrasystoles.

16.3.5. High risk ventricular block

K (Chapter 7)

This group includes:

(a) The appearance of advanced RBBB in patients with sudden dyspnea (possible pulmonary embolism) or anginal pain with ST elevation in precordial leads (possible proximal LAD occlusion or complete occlusion of the main trunk) can lead to a very critical hemodynamic situation, especially in the latter case.

(b) RBBB and LBBB alternance, or RBBB+SAH alternating with RBBB+IPH (Rosenbaum–Elizari syndrome) (Fig. 7.24). In these cases u rgent pacemaker implantation is required.

(c) Masked block. This is characterized by the presence of RBBB in the HP (R in V1) with very left ÂQRS in the FP and without S in I and VL. This pattern is due to bifascicular block (RBBB+SAH) with important LVH. This is due to the fact that the late forces of activation are forward and not directed to the right, but rather to the left. Consequently there is no S in I and VL, although there is terminal R in V1 (Fig. 7.25B).

(d) Generally, in acute and chronic ischemic heart disease and in cardiomyopathies with heart failure, **the presence of branch block, especially LBBB**, is a marker of poor prognosis. In patients with advanced LBBB and left ÂQRS, a terminal R wave in VR suggests that a large dilation in the RV exists (Van Bommel et al., 2011) (see Chapter 7).

L 16.3.6. High risk WPW syndrome

Patients with episodes of very fast AF and very short RR intervals and those who present certain risk factors (fixed pre-excitation in the stress test or very short refractory period in the electrophysio-

logic study (EPS) are at risk of VF (Fig. 8.11) and must undergo ablation of the accessory pathway.

16.3.7. High risk ECG patterns in acute and chronic ischemic heart disease

A. Acute ischemic heart disease   M

• **High risk ACS in relation to the ECG pattern**

   1. ECG pattern of severe and extensive ischemia: ascending S wave being pushed upward by ST elevation and the sum of shifts of ST ≥15 mm (Fig. 9.8).

   2. ECG pattern of STE-ACS due to complete occlusion of the proximal LAD or left main trunk (Fig. 9.11A).

   3. Persistent ST elevation (several days). This is a marker of cardiac rupture.

   4. ECG pattern of left main subocclusion: NSTE-ACS with ST depression in seven or more leads and ST elevation in VR ≥ 1 mm (Fig. 9.21).

   5. Presence of frequent ventricular extrasystoles, atrial fibrillation, or AV block.

   6. Presence of confounding factors (LVH with strain pattern, bundle branch block, pacemaker, etc.)

• **Coronary spasm** with pattern of ST elevation, that looks like TAP pattern, ventricular arrhythmias and/or ST/TQ alternans accompanied by arrhythmia.

B. Chronic ischemic heart disease   N

1. Presence of frequent PVC's in patients with depressed ejection fraction.

2. Presence of sinus tachycardia.

3. Presence of residual ST elevation. It is necessary to rule out ventricular aneurism (Fig. 9.45).

4. Presence of intraventricular conduction disturbances, especially if are viewed.

5. Presence of pacemaker.

6. Presence of atrial fibrillation.

The presence of these patterns as risk markers should be considered in the global clinical setting of patients with acute and chronic ischemic heart disease. In the chronic cases the presence of low ejection fraction and the demonstration of electric instability are especially important. In the acute phase the clinical setting and the hemodynamic

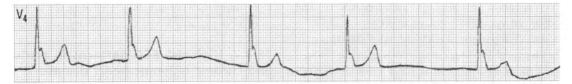

Figure 16.13 Typical ECG pattern of hypothermia. See the evident J wave, the instability of the baseline and the slow heart rate without clear P wave (see text).

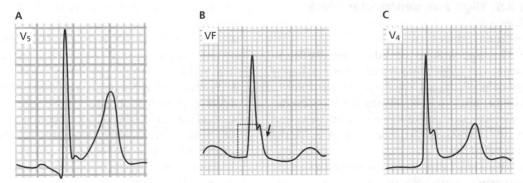

Figure 16.14 Examples of J wave. (A and B) Early repolarization (ER) patterns. (A) ER pattern recorded in mid-left precordial leads with small J wave and rapidly ascending ST-segment. This is a typical benign pattern. (B) Inferior ER pattern with evident J wave (>0,2 mv) and horizontal/descending ST segment. It should be noted that the prevalence of cases of malignant-type ER is very low (see text). (C) Typical pattern of hypothermia with J wave that is seen in many leads (see Fig. 16.13). J wave amplitude was measured from the baseline at PR interval, to the peak of the notch-type J wave (B) or the transition point in case of the slur-type J wave (see Section 16.3.8.2).

situation together with an evaluation of the biomarkers are of great importance.

O **16.3.8. Hypothermia and other ECG patterns with J wave**

16.3.8.1. Hypothermia produces characteristic ECG changes

These include (Fig. 16.13):
- Irregularity of the baseline.
- Bradycardia occasionally with no apparent P wave (undetectable sinus activity, sinoventricular conduction, or escape rhythm).
- Lengthening of the PR and QT intervals.
- Appearance of a clear J wave.
- Risk of serious arrhythmia.

16.3.8.2. Early repolarization (ER)

J wave or slurring appear at the end of QRS, and are recorded especially in V3-V6 and sometimes II, III, VF, I, and VL (see Fig. 16.14). This pattern is usually benign, especially if it is not present in inferior leads. It is frequently seen in athletes and in the presence of high vagal tone, and is usually followed by ascending ST (Fig. 16.14A). The amplitude of the J wave is measured from the high take-off of the J wave to the level of isoelectric line in the PR interval (Fig. 16.14B), or in the case of slurring at the moment of transition point (Nakagama et al., 2014).

It is considered that it may be dangerous if the J-wave is greater than 2 mm, and particularly if it is recorded in the leads of the inferior wall and is followed by a horizontal/descending ST segment. This malignant type of ER is very rare (Fig. 16.14B).

Recently, it has been proposed to combine all processes involving the presence of the J wave, under the term **'J wave syndromes'** (Antzelevitch and Yan, 2010). These authors consider that the electrophysiological explanation of early repolarization (ER) and Brugada syndrome (BS) are similar and that the r′ of BS is a J wave. Therefore, they include BS in J wave syndrome. There are currently some discrepancies about this classification. However, it is true that occasionally both BS and EP patterns appear in the same patient (Sarkozy et al., 2009), which is a marker of bad prognosis.

16.3.9. Ionic disturbances

Ionic disturbances refer especially to abnormalities in blood levels of potassium, which produce the most marked and potentially dangerous ECG changes (Surawicz, 1967). They are often associated with other ionic disturbances (see Bayés de Luna, 2012a).

These ionic abnormalities may be observed, between other situations, after the administration of certain drugs such as diuretics (hypokalemia) and in renal failure (hyperkalemia).

P **1. Hyperkalemia** (Fig. 16.15)
The ECG changes appear progressively in relation to the levels of K.
(a) There is a high and peaked T wave with ST elevation.
(b) In more advanced cases the QRS is wider and the P wave disappears.
(c) The rhythm may progressively slow down (escape rhythm).

Figure 16.15 shows an ECG in a patient with severe renal failure whose abnormalities regress when the problem is solved.

2. Hypokalemia (Fig. 16.16)   Q
The ECG changes include ST depression and a lengthened QT interval, partly because the U wave is mixed with the end of a flat T wave.

16.3.10. Acquired long QT interval

An acquired prolongation of the QT interval is also   R
dangerous and it may provoke serious arrhythmia (pro-arrhythmic effect). The cause of acquired long QT syndrome may be related to ionic and metabolic imbalances, poisoning, or the administration of certain drugs. **The risk of provoking VT/VF is clear when the medication lengthens QT to >60 ms or the QT interval is >500 ms.**

The most common drugs associated with lengthened QT are the following:
1. Antiarrhythmic agents, especially quinidine-like.
2. Antibiotics, such as eritromicine.
3. Fluoroquinolones .
4. Antidepressants: amitriptyline, fluoxetine, etc.
5. Antihistaminic agents: terfenedine (off the market).
6. Digestive tract: cisapride (off the market).

However, with low doses of these drugs, serious problems are very rare. It is useful to monitor the QT interval when these medications are given over long periods of time. See www.qtdrugs.com

16.3.11. Patients with pacemakers

Although the implantation of a pacemaker can save many lives, when implanted in the right ventricle (still the most frequent site), it may cause heart failure over time due to the asynchrony of the contraction of the two ventricles, especially in patients with heart disease or in the elderly. This may require the implantation of a pacemaker in the LV (resynchronization therapy) (see Chapter 13).

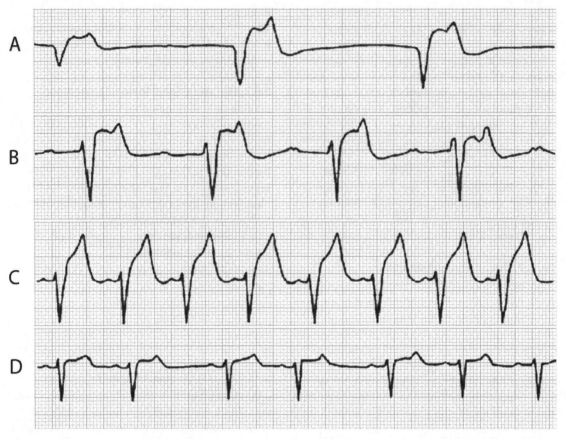

Figure 16.15 An 82-year-old patient with chronic renal failure and significant hyperkalemia (9.2 mEq/l) upon arrival (A) with a diagnosis of a severe renal failure and presyncope. The QRS is very wide and no P waves are seen. This is probably a ventricular escape rhythm, but the possibility of a slow sinus node rhythm with sinoventricular conduction cannot be ruled out, since this kind of conduction disorder may be observed with hyperkalemia (Bellet and Jedlicka, 1969). From (B) to (F), a progressive normalization of the ECG tracing after the improvement of the clinical picture with dialysis. Serum potassium level was normal in (F).

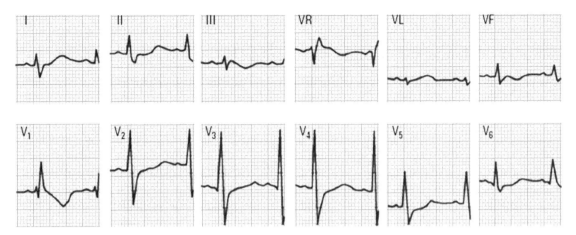

Figure 16.16 This belongs to a 45-year-old patient with advanced mitroaortic heart valve disease treated with excessive doses of digitalis and diuretics. Extracellular K^+ level is 2.3 mEq/l. We can see a long QT and ST depression in many leads especially V2–V4.

Self-assessment

A. What are the typical ECG abnormalities in congenital long QT syndrome?

B. What are the typical ECG abnormalities in short QT syndrome?

C. Describe the two types of Brugada ECG pattern.

D. Explain how the differential diagnosis of the Brugada ECG patterns type II are made.

E. List the ECG characteristics in hypertrophic cardiomyopathy.

F. List the ECG characteristics in ARVD.

G. List the ECG characteristics in non-compacted myocardiopathy.

H. What is the relevance of severe sinus dysfunction?

I. What arrhythmias are related to third-degree interatrial block?

J. Which ECG patterns of ventricular enlargement have a poor prognosis?

K. Which ECG patterns of ventricular block have a poor prognosis?

L. Which ECG patterns in patients with WPW syndrome have a poor prognosis?

M. Which ECG patterns in patients with ACS indicate risk?

N. Which ECG patterns in chronic ischemic heart diseases indicate risk?

O. Describe the typical ECG pattern in hypothermia.

P. Describe the typical ECG pattern in hyperkalemia.

Q. Describe the typical ECG pattern in hypokalemia.

R. Under what circumstances is the acquired long QT syndrome due to drug administration dangerous?

CHAPTER 17

ECG Recordings in Other Heart Diseases and Different Situations

In Chapter 9 we explained the most important aspects of ischemic heart disease, and in Chapter 15 we discussed the important role of the ECG in the diagnosis of precordial pain and other symptoms. In Chapter 16 we described the ECG patterns with a poor prognosis in asymptomatic patients. This includes ECG patterns of genetically induced heart disease and other ECG patterns with poor prognosis, some of which have been described in other parts of this book.

In this chapter we will look very closely at the ECG abnormalities most commonly found in other heart disease cases and different situations, including all types of myocardiopathy seen in patients with systemic or neurodegenerative disease (e.g. amyloidosis or neuromuscular disease).

A 17.1. Valvular heart diseases

The most frequent ECG abnormalities are listed below.

17.1.1. Mitral stenosis
1. P wave of left atrial enlargement (LAE) (Fig. 5.2D).
2. Atrial fibrillation (AF) is very common during the course of the disease.
3. Right ventricular enlargement (RVE) in cases of overload of the right cavities (pulmonary hypertension) (Fig. 6.4A).
4. If tricuspid involvement is present, biatrial enlargement and/or AF may occur (Fig. 5.4).

17.1.2. Mitral regurgitation
1. In advanced cases, signs of LAE and left ventricular enlargement (LVE) are present (Chapters 5 and 6).
2. AF may also occur, but it is less frequent than in mitral stenosis.
3. Apart from LVE, repolarization disturbances may take place, especially in inferolateral leads in patients with mitral valve prolapse.

17.1.3. Aortic valve disease
In the advanced phase of severe stenosis, regurgitation, or double aortic valve disease, we have already commented on the fact that (Figs 6.12A and 6.12B), the ECG generally presents a descending ST and negative asymmetric T wave morphology (strain pattern). This morphology may be modified when associated primary abnormalities exist (Fig. 6.12C).

In severe but not long-lasting cases, the ECG may be nearly normal even when echocardiography reveals LVE. A high voltage R wave with evident 'q' wave and horizontal ST followed by high, peaked, and symmetric T wave, sometimes followed by negative U wave, may be seen in V5–6. This pattern that is seen especially in severe aortic regurgitation that is not long-lasting, evolves with time to a typical pattern of LVE with strain (Fig. 6.12B). The voltage criteria of LVE are usually increased in advanced cases (see Chapter 6).

Isolated aortic valve disease is not usually accompanied by AF. If AF is present, associated mitral valve disease has to be ruled out. At the same time,

ECGs for Beginners, First Edition. Antoni Bayés de Luna.
© 2014 John Wiley & Sons, Inc. Published 2014 by John Wiley & Sons, Inc.

in very advanced cases of calcified aortic stenosis advanced AV block may occur.

17.2. Myocarditis

In the acute phase the following abnormalities may be observed (Fig. 17.1):

1. Sinus tachycardia.
2. Low voltage QRS.
3. Repolarization abnormalities: Flat or negative T wave or ST elevation (differential diagnosis with ACS).
4. Intraventricular conduction disturbances (IVCD) and/or AV block.
5. Pathologic Q, which is often reversible.

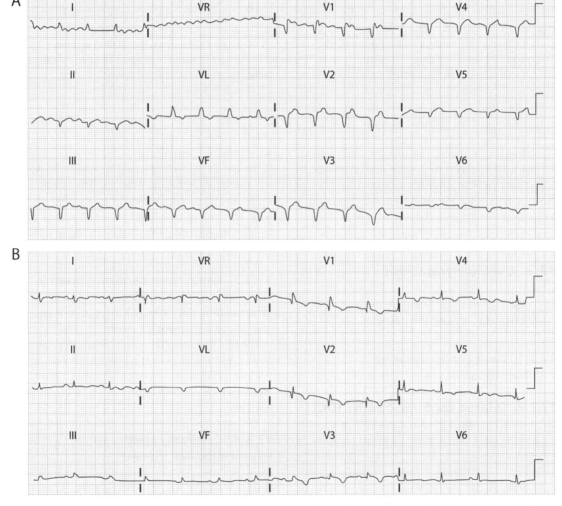

Figure 17.1 (A) A patient with acute myocarditis and ECG with low voltage and signs of right bundle branch block plus superoanterior hemiblock and a Q wave of necrosis in many leads. After the acute phase (B), the Q waves and superoanterior hemiblock disappear. In many leads, a mild and diffuse pattern of negative T wave is present and the low voltage persists.

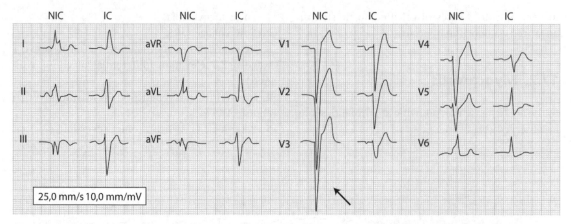

Figure 17.2 ECGs of two patients, one with non-ischemic cardiomyopathy (NIC) and the other with ischemic cardiomyopathy (IC). Both ECGs have a similar QRS width, left ventricular ejection fraction (LVEF) and left ventricular end diastolic diameter (LVEDD). Note the pronounced voltages of right precordial leads, particularly in V2 and V3 (arrow), observable in non-ischemic cardiomyopathy compared to ischemic cardiomyopathy.

During the course of the process, these disturbances usually revert to a large degree, except in cases that evolve to cardiomyopathy. A flat T wave or some type of intraventricular conduction disturbance may remain as a residual pattern.

17.3. Cardiomyopathies

The ECG abnormalities found in different types of cardiomyopathy include the following:

17.3.1. Genetically induced cardiomyopathies (see Chapter 16)

17.3.2. Dilated cardiomyopathy (DC)

The ECG is abnormal in more than 90% of patients if heart failure (HF) is present. It frequently involves:

1. Sinus tachycardia or supraventricular tachyarrhythmia.

2. Different types of intraventricular block. If heart failure is present, LBBB with QRS ≥140 ms requires resynchronization pacemaker implantation.

3. RVE and/or LAE pattern.

4. Ventricular arrhythmia.

5. In the DC of ischemic origin, S wave in V3, in the presence of LBBB, presents less voltage and more slurrings than in idiopathic DC (Fig. 17.2).

6. In the case of LBBB, the presence of terminal R in VR suggests dilation of the RV (Van Bommel et al., 2011) (see Chapter 7) (Fig. 17.3).

17.3.3. Restrictive cardiomyopathy

There are two types: infiltrative (e.g. amyloidosis or sarcoidosis, etc) (Fig. 17.4) or non-infiltrative (e.g. idiopathic or storage disease).

The ECG abnormalities most commonly observed are: (1) pseudonecrosis Q wave; (2) very abnormal P wave; (3) different types of ventricular block; (4) repolarization disturbances; and (5) often atrial fibrillation.

17.3.4. Cardiomyopathy in neuromuscular disease

Examples are Steinert disease, Friedreich disease, Duchene disease, etc. The ECG shows: (1) enlargement; (2) ventricular blocks; (3) Q of pseudonecrosis (Fig. 17.5); (4) R in V1 due to probable right ventricle or septal hypertrophy; and (5) repolarization disturbances.

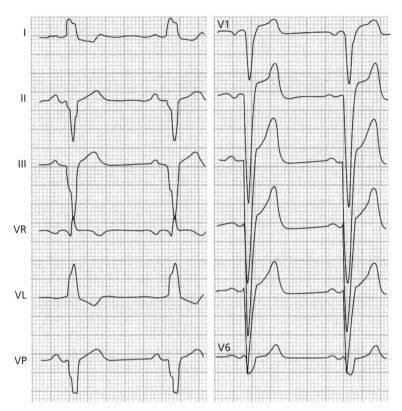

Figure 17.3 ECG of a patient with idiopathic dilated cardiomyopathy with very low ejection fraction and LBBB. See the presence of final tall R wave in VR due to huge right chamber dilation. (Source: Van Bommel, 2011. Reproduced with permission of Elsevier.)

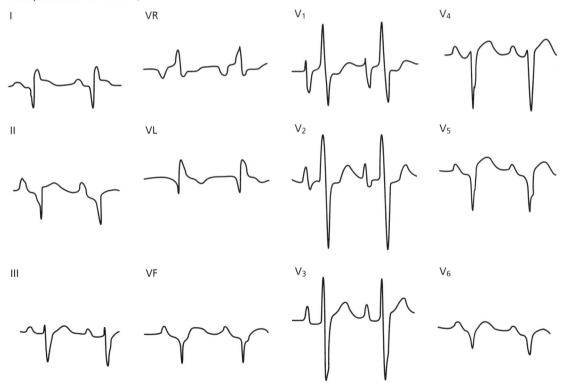

Figure 17.4 A patient with advanced restrictive cardiomyopathy. Note the presence of clear QRS abnormalities simulating lateral necrosis. Evident P wave signs of very important biatrial enlargement are found in this type of cardiomyopathy.

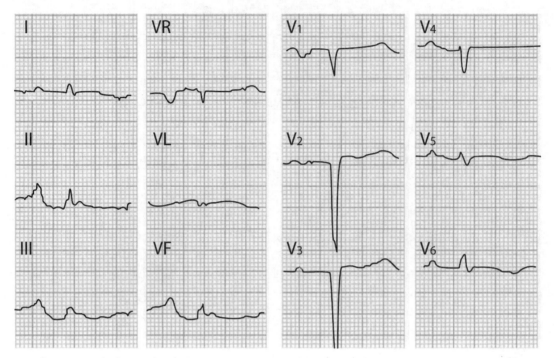

Figure 17.5 Patient of 56 years with cardiac amyloidosis that presents pathologic Q wave, low voltage and abnormal repolarization.

17.4. Diseases of the pericardium

D 17.4.1. Acute idiopathic pericarditis

Four ECG changes have been described that take place over time (Spodick, 1982) (Fig. 17.6):

Phase 1. ST elevation that generally appears as a pattern of early repolarization and evolves to phase 2.

Phase 2. The ST returns to isoelectric line.

Phase 3. The T wave becomes negative.

Phase 4. Return to normal pattern.

However, all of these changes are currently often not observed due to rapid treatment with anti-inflammatory medication.

17.4.2. Pericarditis with important effusion

E Sinus tachycardia and very low QRS voltage are very common, sometimes with slow increase of R voltage in precordial leads. In addition, alternans in the QRS complex may be observed in the presence of pericardial tamponade (Fig. 14.2A).

17.5. Cor pulmonale

The ECG changes indicating RVE that may be seen **F** in **chronic cor pulmonale** (see Fig. 6.4C) and **acute cor pulmonale**, including pulmonary embolism (Figs. 15.3 and 15.4), have been described in Chapter 6.

17.6. Congenital heart disease

The most characteristic abnormalities detected in **G** the most common congenital heart diseases are listed below.

1. Atrial septal defect (ASD) (Fig. 6.6):

   (a) V1 presents in many cases with rSR', ECG pattern similar to partial RBBB that corresponds to RVE with dilation.

   (b) In small ASD the rSR' pattern may be missing.

   (c) Atrial fibrillation (AF) in adults.

   (d) Left ÂQRS in ostium primum ASD.

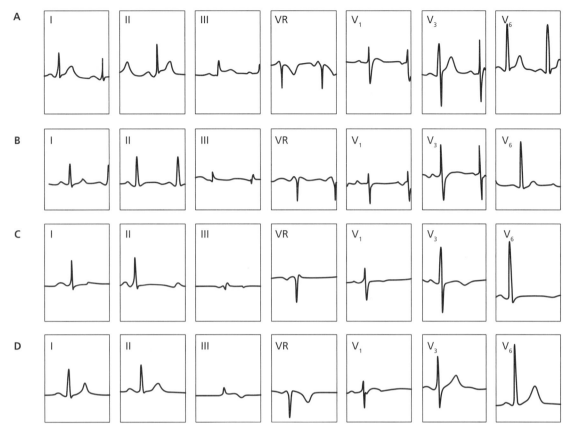

Figure 17.6 A 43-year-old male with acute pericarditis and the four ECG evolutive phases. The A, B, C and D recordings were obtained at days 1, 8, 10, and 90. (A) The ST segment elevation convex respects the isoelectric line. (B) Flattening of the T wave. (C) Inversion of the T wave. (D) Normalization.

2. Ventricular septal defect (VSD) (Fig. 17.7):

(a) In small VSD the ECG is usually normal.

(b) In large VSD signs of biventricular enlargement are seen, sometimes with high RS voltages in mid precordial leads and rSr' in V1.

(c) In severe pulmonary hypertension (Eisenmenger syndrome), R wave may be high in V1.

3. Tricuspid atresia (Fig. 17.8):

(a) Left ÂQRS.

(b) P wave of right atrial enlargement.

4. Ebstein disease (Fig. 17.9):

(a) Atypical RBBB.

(b) High-voltage P wave.

(c) Sometimes delta wave (pre-excitation).

5. Pulmonary stenosis with intact septum (Fig. 6.5):

Depending on severity, various degrees of right ventricular enlargement (RVE), sometimes with R in V_1-V_2, are observed (Fig. 5.4C).

6. Tetralogy of Fallot (Fig. 17.10):

RVE with R in V1, but with RS in V2, is common and differentiates from severe pulmonary stenosis with intact septum. In less severe cases RS with positive T in V1 may be recorded.

7. Stenosis/coarctation of the aorta:

Signs of left ventricular enlargement (LVE) that are more or less relevant according to severity and time of evolution (Fig. 6.12A).

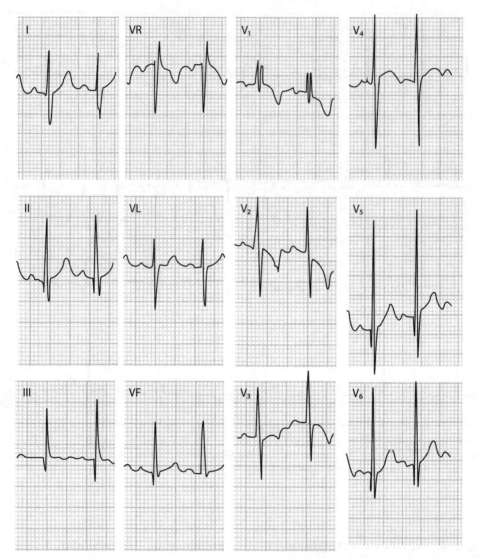

Figure 17.7 Example of biventricular enlargement (see text). An 8-year-old patient with a ventricular septal defect (VSD) and hyperkinetic pulmonary hypertension (Katz–Watchell pattern).

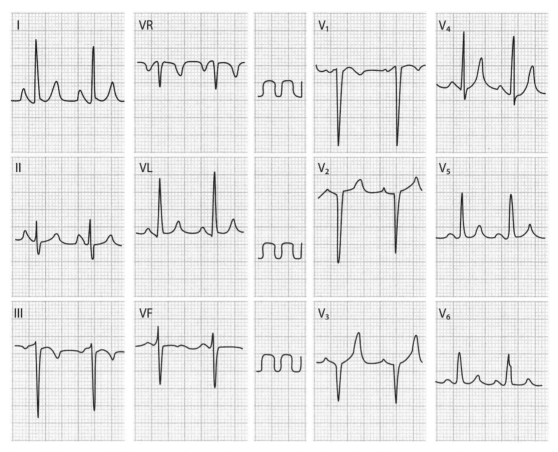

Figure 17.8 A typical ECG of tricuspid atresia. Note the hyperdeviation of the QRS axis to the left and the signs suggestive of right atrial and left ventricular enlargement.

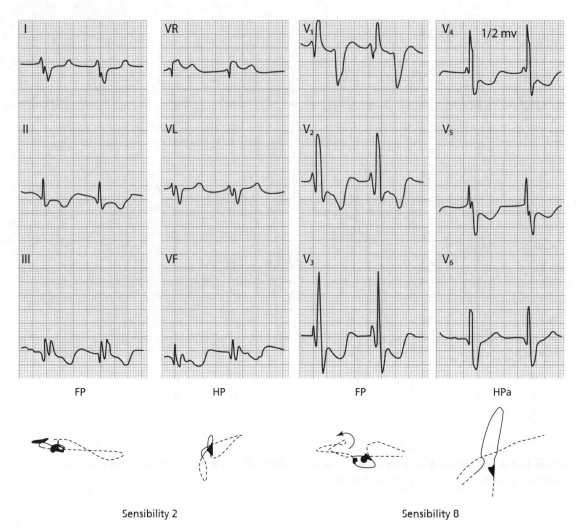

Figure 17.9 ECG and VCG of a child with Ebstein's disease. Note the long PR interval, the high-voltage P wave on the T wave (P +———, mimicking rS morphology in V1) and the atypical right bundle branch block morphology. FP: Frontal plane; HP: horizontal plane.

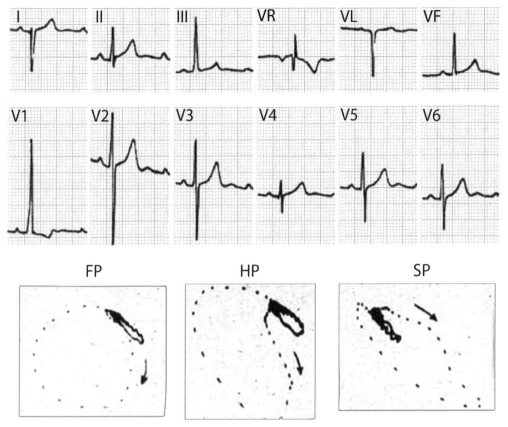

Figure 17.10 A 3-year-old patient with typical tetralogy of Fallot. The ECG corresponds to the Mexican School-named 'RVE with adaptation-type systolic overload' (R in V1 with negative T and rS in V2 with positive T). Note the ECG–VCG correlation.

8. Mirror-image dextrocardia:

Negative P is seen in V1. This may be also seen in the presence of ectopic rhythm, or inversion of right-left arms electrodes (Fig. 3.6).

17.7. Arterial hypertension (AH)

H **Generally, there is a strong relationship between the severity and time of development of AH and the ECG abnormalities.** As previously discussed (Fig. 6.12C), the pattern of left ventricular enlargement (LVE) with strain is seen in advanced cases, and later than LVE is detected by echocardiography. However, the presence of clear signs of LVE indicates a poorer prognosis than the simple presence of LVH in the echocardiogram. Furthermore, the LVE pattern with strain may be reversible with treatment.

The LVE ECG criteria are similar to those described in Chapter 6. The criteria with a higher SE ($\geq$80%) are:

(a) $RV_6 \mid RV_5 > 0.65$.

(b) The global sum of the QRS voltage in the 12 leads >120 mm.

However, the other criteria described in Chapter 6 (Section 6.3.3) are more specific.

As previously stated, the signs of LVE, especially those related to repolarization, may improve with treatment of AH.

Frequently, in cases of mid/moderate AH when the LVE is even absent or not important, the ST/T

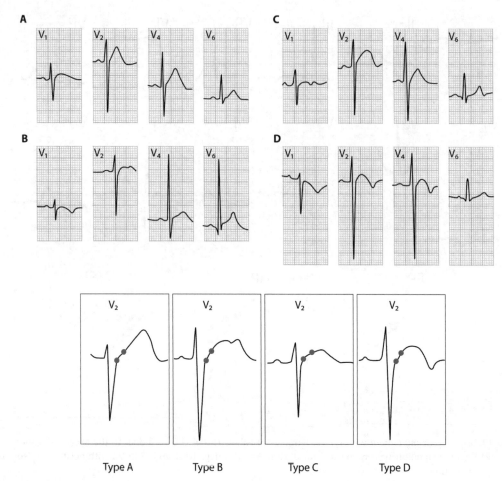

Figure 17.11 Different types of repolarization abnormalities found in athletes. These are usually benign, but it is essential to perform an echocardiogram to rule out hypertrophic cardiomyopathy. Below may be seen (·) the placement in V2 of the two lines (separated by 80 ms) to measure the Corrado index. In all cases the index ST elevation at J point/ ST elevation 80 ms later in <1 in athletes, and in Brugada syndrome is >1 (see Fig. 16.6 and Section 16.2.3.2 in Chapter 16). (See Plate 17.11.)

wave shows mild changes that may also be seen in normal people especially the elderly (rectified ST and symmetric T wave in some leads) (see Fig. 6.11 and Section 4.7.1 in Chapter 4).

17.8. Athletes

It should be remembered that the **ECG changes listed below may be related to physical training** and therefore may disappear or diminish when physical activity is reduced. **Thus, they do not indicate disease.**

1. Sinus bradycardia that is sometimes considerable.

2. First-degree AV block or even Wenckebach-type second-degree AV block when at rest or during sleep.

3. rSr′ pattern in V_1. The differential diagnosis with other processes with r′ in V1, including type 2-Brugada pattern, has to be performed (Fig. 16.5).

4. High R voltage in left precordial leads.

5. Early repolarization pattern (see Chapter 4).

6. Isolated extrasystoles.

   On the contrary, the following ECG abnormalities include:

1. Negative T wave in $\geq$ two contiguous leads (Fig. 17.11).

2. ST depression.

3. Pathologic Q wave.

4. Very abnormal P wave.

5. Right of left advanced BBB.

6. Ruling out Brugada pattern.

7. Ruling out short and long QT.

8. Clear signs of ventricular enlargement (strain).

9. Significant arrhythmia (f.i. >I PVC in 12 lead ECG recording.

   These are non-training related ECG findings and need further evaluation.

17.9. Drugs

J **Many medications can alter the ECG, especially in terms of repolarization** (amiodarone, digitalis). Rarely, these medications **can abnormally, and not homogeneously, prolong repolarization and the QT interval**, producing a dangerous proarrhythmic effect, including SD (Chapter 16 and Bayés de Luna, 2012a).

17.10. Other repolarization disturbances

As previously explained, repolarization may be altered by alcohol or glucose consumption and hyperventilation (Fig. 4.25).

Self-assessment

A. List the most characteristic ECG abnormalities observed in valvular heart diseases.

B. List the most characteristic ECG abnormalities observed in myocarditis.

C. List the most characteristic ECG abnormalities observed in dilated cardiomyopathy.

D. List the most characteristic ECG abnormalities observed in acute idiopathic pericarditis.

E. List the most characteristic ECG abnormalities observed in acute pericarditis with great effusion.

F. List the most characteristic ECG abnormalities observed in acute and chronic cor pulmonale.

G. List the most characteristic ECG abnormalities observed in the more common congenital heart diseases.

H. What are the most common ECG characteristics in arterial hypertension?

I. Describe the ECG changes that may be due to exercise and are not considered pathologic by themselves.

J. Describe the ECG changes that may be due to the administration of different drugs.

CHAPTER 18

Abnormal ECG Without Apparent Heart Disease and Normal ECG in Serious Heart Disease

A I would like to finish this short book which deals with the bases of normal ECG and the clues of ECG diagnosis, with a short chapter devoted to the importance of taking into consideration the clinical context of each patient in interpreting the ECG. For this we will comment on two situations that the physician is faced with: (1) patients without any symptoms or physical signs of heart disease who present an abnormal ECG; and (2) a patient who has a normal (or nearly normal) ECG, but presents with serious heart disease that may be advanced.

We will see how important it is in both cases to know that these situations exist, and that it is important to correlate the ECG with the clinical context of the patient.

18.1. Abnormal ECG in a patient with normal history taking and physical examination

On occasion, an abnormal ECG is recorded (bundle branch block or patterns suggesting chamber enlargement, ischemias, or necrosis, or different types of arrhythmias) in a patient who does not present any symptoms or is not aware that he has this abnormal ECG. The physical examination is also normal. In this situation, we feel that the most important measure to take is to follow the steps outlined below.

1. Do not trust in the automatic interpretation.

All ECGs need a double-check by a physician.

2. Ensure that the ECG recording is correct.

Many patterns compatible with partial RBBB (rSr' in V1) and many other abnormal patterns are due to the erroneous placement of the electrodes (Chapter 3).

3. Complete the medical history again.

Special emphasis must be placed on any symptoms the patients may not have evaluated correctly or not noticed, for example:

(a) High abdominal pain that may be the expression of an apparently silent diaphragmatic infarction, according to the Framingham study. This study showed that the appearance of a Q wave of necrosis from 1 year to the next in the ECG, was due to undiagnosed infarction, especially in diabetics.

(b) Episodes of arrhythmia, especially of atrial fibrillation (AF), or premature beats, or runs of paroxysmal tachycardia that were incorrectly diagnosed, and attributed to emotional palpitations (sinus), or were unnoticed by the patient. In these patients it is important to determine whether emotion or consumption of alcohol or energizing agents could be causing the ECG abnormalities. The presence of asymptomatic arrhythmia, especially if frequent, obliges us to rule out any associated heart disease.

ECGs for Beginners, First Edition. Antoni Bayés de Luna.
© 2014 John Wiley & Sons, Inc. Published 2014 by John Wiley & Sons, Inc.

(c) Erroneous evaluation of dyspnea, which may be due to heart failure or pulmonary embolism, but had been considered to be related with obesity, age, etc.

(d) Erroneous evaluation of syncope or presyncope as due to hypotension or neuro-mediated by vagal reflex when it may be the expression of a serious condition. We must ask patients about a family history of sudden death and inquire more about possible inherited heart disease. We must measure the QT interval carefully, and closely examine the entire ECG recording to rule out Brugada syndrome or any cardiomyopathy of genetic origin (see Chapter 17).

(e) It is necessary to complete the 'bedside diagnosis' with a good physical exam that encompasses inspection, palpation and auscultaton of the heart and the great vessels. This may provide some information, such as the presence of heart murmurs, which may be useful for the global approach of the problem.

(f) Finally it is necessary to follow the systematic method of interpretation explained in Chapter 4.

4. **The cases with abnormal ECG that we have to study more carefully are the following:**

(a) **Presence of abnormal classical parameters: PR and QT intervals, ÂQRS axis, etc.**

B (b) **Presence of Q wave of necrosis in asymptomatic patients.**

Above all, it is important to remember that some deep Q waves may be normal. For example, in lead III a deep Q wave may simulate a myocardial infarction. However, these Q waves are benign and due to positional changes, especially in a horizontal and dextrorotated heart if they disappear with deep breathing (Fig. 4.22).

As previously explained, **the presence of a pathologic Q wave may be due to silent myocardial infarction.** However, an abnormal Q wave in a patient without previous antecedents of ischemic heart disease may be a sign of other conditions that have remained asymptomatic, such as inherited cardiomyopathy (hypertrophic), systemic diseases with myocardial involvement (amyloidosis, sarcoidosis, etc.),

previous myocarditis, neuromuscular disease, or any type of restrictive or hypertrophic cardiomyopathy that has not yet produced symptoms (Chapters 16 and 17).

(c) **Presence of repolarization disturbances.**

Flat/slightly negative T waves seen in many leads may be a sign of **previous pericarditis** that went undetected or **undiagnosed myocarditis.** Naturally, they may be also seen as a **residual pattern of ischemic heart disease.** In these cases some specific lead patterns are usually located, and the T wave may be deeper and present a mirror pattern.

The T wave changes (flat/slightly negative), may be also seen in many other circumstances (Fig. 9.29) and sporadically after consuming alcohol or certain foods, and hyperventilation (Fig. 4.25).

ST changes may be due to multiple causes (Figs 9.20 and 9.28) apart from ischemic heart disease. In acute ischemic heart disease, ST changes occur especially in relation with angina. However they may remain as a residual pattern after the acute phase (see Chapter 9).

(d) **Presence of voltage criteria for LVE.** This may be seen in healthy patients, especially   D in thin young people without ST abnormalities, in the absence of anatomic LVH. However, in some cases especially in the presence of repolarization abnormalities, they may be the expression of undetected true LVH.

(e) **Presence of high R wave or r' in V_1.** This may be a sign of many types of heart disease, but it may also be seen as a normal variant (Table 6.1).

(f) **Presence of advanced bundle branch block in asymptomatic patients.** These cases   F must be studied in depth, especially if the patient is relatively young and the block in located in the left branch. Heart involvement, especially cardiomyopathy due to any etiology, must be ruled out. However, in at least 10% of LBBB patients and in a large number of RBBB patients, it is an isolated manifestation of an exclusive problem in the ventricular conduction system (Lenègre syndrome and Lev syndrome). Nevertheless, it is important to remember the patterns of right or left bundle branch block, that are markers of high risk (Chapter 16).

(g) Presence of active arrhythmias (especially PVCs and/or passive arrhythmias (pauses and/or blocks).

In all these cases it is necessary to rule out the effect of some drugs that may trigger these arrhythmias. It will probably be necessary to perform complementary tests such as Holter ECG, exercise testing and also echocardiography (imaging techniques).

18.2. Normal ECG in patients with advanced cardiovascular disease

Although the ECG is very important in the diagnosis of heart disease, we must not forget that a normal, or apparently normal, ECG may be recorded just before sudden death (SD) of cardiovascular origin. The most common (not exhaustive) severe forms of cardiovascular disease that may be accompanied by a normal ECG are listed below.

1. Acute heart attack.

In the presence of NSTE-ACS, the ECG may appear normal in a small number of cases (see Section 9.3.3.1.4 in Chapter 9). We must also remember that a peaked symmetrical T wave may be the only visible abnormality, especially in V1-V2 in the hyperacute phase of STE-ACS (see Section 9.2.3.1.2 in Chapter 9).

2. Pulmonary embolism.

The cataclysm that is a severe pulmonary embolism may appear suddenly, especially in bedridden patients without evident heart disease and with a previous apparently normal ECG recording. The patient generally presents sinus tachycardia and other ECG abnormalities (Figs 15.3 and 15.4), but elderly patients with deteriorated sinus function and previously abnormal basal ECG, may not present sinus tachycardia, which makes the diagnosis more difficult.

3. Inherited heart diseases.

The ECG may be slightly abnormal or poorly evaluated. This type of disease includes **channelopathies** (Brugada syndrome and long and short QT syndromes) and **genetic cardiomyopathies** (e.g. hypertrophy) (see Chapter 16).

In **hypertrophic cardiomyopathy** the ECG may appear abnormal before the echocardiogram, but in 5% to 10% of cases the ECG may appear to be normal. The same may occur in arrhythmogenic RV dysplasia.

In **Brugada syndrome** the ECG may vary abruptly from normality to type 1 or 2 pattern with certain triggers (e.g. fever, drugs). Furthermore, it may appear normal or nearly normal in the fourth intercostal space (IS) and it may be pathologic in the second IS.

The limits of normality in the **long and short QT syndromes** may require additional tests.

In patients with a family history of inherited channelopathy or cardiomyopathy, a careful analysis and additional tests are required before determining whether an ECG is normal or pathologic.

4. Aortic aneurism with dissection or rupture.

The ECG may be normal or show LVH with strain in V5-V6 that may be confused in V1-V2 with an ST elevation of ACS (mirror pattern) (Fig. 15.2). In young people with normal ECG, a dissection/rupture of an aortic aneurism may be seen especially in case of bicuspid aortic valve.

5. Chronic ischemic patients with or without previous myocardial infarction. In many patients, including postinfarction patients or those who have undergone various bypasses, the ECG is normal or becomes normal over time (Fig. 9.42). Furthermore, rarely the Q wave of necrosis may remain undetected due to a second infarction (Fig. 9.43) or the association of bundle branch blocks..

In these patients, a stress test is useful, as well as a Holter recording, if possible, to identify abnormalities in repolarization or arrhythmias, and an echocardiogram may be used to test contractility and ventricular function. In some cases a coronariography or magnetic resonance (Fig. 9.43) may solve the problem.

6. In some cases of valvular or congenital heart disease that may be severe but not advanced, the ECG may remain normal or show non-evident changes even over years.

7. Other heart diseases with normal ECG. In the first phase of heart failure especially of diastolic **H**

type, and also often in pericarditis, cardiomyopathies, cardiac tumors etc, a normal ECG may be recorded.

The ECG in the clinical context of the patient

It is quite obvious, based on the above, that an ECG must be evaluated within a clinical context.

Therefore we would like to emphasize that a normal ECG is not a guarantee of cardiovascular health, nor is a pathologic ECG an unequivocal sign of heart disease.

This must always be remembered when interpreting the ECG.

Self-assessment

A. List the steps to follow in the evaluation of isolated abnormal ECG.

B. Describe the procedure used to evaluate asymptomatic patients with abnormal Q.

C. Describe the procedure used to evaluate patients with ST-T abnormalities.

D. Is it possible to observe the voltage criteria for increased LVE in healthy individuals?

E. List the normal and pathologic causes for prominent R in V1 (Table 6.1).

F. How should advanced branch block in asymptomatic patients be interpreted?

G. List five serious conditions in which a normal ECG may be observed in patients with cardiovascular involvement, including severe cases.

H. What is the golden rule to be used when interpreting the ECG recording?

Bibliography

Anttonen O, Junttila J, Maury F, et al. Differences in 12-lead ECG between symptomatic and asymptomatic subjects with short QT interval. Heart Rhythm 2009;6: 267.

Antzelevitch C, Yan GX. J wave syndromes. Heart Rhythm 2010;7:549.

Ashman R, Hull E. Essentials of Electrocardiography. The McMillan Co, New York, 1941.

Baranchuk A, Anselm DD. Brugada phenocopy: redefinition and updated classification. Am J Cardiol 2013;111:453.

Baranchuk A, Bayés de Luna A, Fiol M, et al. Differential diagnosis of ECG pattern with r' in V_1. Ann Non Inv ECG, 2014 (submitted).

Bayés de Luna A. Clinical Arrhythmology. Wiley-Blackwell, Oxford, 2011.

Bayés de Luna A. Clinical Electrocardiography. A Textbook, 4th edn. Wiley-Blackwell, Oxford, 2012a.

Bayés de Luna A, Baranchuk A, Brugada J, et al. New ECG consensus document on Brugada syndrome. J Electrocardiol 2012b;45;437.

Bayés de Luna A, Carreras F, Cladellas M, et al. Holter ECG study of the electrocardiographic phenomena in Prinzmetal angina attacks with emphasis on the study of ventricular arrhythmias. J Electrocardiol 1985b;18:267.

Bayés de Luna A, Carrió I, Subirana T, et al. Electrophysiological mechanisms of the S_I S_{II} S_{III} electrocardiographic morphology. J Electrocardiol 1987;20:38.

Bayés de Luna A, Cino J, Goldwasser D, et al. New electrocardiografic diagnostic criteria for the pathologic R waves in leads V1 and V2 of anatomically lateral myocardial infarction. Electrocardiology 2008a;41:413.

Bayés de Luna A, Cino J, Pujadas S, et al. Concordance of electrocardiographic patterns and healed myocardial infarction location detected by cardiovascular magnetic resonance. Am J Cardiol 2006b;97:443.

Bayés de Luna A, Cladellas M, Oter R, et al. Interatrial conduction block and paroxysmal arrhythmias. Eur Heart J 1988;9:1112.

Bayés de Luna A, Coumel P, Leclercq J. Ambulatory sudden cardiac death: mechanisms of production of fatal arrhythmia on the basis of data from 157 cases. Am Heart J 1989;117:151.

Bayés de Luna A, Fiol-Sala M. Electrocardiography in ischemic heart disease. Clinical and imaging correlations and prognostic implications. Blackwell-Futura, Oxford, 2008b.

Bayés de Luna A, Fort de Ribot R, Trilla E, et al. Electrocardiographic and vector cardiographic study of interatrial conduction disturbances with left atrial retrograde activation. J Electrocardiol 1985a;18:1.

Bayés de Luna A, Guindo J, Homs E, et al. Active versus passive, rhythm as explanation of bigeminal rhythm with similar P wave. Chest 1991;99;735.

Bayés de Luna A, Pérez Riera A, Baranchuck A, et al. ECG manifestation of the middle fibers/Leith septal fascicle block. A consensus paper. J Electrocardiol 2012d;45;455.

Bayés de Luna A, Platonov P, Cosio FG, et al. Interatrial blocks. A separate entity from left atrial enlargement: a consensus paper. J Electrocardiol 2012c;45:454.

Bayés de Luna A, Wagner G, Birnbaum Y, et al. A new terminology for left ventricular walls and location of myocardial infarcts that present Q wave based on the standard of cardiac magnetic resonance imaging. A statement for healthcare professionals from a committee appointed by the International Society for Holter and Noninvasive Electrocardiology. Circulation 2006a;114:1755.

Bayés Genis A, Lopez L, Viñolas X, et al. Distinct LBBB pattern in ischemic and non-ischemic dilated CM. Eur J Heart Failure 2003;5:165.

Bellet S, Jedlicka J. Sinoventricular conduction and its relation to sinoatrial conduction. Am J Cardiol 1969;24:831.

Birnbaum Y, Bayés de Luna A, Fiol M, et al. Common pitfalls in the interpretation of ECGs from patients with acute coronary syndromes with narrow QRS:A consensus report. J Electrocardiol 2012;45:463.

Birnbaum Y, Sclarovsky S, Blum, et al. Prognostic significance of the initial electrocardiographic pattern in a first acute anterior wall myocardial infarction. Chest 1993;103;1681.

Breithardt G, Shanesa M, Borgraffe M, Hindricks G, Josephson M (eds). Cardiac mapping. Wiley-Blackwell, Oxford, 2012.

Brugada P, Brugada J. Right bundle branch block, persistent ST segment elevation and sudden cardiac death: a distinct clinical and electrocardiographic syndrome. A multicenter report. J Am Coll Cardiol 1992;20:1391–1396.

Brugada P, Brugada J, Mont L, et al. A new approach to the differential diagnosis of a regular tachycardia with a wide QRS complex. Circulation 1991;83:1649.

Burke A, Farb A, Malcom GT, et al. Coronary risk factors and plaque morphology in men with coronary disease who die suddenly. N Engl J Med 1997;336:1276.

Camm J, Saksena S. Electrophysiological disorders of the heart. Elsevier, Oxford, 2012.

Cerqueira MD, Weissman NJ, Disizian V. Standardized myocardial segmentation and nomenclature for tomographic imaging of the heart: a statement for healthcare professionals from the Cardiac Imaging Committee of the Council on Clinical cardiology of the American Heart Association. Circulation 2002;86;341.

Chevallier S, Forclaz A, Tenkorang J, et al. New electrocardiographic criteria for discriminating between Brugada types 2 and 3 patterns and incomplete right bundle block. J Am Coll Cardiol 2011;58:2290.

Chung EK. Aberrant atrial conduction. Br Heart J 1972;34:341.

Conde D, Baranchuk A. Interatrial block as anatomical-electrical substrate for supraventricular arrhythmias: Bayeś syndrome. Arch Cardiol Mex 2014;84:32.

Cooksey JD, Dunn M, Marrie E. Clinical Vectorcardiography and Electrocardiography. Year Book Medical Publishers, 1977.

Corrado D, Pelliccia A, Heibuchedl H, et al. Recommendations for interpretation of 12-lead electrocardiograms in the athlete. Eur Heart J 2010;31:243.

Coumel P, Fidelle F, Cloup M, et al. Les tachycardies reciproques a evolution prolongue cher l'enfant. Arch Mal Coeur 1974;67;23.

Das MK, Khan B, Jacob S, et al. Significance of a fragmented QRS complex versus a Q wave in patients with coronary artery disease. Circulation 2006;113:2495.

Desserte F. La tachycardia ventriculaire a dues foyers opposes variables. Arch Mal Coeur 1966;59;263.

De Winter RJ, Verouden NJ, Wellens HJ, et al. A new ECG sign of proximal LAD occlusion. N Engl J Med 2008;359:2071.

Durrer D, Van Dam R, Freud G, et al. Total excitation of the isolated human heart. Circulation 1970;41;899.

Elizari M, Chiale P. The ECG features of complete and partial left anterior and left posterior hemiblocks. J Electrocardiol 2012;45;528.

Farré J, Ross D, Wiener I, et al. Reciprocal tachycardias using accessory pathways with long conduction times. Am J Cardiol 1979;44:1099.

Fiol M, Carrillo A, Cygankiewicz I, et al. A new electrocardiographic algorithm to locate the occlusion in left anterior descending coronary artery. Clin Cardiol 2009;32:E1.

Fiol M, Carrillo A, Rodríguez A, et al. Electrocardiographic changes of ST-elevation myocardial infarction in patients with complete occlusion of the Leith main trunk without collateral circulation: Differential diagnosis and clinical considerations. J Electrocardiol 2012;45;487.

Fiol-Sala M, Cygankiewicz I, Carrillo A, et al. Value of electrocardiographic algorithm based on 'ups and downs' of ST in assessment of a culprit artery in evolving inferior wall acute myocardial infarction. Am J Cardiol 2004;94:709.

Fish C, Knobel S. Electrocardiography of Clinical Arrhythmias. Futura, London, 2000.

Garcia Cosio F, Goicolea A, López-Gil M, et al. Atrial endocardial mapping in the rare form of atrial flutter. Am J Cardiol 1990;66;715.

Garcia Niebla J, Llontop-Garcia P, Valle-Rocero, et al. Technical mistakes during the acquisition of an ECG. ANE 2009;14:989.

Gerstch M. The ECG: A Two Step Approach for Diagnosis. Springer, New York, 2004.

Gettes L, Kligfield P. Should electrocardiogram criteria for the diagnosis of left bundle-branch block be revised? J Electrocardiol 2012;45:500.

Haïsaguerre M, Jaïs P, Shah DC, et al. Spontaneous initiation of atrial fibrillation by ectopic beats originating in the pulmonary veins. N Engl J Med 1998;339–659.

Hathaway WR, Peterson ED, Wagner GS, et al. Prognostic significande of the initial electrocardiogram in patients with acute myocardial infarction. GUSTO-I Investigators. Global Utilization of Streptokinase and t-PA for Occluded Coronary Arteries. JAMA 1998;279:387.

Investigators. Global Utilization of Streptokinase and t-PA for Occluded Coronary Arteries. JAMA 1998;279: 387.

Issa Z, Miller J, Zipes D. Clinical Arrhythmology and Electrophysiology. Wolters-Kluwer, Philadelphia, 2008.

Jain R, Dalal D, Daly A, et al. Electrocardiographic features of arrhythmogenic right ventricular dysplasia. Circulation 2009;12:477.

Josephson ME. Clinical Cardiac Electrophysiology. Wolters-Kluwer, Philadelphia, 2008.

Kosuge M, Ebene T, Hubi K, et al. An early and simple predictor of severe left main and/or three-vessel diseases in patients with non-ST segment elevation acute coronary syndrome. Am J Cardiol 2011;107:495.

Lown B, Wolf M. Approaches to sudden death from coronary heart disease. Circulation 1971;44:130.

Macfarlane PW, Lawrie TDV (eds) Comprehensive Electrocardiology. Pergamon Press, Oxford, 1989.

Macfarlane PW, Van Oosterom A, Pahlm O, Kligfield P, Janse M, Camm J (eds). Comprehensive Electrocardiology, 2nd edn. Springer-Verlag, London, 2011.

Marcus FI, McKenna WJ, Sherrill D, et al. Diagnosis of arrhythmogenic right ventricular cardiomyopathy/dysplasia. Proposed modification of the task force criteria. Circulation 2009;415:213.

Maron BJ. Contemporary insights and strategies for risk stratification and prevention of sudden death in hypertophic cardiomyopathy. Circulation 2010;121: 445.

Maron BJ, Gottdiener JS, Epstein SE. Patterns and significance of distribution of left ventricular hypertrophy in hypertrophic cardiomyopathy. A wide angle, two dimensional echocardiographic study of 125 patients. Am J Cardiol 1981;48:418.

McKenna WJ, Behr ER. Hypertrophic cardiomyopathy: management, risk stratification and prevention of sudden death. Heart 2002;87:169.

Migliore F, Zorzi A, Perazzolo Marra M, et al. Myocardial edema underlies dynamic T-wave inversion (Wellens' ECG pattern) in patients with reversible left ventricular dysfunction. Heart Rhythm 2011;8:1629.

Moe GM, Méndez C. Physiological basis of reciprocal rhythm. Prog Cardiovasc Dis 1966;8:561.

Moon JC, De Arenaza DP, Elkington AG, et al. The pathologic basis of Q-wave and non-Q-wave myocardial infarction: a cardiovascular magnetic resonance study. J Am Coll Cardiol 2004;44:554.

Moss A, Robinson J. Clinical features of idiopathic QT syndrome. Circulation 1992;85(suppl):1140.

Nakagama M, Tsunemitsu C, Kata S, et al. Effect of ECG filter on J-wave J. ECG 2014:47;7.

Nielsen JC. On behalf of DANPACE investigators. 2010 http://escardio.org/congresses/esc-2010/congress reports/page798.IDANPACE.aspx.

Nikus K, Pahlm O, Wagner G, et al. Electrocardiographic classification of acute coronary syndromes: a review by a committee of the International Society for Holter and Non-Invasive Electrocardiology. J Electrocardiol 2010;43:91.

Padalinam BJ, Manfrech JA, Steinberg JA, et al. Differentiating junctional tachycardia and AV node reentrant tachycardia based on response to atrial pacing. J Am Coll Cardiol 2008;52;1711.

Pava L, Perafán P, Badiel M, et al. R-wave peak time at DII: A new criterion for differentiating between wide complex QRS tachycardias. Heart Rhythm 2010;7:922.

Plas F. Guide du Cardiologie du Sport. Bailliere, Paris, 1976.

Pride YB, Tung P, Mohanavelu S, et al. TIMI Study Group. Angiographic and clinical outcomes among patients with acute coronary syndromes presenting with isolated anterior ST-segment depression: a TRITON-TIMI 38 (Trial to Assess Improvement in Therapeutic Outcomes by optimizing Platelet Inhibition With Prasugrel-Thrombolysis in Myocardial Infarction 38) substudy. JACC Cardiovasc Interv 2010;3:806.

Rosenbaum MB, Elizari M, Lazzari JO, et al. The mechanism of intermittent bundle branch block. Relationship to prolonged recovery, hipopolarization and spontaneous diastolic depolarization. Chest 1973;63: 666.

Rosenbaum MB, Elizari MV, Lazzari JO. Los hemibloqueos. Editorial Paidos. Buenos Aires, 1968.

Rovai D, Di Bella G, Rossi G, et al. Q-wave prediction of myocardial infarct location, size and transmural extent at magnetic resonance imaging. Coron Art Dis 2007;18:381.

Sarkozy A, Cherchia G, Paparella G, et al. Inferior and lateral ECG repolarization abnormalities in Brugada syndrome. Circ Arrhythmic Electrophysiol 2009;2:154.

Schwartz PJ, Moss AJ, Vincent GM, Crampton RS. Diagnostic criteria for the long QT syndrome. An update. Circulation 1993;88:782.

Serra G, Baranchuk A, Bayés de Luna A, et al. New electrocardiographic criteria to differentiate the Type-2 Brugada pattern from electrocardiogram of healthy athletes with r'-wave in leads V1/V2. Europace, 2014. March 6.

Seurer G, Gursoy S, Frei B, et al. The differential diagnosis on the ECG between ventricular tachycardia and pre-excited tachycardia. Clin Cardiol 1994;17:306.

Sgarbossa EB, Pinski SL, Barbagelata A, et al. Electrocardiographic diagnosis of evolving acute myocardial infarction in the presence of left bundle branch block. GUSTO-1 (Global Utilization of Streptokinase and Tissue Plasminogen Activator for Occluded Coronary Arteries) Investigators. N Engl J Med 1996;334: 481.

Singer D, Ten Eick R. Aberrancy: electrophysiological aspects. Am J Cardiol 1971;28:381.

Sodi Pallares D, Bisteni A, Medrano G. Electrocardiografia y vectorcardiografia deductiva. La Prensa Médica Mexicana, 1967.

Spodick DH. Acute pericarditis; ECG changes. Primary Cardiol 1982;8:78.

Spodick DH, Ariyarajah V. Interatrial block: a prevalent, widely neglected and portentous abnormality. J Electrocardiol 2008;41:61.

Strauss DG, Selvester RH, Wagner GS. Defining left bundle branch block in the era of cardiac resynchronization therapy. Am J Cardiol 2011;107:927.

Subirana VT, Juan-Babot JO, Puig T, et al. Specific characteristics of sudden death in a Mediterranean Spanish population. Am J Cardiol 2011;107:622.

Surawicz B. Relationship between electrocardiogram and electrolytes. Am Heart J 1967;73:814.

Surawicz B, Knilans TK. Chou's Electrocardiography in Clinical Practice, 6th edn. WB Saunders Company, 2009.

Surawicz B, Uhley H, Brown R, et al. Task force I, Standarization of terminology and interpretation. Am J Cardiol 1978;41:130.

Thygessen K, Alpert J, Jaffe AS, et al. Third universal definition of myocardial infarction. Eur Heart J 2012;33: 2551.

Van Bommel R, Marsan N, Delgado V, et al. Value of the surface ECG in detecting right ventricular dilatation in the presence of left bundle branch block. Am J Cardiol 2011;107:736.

Van der Weg K, Bekkers S, Winkens B, et al. On behalf of MAST. The R in V1 in non-anterior wall infarction indicates lateral rather than posterior involvement. Results from ECG/MRI correlations. Eur Heart J 2009;30 (suppl);P2981K.

Vereckei A, Duray G, Szénasi G, et al. New algorithm using only lead a VR for differential diagnosis of wide QRS complex tachycardia. Heart Rhythm 2008;5:89.

Villafane J, Atalla F, Golob M et al. Longterm follow-up of a pediatric cohort of short QT syndromes. J Am Coll Cardiol 2013;61:1183.

Wagner BS. Marriott's Practical Electrocardiography, 10th edn. Lippincott Williams & Wilkins, 2001.

Wellens HJ. The value of the right precordial leads of the electrocardiogram. N Engl J Med 1999;340: 381.

Willems JL, Robles E, Bernard R, et al. Criteria for intraventricular conduction disturbances and preexcitation. WHO/WHF. J Am Coll Cardiol 1985;5:1261.

Zareba W. Cardiac resynchronization therapy: Forget QRS duration but do not forget QRS morphology. J Cardiol 2013;46:145.

Zareba W, Cygankiewicz I. Long QT syndrome and short QT syndrome. Prog Cardiovasc Dis 2008;51:264.

Zareba W, Moss AJ, Schwartz PJ, et al. Influence of genotype of long-QT syndrome Registry Research Group. N Engl J Med 1998;339:960.

Index

Page numbers in *italics* denote figures, those in **bold** denote tables.

ECGs for Beginners, First Edition. Antoni Bayés de Luna.
© 2014 John Wiley & Sons, Inc. Published 2014 by John Wiley & Sons, Inc.